WOLFSON INSTITUTE OF PREVENTIVE MEDICINE

OXFORD MEDICAL PUBLICATIONS

UK SMOKING STATISTICS

Second edition

3

The preparation of this book was financially supported by the
Imperial Cancer Research Fund

UK SMOKING STATISTICS

Second edition

Edited by

Nicholas Wald
and
Ans Nicolaides-Bouman

Wolfson Institute of Preventive Medicine,
St. Bartholomew's Hospital Medical College, London

London
WOLFSON INSTITUTE OF PREVENTIVE MEDICINE

Oxford New York Tokyo
OXFORD UNIVERSITY PRESS

1991

Wolfson Institute of Preventive Medicine, Charterhouse Square, London EC1M 6BQ

Oxford University Press, Walton Street, Oxford OX2 6DP
Oxford New York Toronto
Delhi Bombay Calcutta Madras Karachi
Petaling Jaya Singapore Hong Kong Tokyo
Nairobi Dar es Salaam Cape Town
Melbourne Auckland
and associated companies in
Beirut Berlin Ibadan Nicosia

Oxford is a trade mark of Oxford University Press

Published in the United States
by Oxford University Press, New York

Library of Congress Cataloguing in Publication Data
(Data available)
ISBN 0 19 261680 3

Printed in Great Britain by
Bookcraft Limited, Midsomer Norton

Preface to the first edition

This book is a compilation of statistics about smoking in the United Kingdom. The Tobacco Research Council published statistics on smoking habits in the United Kingdom until 1975. Since then the principal published sources of data on smoking have been the reports of the General Household Survey; the tar, nicotine, and carbon monoxide tables issued by the Health Departments of the United Kingdom; and the market shares of manufactured cigarette brands, published in tobacco trade journals. It is the purpose of this book to provide a comprehensive description of smoking in the United Kingdom by amalgamating published and unpublished data from various sources, including those that were previously used to produce the annual Tobacco Research Council statistics, and those from National Opinion Polls.

Data on tobacco sales were first available at the end of the last century, and estimates of the consumption of tobacco by men and women have been made since 1905. From about 1950 onwards, surveys provide more detailed information on smoking habits classified according to age, social class, and type of cigarette smoked.

From 1972 the tar and nicotine yields of cigarettes, and later also the carbon monoxide yields, have been tested regularly by the Laboratory of the Government Chemist. A study that examined stored cigarettes makes it possible to describe the sales-weighted mean yields of these three smoke components from as far back as 1934.

Also included are data on smoking habits in different regions of the United Kingdom, data on the taxation of tobacco obtained from HM Customs and Excise, and on the smoking habits of British children assessed from various surveys conducted since 1965.

The figures are intended to provide an easily interpretable summary of the data presented in the tables and the commentary has been deliberately kept to a minimum.

The tables and text in this monograph have been compiled by Stephanie Kiryluk and Nicholas Wald, with assistance from the other editors.

February 1987   The Editors

Preface to the second edition

This edition replaces the previous edition by providing all the information included in the first edition (apart from Tables 11.8 and 11.9, extracts from *Hansard*, which have been replaced by more recent answers to parliamentary questions) as well as more recent data. Consequently, there is no need for cross referencing between the two editions.

The two main primary sources of data on smoking habits are the General Household Survey carried out every two years and the annual survey carried out on behalf of the tobacco industry. The last year for which data are available from the General Household Survey is 1988 and this book includes some previously unpublished material from this Survey. The Tobacco Advisory Council which had previously kindly agreed to us publishing their tobacco industry data have declined to make these available since 1987. The General Household Survey therefore, is the only main national source of Smoking Statistics in the UK and in this volume we have sought to obtain additional unpublished material in order to fill some of the gaps created by the absence of the tobacco industry data.

This edition includes a new chapter on smoking among pregnant women. Most of the table and figure numbers are the same as the corresponding ones in the previous edition.

The first edition was edited by N. Wald, S. Kiryluk, S. Darby, R. Doll, M. Pike, and R. Peto and we are grateful to the other editors of the first edition for their contribution.

April 1991   Nicholas Wald
                                                                          Ans Nicolaides-Bouman

Acknowledgments

We are grateful to Stephanie Kiryluk whose work in the first edition laid the foundations for this edition. We would like to acknowledge the help given by the Department of Health and Social Security, HM Customs and Excise, the Central Statistical Office, the Laboratory of the Government Chemist, National Opinion Polls Market Research Limited, the Office of Population Censuses and Surveys, Peter Lee and the Tobacco Advisory Council , Geoffrey Hardman, and Joy Townsend. We thank Kristie Kryston who assisted in the preparation of this edition and Stephanie Kiryluk, Sir Richard Doll, and Barbara Forey for their comments on its contents. We also thank the Imperial Cancer Research Fund for their financial support of Ans Nicolaides-Bouman in connection with the production of this book.

Contents

Tables

The title of each table, with the population to which the table applies and the source of the data. An explanation of the abbreviations for the sources of data is given on page xxv.

Tables

Figures

Figures   **xxiii**

Explanatory notes

Abbreviations

The following abbreviations are used:
GHS   General Household Survey
LGC   Laboratory of the Government Chemist
NOP   National Opinion Polls Market Research Ltd.
TAC   Tobacco Advisory Council
TRC   Tobacco Research Council
TAC is used at the foot of the tables to indicate data collected by the Tobacco Advisory Council and/or the Tobacco Research Council.

Symbols used in the tables

```
..      Data not available
0       Nil or less than 0.5
0.0     Nil or less than 0.05
```
Occasionally tables contain blanks where zeros would be expected, e.g. data for women in years before women started to smoke in appreciable numbers.

Population covered by the data

Some of the tables and figures in this book relate to the United Kingdom (England, Wales, Scotland, and Northern Ireland), and some to Great Britain (England, Wales, and Scotland). The relevant tables and figures are marked United Kingdom and Great Britain respectively.

Data applying to the United Kingdom

The following data relate to the United Kingdom:
(i)   Total sales of tobacco
(ii)   Tobacco tax revenue
(iii)   Type of cigarette sold (plain or filter)
(iv)   Cigarette yields (tar, nicotine, carbon monoxide, and other noxa)
(v)   Some of the data whose source is the TAC
(vi)   Retail prices index from the Central Statistical Office

Data applying to Great Britain

The following data relate to Great Britain:
(i)   All those from the GHS and NOP surveys
(ii)   Most of the data with TAC as the source
Much of the TAC survey data has been adjusted for under-reporting, the adjustment being derived from total United Kingdom sales data. Data from surveys that were conducted in Great Britain, but adjusted for under-reporting using United Kingdom sales data are marked 'Great Britain, sales adjusted'. The method of adjustment is decribed on page xxxii.

Sources of data

1. Tobacco Research Council (TRC)/Tobacco Advisory Council (TAC)

The Tobacco Research Council was renamed the Tobacco Advisory Council in 1976. From 1948 to 1987, the TRC/TAC commissioned an annual survey on smoking habits in Great Britain from Research Services Ltd., a market research company. The results of the surveys were published at intervals between 1957[a] and 1976[b] by the TRC and until 1985 in the first edition of UK Smoking Statistics. This edition also includes the results of the surveys carried out in 1986 and 1987. In 1988 no survey was carried out. In 1989 the TAC did commission a survey as they had done for previous years, but declined to make available the results. The TAC did agree, however, to supply annual sales data of tobacco products to the trade from 1979 to 1989. These are included in this edition.

Most of these surveys interviewed about 10 000 people. Quota sampling has been used to select subjects, with the number of subjects required in specific sex, age, social class, regional, and occupational groups determined in advance, so that the final sample obtained reflected the proportions in these particular groups in the general population. Interviewers are free to interview anyone who fits their quota at home or at work, with a limit placed on the number of interviews that can be conducted in any one place of work. Since the survey results for younger people are frequently grouped by finer age groups than is the case for older people, additional subjects have been interviewed in the 16-34 year age group (to reduce random sampling errors) and the figures subsequently weighted, where appropriate, to retain the correct proportions in the total sample. The survey data have been adjusted against sales figures for under-reporting as described on page xxxii.

2. General Household Survey (GHS)

The General Household Survey[c] is an annual survey conducted by the Social Survey Division of the Office of Population Censuses and Surveys, sponsored by the Central Statistical Office. It provides information on social policy issues for central government in five areas, namely population, housing, employment, education, and health.

The GHS started in 1971. The GHS sample comprises private households in Great Britain, the information being collected week by week throughout the year. Interviews are sought with all adult members (aged 16 years and over) of a sample of private households, selected from the Electoral Register from 1971 to 1983, and from the Postcode Address File from 1984 to 1988.

About 14 000 households were selected for interview annually until 1982, after which the number was reduced to around 12 000. Responses have been received from about 83 per cent of households in each survey. The number of persons interviewed has been approximately equal to twice the number of households responding. In some circumstances, when a particular member of a household could not be contacted, a proxy interview with a near relative in the same household has been conducted. This has occured in approximately 5 per cent of households.

Questions on smoking habits were included in the five annual surveys from 1972 to 1976, and in every second year thereafter. Data from surveys conducted in 1973 and 1975 are not included in this book. The GHS provides data on the percentage of smokers in the population and their tobacco consumption, subdivided by sex, age, type of product, and socio-economic group. Since 1984 a question was asked in the GHS to identify the tar level of cigarettes smoked. Consumption figures are not adjusted against sales figures.

Some previously unpublished material from the 1988 survey has been included (Tables 6.10 and 7.3).

3. National Opinion Polls Market Research Ltd. (NOP)

National Opinion Polls Market Research Ltd. have been commissioned by the Office of Population Censuses and Surveys on behalf of the Department of Health and Social Security to carry out a survey[d] on smoking habits and attitudes in Great Britain once or twice yearly since 1971. On each occasion, a random sample of about 4000 adults (about 2000 prior to 1974) has been interviewed. The sample used has been a two-stage stratified random sample, electors' names being drawn at random from the Electoral Register for a selection of parliamentary constituencies. At the household of each selected elector, one non-elector has been interviewed if any non-electors aged 16 and over were present in the household. Questions about type of tobacco product and amount smoked have been asked on each occasion. On some occasions additional questions, for example on the effect of advertising, or attitudes to smoking in public places, were also asked. NOP consumption figures are not adjusted against sales figures.

4. Laboratory of the Government Chemist (LGC)

Since 1972 the Laboratory of the Government Chemist has been commissioned by the Department of Health and Social Security to conduct surveys of the tar and nicotine yields, and later the carbon monoxide yields, of manufactured cigarettes sold in the United Kingdom. Manufactured cigarettes comprising about 90 per cent of the market have been tested in each survey. The testing period for each survey spans six months, with a gap of one month unsampled before sampling for the next survey begins. The Health Departments of the UK have issued tables[e] of the tar and nicotine yields of manufactured cigarettes resulting from these surveys from 1972 until 1989 (except for 1984 and part of 1987), with the addition of carbon monoxide from Survey 16 (1981-82). These tables are reproduced in full with a summary of the tar, nicotine, and carbon monoxide yields for the main brands of cigarettes from 1972 until 1989.

At the request of the Independent Scientific Committee on Smoking and Health, the

LGC determined the yields of a variety of other analytes (thought potentially injurious to health) in the mainstream smoke of key UK brands of cigarettes. Details of the results are also included.

In a study by Wald, Doll, and Copeland[f] old cigarettes manufactured in the United Kingdom between 1934 and 1979 were obtained. The tar, nicotine, and carbon monoxide yields of these cigarettes were analysed by the LGC and sales-weighted yields were calculated. The annual sales-weighted yields can now be extended to 1988 and are included in this book.

5. Maxwell's tables (*World Tobacco*) and *Tobacco* publications

Maxwell's international estimates of the market share of brands of manufactured cigarettes have been published annually in the journal *World Tobacco*[g] since 1964. Over the years the total market share covered by the tables has increased to about 90 per cent. Since the early 1970s the journal *Tobacco*[h] has carried out an anonymous tabulation entitled 'Brand Shares of the UK Cigarette Market' each year. The market shares quoted by these two publications are fairly consistent.

6. Customs and Excise

Data on rates of duty and receipts from duty on tobacco and tobacco products are available annually from HM Customs and Excise[i].

7. *Hansard*

Information on tobacco revenue and price can be obtained from the replies to parliamentary questions recorded in *Hansard* periodically[j]. Some recent replies to written parliamentary questions have been included in this book to replace Tables 11.8 and 11.9 from the first edition.

8. Central Statistical Office

Data on the Retail Price Index (all items, RPI) and the retail price index for cigarettes are available monthly from the Central Statistical Office[k]. (The data from Table 11.10 on retail prices was taken from *Hansard* in the first edition of this book, but is now supplied by the Central Statistical Office.)

9. Children and smoking

A number of surveys of the smoking habits of British children have been conducted since 1965. These are summarized, with references, in Section 12.

10. Pregnant women and smoking

Surveys of the smoking habits of pregnant women in Britain are included, with references, in Section 13.

Definitions and classifications

The definitions and categories (of, say, cigarette consumption) vary according to the data used. The source is indicated on each tabulation and the appropriate definitions and categories can be determined from the following notes.

Data from the Tobacco Advisory Council, the General Household Survey, and National Opinion Polls Market Research Ltd. are placed in that order within each section or subsection of the book.

1. Definition of an adult

When census data have been used to estimate the population on which per person consumption has been calculated, an adult is defined as a person aged 15 or over (15+).

In most tables, estimates are based on survey data, and in these tables an adult is defined as a person aged 16 or over (16+). The age group used is stated in the tables where appropriate.

2. Age groups

TAC
The TAC used various age groups at different times. One of the main changes occurred in 1976, and this led to a break in continuity of the analysis of trends. The age groups used by the TAC are as follows, in years:
Before 1976
     16-19, 20-24, 25-34, 35-59, 60+
     16-19, 20-24, 25-34, 35-49, 50-59, 60+
1976 and thereafter
     16-24, 25-34, 35-49, 50-64, 65+.

In both periods (before 1976 and thereafter) some tables are given for ages 16-19, then five-year age groups from 20-24 to 75-79, and 80+ years.

When available, 1975 data are presented for both sets of age groups to indicate the effects of switching from one set to another. Discontinuity in the analysis of trends due to the use of different age groupings is indicated on the graphs.

GHS
The GHS has used consistent age groups, namely, in years:
     16-19, 20-24, 25-34, 35-49, 50-59, 60+.

NOP
NOP has used consistent age groups, namely, in years:
     16-24, 25-34, 35-44, 45-54, 55-64, 65+.

3. Definition of smoking

Much of the data from the Tobacco Advisory Council is concerned with the smoking of manufactured cigarettes, whereas the General Household Survey considers the smoking of all cigarettes, without differentiating between manufactured and hand-rolled.

TAC

'Smokers' are people who answer 'Yes' to at least one of the following questions:
'Do you smoke packeted cigarettes?'
'Do you smoke hand-rolled cigarettes?'
'Do you smoke a pipe?' (not asked of women)
'Do you smoke as much as one cigar or miniature cigar a week?'

Manufactured cigarette smokers, hand-rolled cigarette smokers, pipe smokers, and cigar smokers are defined according to the above questions.

'Ex-smokers' are people who are not 'smokers' but who claim to have smoked in the past at least a cigarette a day, or a pipe a day, or a cigar a week, for as long as a year. People who 'have never smoked' are people who have never smoked cigarettes, pipe, or cigars at this rate.

For all these definitions, pipe applies only to men. The category 'cigars' includes cigars of all sizes and cigarillos.

TAC figures prior to 1964 do not include smokers of cigars only.

Cigarette consumption is estimated from answers to the following question:
'How many cigarettes did you smoke yesterday?' (On Mondays, twice the usual number of people are interviewed, and half are asked 'How many cigarettes did you smoke on Saturday?')

GHS

'Smokers' are people who answer 'Yes' to at least one of the following questions:
'Do you smoke cigarettes at all nowadays?'
'Do you smoke a pipe at all nowadays?' (not asked of women)
'Do you smoke cigars of any kind at all nowadays?' (1974, 1976)
'Do you smoke at least one cigar of any kind per month nowadays?' (1972, 1978, 1980, 1982, 1984, 1986, 1988)

'Ex-smokers' are defined as persons who do not smoke cigarettes or a pipe or cigars of any kind at all nowadays, and who answer 'Yes' to at least one of the following questions:
'Have you ever smoked cigarettes regularly?'
'Have you ever smoked a pipe regularly?' (not asked of women)
'Have you ever smoked cigars of any kind regularly?' (1974, 1976)
'Have you ever regularly smoked at least one cigar of any kind per month?' (1972, 1978, 1980, 1982, 1984, 1986, 1988)

People who have 'never smoked' are persons who answer 'No' to the above questions. Cigarette, pipe, and cigar smoking are defined by answers to the above questions.

Cigarette consumption is estimated from answers to the following questions:
'About how many cigarettes a day do you usually smoke at weekends?'
'And about how many cigarettes a day do you usually smoke on weekdays?'

NOP

Smokers are people who answer 'Yes' to at least one of the following questions:
'Do you regularly smoke one or more of these?
(i)   Cigarettes - at least one a day, on average, over a year
(ii)   Cigars - at least three a week, on average, over a year
(iii) Pipe - at least one pipe a day, on average, over a year'

Manufactured cigarette consumption is estimated from replies to:
'How many packeted cigarettes did you smoke yesterday?'

4. Classification of social class

TAC

The TAC uses the Registrar General's social class classification[1], which is based on occupation, as follows:

Class I   Professional occupations
Class II   Managerial and lower professional occupations
Class IIINM   Non-manual skilled occupations
Class IIIM   Skilled manual occupations
Class IV   Partly skilled occupations
Class V   Unskilled occupations
Class VI   Unoccupied.

Those who have been unemployed for less than two months are classified according to their previous occupation. Those who have been unemployed for more than two months are classified as unoccupied. The retired are classified according to their previous occupation.

For married women, social class is determined by their husband's occupation. Single women (including divorcees and widows) are classified by their own occupation.

GHS

The GHS uses the more recent classification by Socio-Economic Group (SEG)[1], consisting of 17 categories based on employment status and occupation. These categories are then combined as follows:

	SEG numbers
Professional	3,4
Employers and managers	1,2,13
Intermediate and junior non-manual	5,6
Skilled manual and own-account non-professional	8,9,12,14
Semi-skilled manual and personal service	7,10,15
Unskilled manual	11.

Persons whose occupations were inadequately described (SEG 17), members of the Armed Forces (SEG 16), and persons who have never worked have been included in the tables only in the totals. SEG classification is determined by a person's present job, or, for those not currently working, by their last job, except that married women whose husbands are in the household are classified according to their husband's present or last job.

NOP

NOP uses the Institute of Practitioners in Advertising system of coding, commonly used for market research. Social class categories are based on the head of household's occupation as follows:

Class A   Higher managerial, administrative, or professional
Class B   Intermediate managerial, administrative, or professional
Class C1 Supervisory or clerical, and junior managerial, administrative, or professional
Class C2 Skilled manual workers

Class D   Semi- and unskilled manual workers

Class E   State pensioners or widows (no other earners), casual or lowest grade workers, long-term unemployed (no other earners).

Adjustment for under-reporting

Some smokers tend to under-report their cigarette consumption, while some do not admit to smoking when questioned in surveys. This leads to a short fall when estimates from survey data are compared with known sales totals. The TAC have adjusted their survey findings for under-reporting as described below. Tables and figures that contain data that have been adjusted for under-reporting are marked 'sales-adjusted'. No such adjustment has been applied by the GHS or NOP to their data.

Adjustment of TAC survey findings

The TAC figures derived from their annual survey based on personal interviews were adjusted to take into account known sales to the public as follows.

1. Manufactured cigarettes

The consumption of manufactured cigarettes was estimated from the survey findings. This figure was then compared with the sales estimate for the period of the survey, the under/overstatement calculated, and an adjusting factor applied accordingly.

The adjustment was only applied to cigarette consumption until 1969, when it was split between smokers and consumption. The apportionment of the factor to smokers or consumption was based on information derived from other surveys. From 1978 onwards the same adjusting factor was aplied to numbers of smokers and to consumption. When the adjustment was applied, no attempt was made to correct individual age or sex groups differently.

In the case of manufactured cigarettes, the understatement averaged 5 per cent since the survey first began. The adjustment of the data has a relatively small effect on the published figures, only increasing the overall proportion of manufactured cigarette smokers by around 1 per cent, and average daily consumption by about half a cigarette per day.

2. Tobacco for hand rolling

The adjusting factors for hand-rolled tobacco were calculated in the same way as for manufactured cigarettes.

3. Pipe tobacco

In the case of pipe tobacco, the level of understatement has been small, and therefore the adjustment was applied only to consumption.

4. Cigars

No adjustment was applied to data on cigars.

A note on some differences between the TAC and GHS surveys

A comparison of the TAC and GHS data on cigarette consumption for 1972-86 shows that, while the trends for these years are similar within each survey, the GHS estimates of consumption of cigarettes (manufactured and hand-rolled) per cigarette smoker are between 12 per cent and 19 per cent lower than the TAC estimates on consumption of manufactured cigarettes per manufactured cigarette smoker. Thus the understatement of consumption per smoker is greater in the GHS than the TAC surveys, even allowing for the fact that the TAC data are sales-adjusted. The data on percentage of cigarette smokers are less discrepant.

The 1972 General Household Survey states that 'it is likely that the GHS data understate tobacco consumption, and possibly, though to a lesser extent, the number of smokers in adult age groups as well as amongst adolescents'. Possible reasons for the understatement include the fact that the GHS questions on smoking follow a section on health, and also that some people may be reluctant to disclose the extent of their smoking in front of other family members who may be present at the interview. Differences in the wording of the question on consumption in the GHS and TAC surveys (TAC asks about the number of cigarettes smoked yesterday whereas GHS asks about the number of cigarettes usually smoked), and the fact that the TAC survey is only concerned with smoking whereas the GHS survey covers many other areas, may also help to explain the discrepancy mentioned above. The similarity in the trends displayed by the two surveys implies that both surveys can be used individually to compare changes over time. Care should, however, be taken when switching from the TAC to the GHS results and vice versa.

References

a. Todd, G.F. (ed.) 'Statistics of smoking in the United Kingdom'. (Research Paper 1) 1st edition. London: Tobacco Research Council, 1957.

b. Lee, P.N. (ed.) 'Statistics of smoking in the United Kingdom'. (Research Paper 1) 7th edition. London: Tobacco Research Council, 1976. (Most TAC data included in this book for 1976-87 are previously unpublished.)

c. Office of Population Censuses and Surveys. HMSO. 'General Household Survey 1972': 1975. 'General Household Survey 1974': 1977. 'General Household Survey 1976': 1978. 'General Household Survey 1978': 1980. 'General Household Survey 1980': 1982. 'General Household Survey 1982': 1984. 'General Household Survey 1984': 1986. 'General Household Survey 1986': 1989. 'General Household Survey 1988': 1990.

d. National Opinion Polls Market Research Limited. 'Smoking Habits. A Report on a Survey Carried out by NOP Market Research Limited for the Office of the Population Censuses and Surveys'. Unpublished reports, January 1974, January 1975, April 1976, January 1977, January 1978, January 1979, January 1980, January 1981, December 1982, December 1983, December 1984, December 1985, December 1986, December 1987, December 1988.

e. 'Tar and Nicotine Yields of Cigarettes'. Leaflets issued by the Health Departments of the United Kingdom, April 1973, February 1974, September 1974, May 1975, January 1976, August 1976, March 1977, October 1977, July 1978, January 1979, October 1979, May 1980, March 1981, October 1981, April 1982.

'Tar, Carbon Monoxide and Nicotine Yields of Cigarettes'. Leaflets issued by the Health Departments of the United Kingdom, November 1982, May 1983, October 1983, June 1984, January 1986, July 1986, January 1988, September 1989 (London Gazette), June 1990, August 1990 (London Gazette).

f. Wald, N., Doll, R., and Copeland, G. 'Trends in the tar, nicotine, and carbon monoxide yields of UK cigarettes manufactured since 1934'. *British Medical Journal*, 1981, **282**: 763-5.

g. Maxwell, J.C. 'How the Brands ranked. Maxwell International Estimates'. *World Tobacco* 1973; **41**:54 1974; **45**:48-9 1975; **50**:47-8 1976; **53**:88 1977; **57**:66 1978; **61**:76 1979; **65**:68 1980; **69**:62 1981; **73**:105 1982; **77**:57 1983; **81**:57 1984; **85**:49 1985; **90**:41 1986; **94**:18 1988;**106**:51.

h. Anonymous. 'Brand shares of the UK cigarette market'. *Tobacco* July, 1973:26 July, 1974:39 July, 1975:19 July, 1976:40-1 August, 1977:18-19 August, 1978:18-19 August, 1979:20-1 August, 1980:28-9 August, 1981:24-5 August, 1982:18-19 September, 1983:20-1 September, 1984:7 September, 1985:4-5 August, 1986:7-9 August, 1987:15-17 August, 1988:7-9 August, 1989:10-11.

i. The Report of the Commissioners of Her Majesty's Customs and Excise for the year ended 31st March, HMSO. 1913; table 61, page 51 1928; table 59, page 80 1938; table 56, page 79 1948; table 60, page 87 1958; table 41, page 85 1968; table 39, page 84 1969; table 38, page 83 1978; table 14, page 51 1979; table 11, page 48 1985; table 15, page 50, table 16, page 51, table 17, page 52 1989; table E1, page 58, table E2, page 59, table E4, page 60.

j. *The House of Commons Official Report (Hansard)*. HMSO, Vol. **147**, c620W Vol. **149**, c60W.

k. The Retail Price Index (RPI) and the retail price index for cigarettes, 1962-1989. As published by the Central Statistical Office.

l. Office of Population Censuses and Surveys. 'Classifications of occupations 1980'. HMSO, 1980.

The use of tobacco spread from America to other countries during the sixteenth century. The first factories making cigarettes by machine were set up in Havana in 1853, in London in 1856, and in the USA in 1872. However, during the nineteenth century, tobacco for pipes and chewing, and tobacco for cigars and snuff, accounted for virtually all the tobacco sold. From 1895 sales of manufactured cigarettes increased rapidly, so that by 1919 they comprised more sales by weight than all other forms of tobacco combined. Filter cigarettes, although available from the 1930s, did not become popular until the 1960s when they quickly replaced plain cigarettes. Hand-rolled cigarettes have accounted for only about 6 per cent of total annual cigarette sales by weight during the last 30 years.

Since the early 1960s there has been a decline in the total weight of tobacco sold as manufactured cigarettes or for hand-rolling. The decline was initially due to the introduction of filters, reducing the amount of tobacco used in each cigarette. The total numbers of cigarettes consumed (manufactured and hand-rolled) started to decline in the mid-1970s and fell by some 25 per cent over the next 10 years. Since the mid-1980s, though the decline in hand-rolled cigarette consumption has continued, there has been little change in the number of manufactured cigarettes sold. The sales of cigars, measured either by weight or numbers, increased until the mid-1970s and decreased somewhat thereafter. Sales of pipe tobacco have been in continuous decline for many years. Assessment of recent trends is not materially affected by the switch from estimates of sales to the public to estimate of sales to the trade (see note 2 on page 2).

Smoking was mainly a male habit until manufactured cigarettes became popular among women during the Second World War. Women therefore lagged some 40 years behind men in adopting the cigarette-smoking habit. After 1981 women were smoking over 45 per cent of all manufactured cigarettes. Other forms of tobacco have never been popular with women in the United Kingdom.

As total consumer sales data after 1987 were not provided to us by the TAC, and no data on sales were collected by the GHS, an estimate of the sales of manufactured cigarettes was calculated for 1988 to maintain continuity of sales data - one of the most useful measures of tobacco consumption. The sales figure for 1988 was estimated from a linear regression of the percentage difference between annual cigarette consumption (*Source*: GHS) and annual sales of manufactured cigarettes (*Source*: TAC) on time, 1972 to 1986 at two-year intervals (see Table 1.6). Although the GHS consumption figures are lower than the TAC sales figures (see note 12 for an explanation), a similar decline in the consumption and sale of cigarettes has occurred since the mid-1970s.

Notes for Section 1

1. The sales data were calculated by TAC from sales to the public of home-manufactured and imported tobacco goods, using the following sources of information:
   (i) Todd, G.F. 'The Statistical History of the Tobacco Trade, 1870-1920' (mimeographed for private circulation, 1947), tables 9, 26(a), (b), (c), (d).
   (ii) For the years 1920 to 1987, figures of sales of home-manufactured tobacco goods have been estimated from trade sources, and figures of imports have been taken from the 'Annual Statements of the Trade of the UK'.

2. The sales data from 1979 to 1989 (Table 1.3) are based on UK manufacturers sales to the wholesale and retail trade and estimates of sales of imported goods. Although sales to the trade are closely in line with sales to the public on a long-term basis, differences arise because of timing, in particular due to increased sales to the trade prior to the Chancellor's budget, and may be affected as in 1987 by the period of pre-budget restrictions imposed by HM Customs and Excise.

3. Sales for the years 1914-1919 exclude duty-free supplies to HM Forces.

4. Sales in the Irish Republic are excluded from 1924 onwards.

5. Imported cigarettes are included in the category 'Tobacco, Cigars, and Snuff' prior to 1900.

6. Imports exclude duty-free supplies imported by overseas organizations for their armed forces in the UK, but include private gift parcels from individuals abroad to these forces.

7. The average weight of a cigarette varies, depending on a number of factors such as size and whether it has a filter. Numbers of cigarettes sold during the years 1905-1919 were estimated from cigarette sales in pounds weight by using a conversion factor of 1g=1 cigarette.

8. The weight of 'filter cigarettes' sold represents the weight of tobacco in cigarettes tipped with a plug made of cellulose acetate fibre or some material other than tobacco.

9. The weight of tobacco sold has been divided into 'pipe tobacco' and 'hand-rolling tobacco' according to estimates of the amounts actually used in these ways. Numbers of hand-rolled cigarettes have been estimated from sales of tobacco and consumer survey findings.

10. 'Cigarillos' are product manufactured from cigar tobacco and are of approximately cigarette size, wrapped either in paper saturated with tobacco sauce or in processed tobacco sheet of natural tobacco colour.

11. The sales of plain and filter cigarettes and of tobacco sold for hand-rolling and the proportions of total consumption by men and by women have been estimated by Imperial Tobacco Limited.

12. There are at least three factors involved in the difference between the GHS consumption figures and the TAC sales figures: (i) the underestimate of smoking from GHS surveys (see page xxxiii), (ii) GHS surveys do not cover Northern Ireland, whereas TAC sales data include sales to Northern Ireland, and (iii) GHS data include hand-rolled cigarettes.

Table 1.1 Total annual sales of tobacco products (thousands of tonnes manufactured weight), 1870-1987
United Kingdom

Year	Manufactured cigarettes	Tobacco, cigars, and snuff	All tobacco products
1880-84	0.0	29.4	29.4
1885-89	0.0	30.8	30.8
1890-94	0.5	34.1	34.6
1895-99	2.8	35.7	38.4
1900-04	7.2	34.5	41.7
1905-09	13.3	30.4	43.7
1910-14	19.4	27.3	46.7
1915	24.6	28.5	53.1
1916	24.1	26.5	50.6
1917	25.0	26.9	51.9
1918	25.8	27.5	53.3
1919	36.2	35.1	71.3

Year	Manufactured cigarettes			Tobacco			Cigars and snuff			All tobacco products
	Plain	Filter	Total	Pipe	Hand-rolling	Total	Cigars and cigarillos	Snuff	Total	
1920	36.4	0.0	36.4	..	..	31.9	..	..	1.2	69.5
1921	35.4	0.0	35.4	..	..	31.3	..	..	1.2	67.9
1922	34.0	0.0	34.0	..	..	30.4	..	..	1.2	65.6
1923	34.1	0.0	34.1	..	..	28.6	..	..	1.2	63.9
1924	34.1	0.0	34.1	..	..	26.3	..	..	1.2	61.6
1925	36.3	0.0	36.3	..	..	26.4	..	..	1.2	63.9
1926	37.7	0.0	37.7	..	..	25.4	..	..	1.2	64.3
1927	40.4	0.0	40.4	..	..	25.0	..	..	1.2	66.6
1928	43.3	0.0	43.3	..	..	24.9	0.6	0.5	1.1	69.3
1929	45.9	0.0	45.9	..	..	24.2	0.6	0.5	1.1	71.2
1930	48.5	0.0	48.5	..	..	23.4	0.6	0.4	1.0	72.9
1931	49.2	0.1	49.3	21.9	0.7	22.6	0.6	0.4	1.0	72.9
1932	49.4	0.2	49.6	19.8	1.6	21.4	0.5	0.4	0.9	71.9
1933	51.8	0.2	52.0	18.3	2.4	20.7	0.5	0.4	0.9	73.6
1934	53.8	0.2	53.9	17.5	3.4	20.8	0.5	0.4	1.0	75.7
1935	57.3	0.2	57.5	17.1	3.3	20.4	0.6	0.5	1.0	79.0
1936	61.7	0.3	62.1	16.8	3.3	20.0	0.6	0.5	1.0	83.1
1937	66.3	0.4	66.7	16.4	3.2	19.6	0.6	0.5	1.1	87.4
1938	70.2	0.5	70.7	16.3	3.2	19.5	0.6	0.5	1.0	91.2
1939	73.3	0.5	73.8	15.6	3.3	18.9	0.5	0.5	1.0	93.7
1940	72.6	0.5	73.1	..	..	18.2	0.4	0.5	0.8	92.1
1941	80.8	0.5	81.3	..	..	19.5	0.4	0.5	0.9	101.7
1942	84.9	0.5	85.4	..	..	19.9	0.5	0.5	1.0	106.3
1943	85.3	0.5	85.9	..	..	17.6	0.5	0.5	1.0	104.4
1944	85.5	0.6	86.1	..	..	17.0	0.4	0.5	1.0	104.0
1945	94.2	0.6	94.8	..	..	17.4	0.4	0.5	0.9	113.1
1946	100.1	0.6	100.7	14.8	4.1	18.9	0.4	0.5	0.8	120.4
1947	87.1	0.5	87.6	12.5	4.5	17.1	0.5	0.4	0.9	105.6
1948	82.9	0.6	83.5	13.4	5.2	18.6	0.4	0.4	0.8	102.8
1949	79.8	0.9	80.7	12.2	6.4	18.6	0.4	0.3	0.7	99.9

Table 1.1 (*continued*)   Total annual sales of tobacco products (thousands of tonnes manufactured weight), 1870-1987
United Kingdom

Year	Manufactured cigarettes			Tobacco			Cigars and snuff				All tobacco products
	Plain	Filter	Total	Pipe	Hand-rolling	Total	Cigars and cigarillos		Snuff	Total	
1950	81.0	1.4	82.4	11.5	5.9	17.4	0.4		0.3	0.7	100.5
1951	85.8	0.8	86.5	10.4	5.9	16.3	0.4		0.3	0.7	103.5
1952	87.2	0.8	88.0	10.4	6.3	16.6	0.4		0.3	0.7	105.4
1953	89.2	0.9	90.1	10.1	6.2	16.2	0.4		0.4	0.7	107.0
1954	91.2	1.4	92.5	9.9	6.1	16.0	0.4		0.3	0.7	109.3
1955	94.1	1.6	95.8	9.3	6.0	15.3	0.4		0.3	0.7	111.8
1956	95.2	2.6	97.8	8.8	5.8	14.7	0.5		0.3	0.8	113.2
1957	95.8	4.6	100.4	8.9	6.0	14.9	0.5		0.3	0.9	116.1
1958	93.8	8.3	102.1	8.6	6.6	15.2	0.6		0.3	0.9	118.3
1959	93.4	11.0	104.5	8.3	7.0	15.3	0.7		0.3	1.0	120.7
1960	93.7	14.8	108.5	7.9	7.1	15.1	0.7		0.3	1.0	124.6
1961	91.6	18.7	110.3	7.4	7.3	14.7	0.7		0.3	1.0	126.0
1962	80.8	23.9	104.7	7.8	7.2	15.0	0.9		0.3	1.1	120.8
1963	76.5	31.3	107.9	7.3	7.6	14.9	1.0		0.2	1.2	123.9
1964	65.0	39.7	104.7	7.1	7.7	14.7	1.2		0.2	1.5	120.9
1965	51.4	48.7	100.1	6.6	7.3	13.9	1.3		0.2	1.5	115.6
1966	44.3	57.0	101.3	6.4	7.1	13.5	1.6		0.2	1.8	116.6
1967	38.7	61.7	100.4	6.3	7.1	13.4	1.8		0.2	2.0	115.8
							Cigars	Cigarillos			
1968	33.7	66.2	99.9	6.0	7.0	13.0	1.6	0.3	0.2	2.1	114.9
1969	28.6	69.6	98.2	5.9	6.8	12.8	1.6	0.2	0.2	2.1	113.1
1970	25.3	72.4	97.7	5.8	6.5	12.3	1.9	0.2	0.2	2.2	112.2
1971	22.6	70.0	92.6	6.0	5.9	11.9	2.6	0.1	0.2	2.9	107.4
1972	21.8	76.2	98.1	5.7	6.2	11.8	2.8	0.1	0.2	3.1	113.0
1973	21.1	82.7	103.8	5.6	6.1	11.7	3.1	0.1	0.2	3.4	119.0
1974	19.1	83.2	102.3	5.4	6.1	11.5	3.1	0.1	0.2	3.4	117.3
1975	15.7	80.7	96.4	5.0	6.5	11.5	3.2	0.1	0.2	3.5	111.4
1976	13.8	79.4	93.2	5.0	6.5	11.5	3.1	0.1	0.1	3.3	108.0
1977	10.7	79.0	89.7	4.9	6.5	11.4	3.0	0.1	0.1	3.2	104.3
1978	10.3	88.6	98.9	4:6	6.1	10.7	3.1	0.1	0.1	3.3	112.9
1979	9.1	89.5	98.6	4.2	5.7	9.9	3.1	0.1	0.1	3.3	111.8
1980	7.5	89.7	97.2	4.0	5.6	9.6	2.9	0.1	0.1	3.1	109.9
1981	6.2	83.2	89.4	3.8	6.2	10.0	2.8	0.1	0.1	3.0	102.4
1982	4.9	77.7	82.6	3.5	6.2	9.7	2.7	0.0	0.1	2.8	95.1
1983	4.3	78.7	83.0	3.3	5.8	9.1	2.6	0.0	0.1	2.7	94.8
1984	3.7	77.9	81.6	3.2	5.3	8.5	2.7	0.0	0.1	2.8	92.9
1985	3.1	78.0	81.1	3.0	5.0	8.0	2.6	0.0	0.1	2.7	91.8
1986	2.7	77.1	79.8	2.8	4.8	7.6	2.6	0.0	0.1	2.7	90.1
1987	2.2	77.2	79.4	2.5	4.8	7.3	2.7	0.0	0.1	2.8	89.5

Source: TAC

Fig. 1.1 Total annual sales of all tobacco products and of manufactured cigarettes by weight, 1870-1987 (5-year averages plotted)
United Kingdom. *Source*: TAC

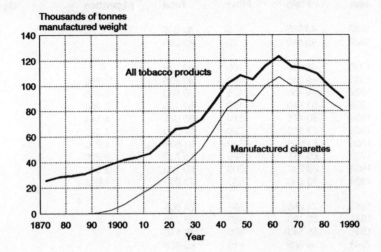

Table 1.2 Total annual sales of cigarettes and cigars (numbers in millions), 1905-1987
United Kingdom

Year	Manufactured cigarettes			Hand-rolled cigarettes	Cigars and cigarillos
	Plain	Filter	Total		
1905	11 200	0	11 200	..	..
1906	12 400	0	12 400	..	..
1907	13 600	0	13 600	..	..
1908	14 400	0	14 400	..	..
1909	14 800	0	14 800	..	..
1910	16 400	0	16 400	..	..
1911	18 200	0	18 200	..	..
1912	19 500	0	19 500	..	..
1913	20 700	0	20 700	..	..
1914	22 400	0	22 400	..	..
1915	24 600	0	24 600	..	..
1916	24 100	0	24 100	..	..
1917	25 100	0	25 100	..	..
1918	25 800	0	25 800	..	..
1919	36 200	0	36 200	..	..
1920	36 240	0	36 240	..	..
1921	35 185	0	35 185	..	..
1922	33 730	0	33 730	..	..
1923	33 725	0	33 725	..	..
1924	33 835	0	33 835	..	..
1925	36 030	0	36 030	..	..
1926	37 435	0	37 435	..	..
1927	40 030	0	40 030	..	..

Year	Manufactured cigarettes			Hand-rolled cigarettes	Cigars and cigarillos
	Plain	**Filter**	**Total**		
1928	43 035	0	43 035	..	135
1929	45 510	25	45 535	..	135
1930	48 235	100	48 335	..	140
1931	49 045	190	49 235	896	150
1932	49 455	175	49 630	2 016	135
1933	51 940	190	52 130	2 968	135
1934	53 415	210	53 625	4 144	145
1935	57 110	220	57 330	4 040	155
1936	61 295	340	61 635	4 030	165
1937	65 415	420	65 835	3 900	170
1938	69 240	500	69 740	3 940	170
1939	73 240	570	73 810	4 088	175
1940	74 255	550	74 805	..	125
1941	82 180	580	82 760	..	155
1942	85 540	570	86 110	..	150
1943	84 865	610	85 475	..	155
1944	83 885	640	84 525	..	130
1945	92 660	640	93 300	..	120
1946	98 345	670	99 015	5 040	100
1947	86 975	550	87 525	5 600	125
1948	83 540	640	84 180	6 624	110
1949	80 900	1 050	81 950	8 064	105
1950	83 435	1 710	85 145	7 488	115
1951	88 435	900	89 335	7 696	120
1952	89 520	880	90 400	8 170	125
1953	91 655	1 040	92 695	8 051	130
1954	93 680	1 550	95 230	8 424	140
1955	96 800	1 870	98 670	8 237	150
1956	96 510	3 050	99 560	8 192	180
1957	96 880	5 370	102 250	8 448	210
1958	94 320	9 700	104 020	9 344	250
1959	93 700	12 900	106 600	9 856	290
1960	93 400	17 500	110 900	10 299	315
1961	91 300	22 100	113 400	10 496	315
1962	81 300	28 600	109 900	11 300	390
1963	77 400	37 800	115 200	11 169	445
1964	66 600	47 800	114 400	11 546	590
1965	52 600	59 400	112 000	11 742	700
1966	46 300	71 300	117 600	11 178	900
1967	40 600	78 500	119 100	11 103	1 135

Year	Plain	Filter	Total	Hand-rolled cigarettes	**Cigars**	**Cigarillos**
1968	35 700	86 100	121 800	11 359	835	345
1969	30 600	94 300	124 900	11 165	845	290
1970	27 800	100 100	127 900	10 875	975	215
1971	24 700	97 700	122 400	9 915	1 360	195
1972	23 900	106 600	130 500	10 689	1 410	165
1973	23 300	114 100	137 400	10 383	1 545	170
1974	21 250	115 750	137 000	10 088	1 600	165
1975	17 750	114 850	132 600	10 924	1 640	160
1976	15 600	115 000	130 600	11 500	1 580	145

Table 1.2 (*continued*) Total annual sales of cigarettes and cigars (numbers in millions), 1905-1987
United Kingdom

Year	Manufactured cigarettes			Hand-rolled cigarettes	Cigars and cigarillos	
	Plain	Filter	Total		Cigars	Cigarillos
1977	12 550	113 350	125 900	11 100	1 570	120
1978	12 000	113 200	125 200	10 550	1 610	120
1979	10 600	113 700	124 300	9 500	1 650	105
1980	8 750	112 750	121 500	9 400	1 610	85
1981	7 050	103 250	110 300	11 500	1 540	70
1982	5 750	96 250	102 000	11 700	1 465	55
1983	5 000	96 600	101 600	11 200	1 445	50
1984	4 300	94 700	99 000	9 850	1 400	45
1985	3 600	94 150	97 750	9 500	1 380	40
1986	3 100	92 400	95 500	9 000	1 420	30
1987	2 650	92 350	95 000	8 900	1 490	25

Source: TAC

Fig 1.2   Total annual sales of plain and filter manufactured cigarettes in numbers, 1905-1987 (5-year averages plotted)
United Kingdom. *Source*: TAC

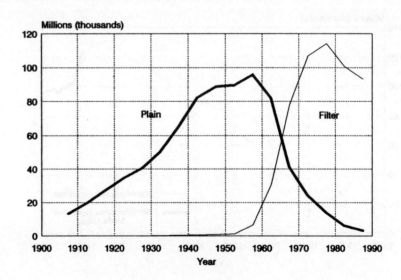

Year	Cigarettes	Cigars	Cigarillos	Pipe	Hand-rolled cigarettes
	(numbers in millions)			(thousands of tonnes weight)	
1979	124 110	1 640	105	4.0	5.7
1980	121 460	1 630	85	3.8	5.7
1981	110 090	1 530	70	3.6	6.3
1982	101 500	1 460	55	3.3	6.3
1983	102 150	1 440	50	3.1	6.0
1984	99 220	1 400	45	3 0	5.5
1985	98 310	1 380	40	2.9	5.1
1986	95 110	1 420	30	2.7	4.8
1987	98 380	1 510	26	2.5	4.8
1988	97 300	1 520	23	2.3	4.5
1989	97 300	1 500	14	2.1	4.3

Source: TAC

Fig 1.3 Total annual sales of manufactured cigarettes in numbers, 1905-1987 (5-year averages plotted) and total annual sales of manufactured cigarettes to the trade in numbers, 1979-1989
United Kingdom. *Source*: TAC

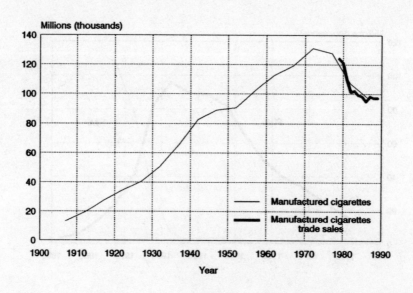

Year	Manufactured cigarettes		All tobacco[1] products
	Men	**Women**	**Men**
1905	11.2	..	42.8
1906	12.4	..	43.1
1907	13.6	..	44.5
1908	14.4	..	44.5
1909	14.8	..	43.5
1910	16.4	..	44.6
1911	18.1	..	46.0
1912	19.5	..	46.0
1913	20.6	..	47.3
1914	22.3	..	49.6
1915	24.6	..	53.1
1916	24.1	..	50.6
1917	25.0	..	51.9
1918	25.8	..	53.3
1919	36.2	..	71.3
1920	36.4	0.0	69.5
1921	35.2	0.3	67.6
1922	33.4	0.6	65.0
1923	33.2	0.8	63.0
1924	32.8	1.2	60.4
1925	34.7	1.6	62.3
1926	35.8	1.9	62.4
1927	38.1	2.3	64.3
1928	40.6	2.8	66.5
1929	42.7	3.3	68.0
1930	44.9	3.6	69.3
1931	45.2	4.1	68.8
1932	45.1	4.4	67.4
1933	47.1	4.9	68.7
1934	48.5	5.4	70.3
1935	51.4	6.1	72.9
1936	55.2	6.9	76.2
1937	59.0	7.7	79.7
1938	62.1	8.6	82.6
1939	64.4	9.5	84.2
1940	61.6	11.5	80.6
1941	66.1	15.2	86.5
1942	66.8	18.6	87.7
1943	65.0	20.9	83.6
1944	62.7	23.4	80.6
1945	69.4	25.4	87.7
1946	77.2	23.5	96.9
1947	66.5	21.1	84.5
1948	64.6	18.8	84.0
1949	60.6	20.1	79.8

Table 1.4 (*continued*) Total annual consumption of tobacco products (thousands of tonnes manufactured weight) by men and women, 1905-1987
United Kingdom

| Year | Manufactured cigarettes | | All tobacco[1] products |
	Men	Women	Men
1950	60.7	21.7	78.7
1951	64.0	22.5	81.0
1952	64.8	23.2	82.1
1953	65.8	24.3	82.7
1954	67.1	25.4	83.8
1955	68.9	26.9	84.9
1956	68.4	29.3	83.9
1957	69.3	31.1	85.0
1958	70.5	31.6	86.7
1959	71.8	32.6	88.1
1960	75.4	33.1	91.4
1961	75.1	35.2	90.8
1962	71.1	33.6	87.2
1963	71.5	36.3	87.6
1964	69.3	35.4	85.5
1965	65.0	35.2	80.4
1966	64.1	37.2	79.4
1967	64.5	35.9	80.0
1968	64.8	35.1	79.9
1969	61.2	37.0	76.1
1970	61.2	36.5	75.8
1971	57.7	34.9	72.5
1972	61.1	37.0	76.0
1973	62.5	41.3	77.7
1974	60.2	42.1	75.1
1975	57.0	39.5	72.0
1976	52.9	40.3	67.8
1977	49.8	39.9	64.4
1978	55.2	43.8	69.2
1979	55.2	43.4	68.4
1980	54.6	42.6	67.4
1981	47.9	41.5	60.9
1982	44.2	38.4	56.7
1983	43.9	39.1	55.7
1984	44.6	37.0	55.9
1985	42.5	38.6	53.2
1986	42.0	37.8	52.3
1987	41.8	37.6	51.9

1 Forms of tobacco other than manufactured cigarettes have never been popular with women in the United Kingdom, and so data on all tobacco products for women have not been presented in this table. In most years, the figure for all tobacco products for women is equal to that for manufactured cigarettes.

Source: TAC

Table 1.5   Total annual consumption of cigarettes (manufactured and hand-rolled), numbers in millions, 1972-1988

Men and women aged 16 and over, Great Britain

Year	Estimated size of population (i)	Percentage who smoke cigarettes (ii)	Cigarettes smoked number/year (iii)	Annual consumption of cigarettes (in millions) (i)x(ii)x(iii)		Year	Total annual consumption of cigarettes (in millions)
Men							
1972	19 411900	52	6 240	62 988			
1974	19 570300	51	6 500	64 876			
1976	19 765700	46	6 708	60 991			
1978	20 003600	45	6 604	59 447			
1980	20 318800	42	6 448	55 027			
1982	20 544900	38	6 292	49 122			
1984	20 843600	36	5 980	44 872		1972	102 551
1986	21 103200	35	5 980	44 169		1974	107 861
1988	21 334800	33	6 240	43 933		1976	104 101
						1978	101 913
Women						1980	98 465
1972	21 329500	41	4 524	39 563		1982	86 735
1974	21 449100	41	4 888	42 986		1984	80 980
1976	21 601200	38	5 252	43 111		1986	79 887
1978	21 853200	37	5 252	42 466		1988	79 513
1980	22 134400	37	5 304	43 438			
1982	22 366400	33	5 096	37 613			
1984	22 603300	32	4 992	36 107			
1986	22 842600	31	5 044	35 718			
1988	23 038300	30	5 148	35 580			

Source: Office of Population Censuses and Surveys (unpublished data) Crown Copyright reserved with respect of data included in this table. Published by permission of the Controller of Her Majesty's Stationery Office GHS

Table 1.6 Total annual sales of manufactured cigarettes in the UK, 1972-1986, and the estimated sales for 1988, numbers in millions

Year	Total annual consumption of cigarettes[1] Great Britain (GHS) (in millions)	Total annual sales of manufactured cigarettes UK (TAC) (in millions)	Difference between annual cigarette consumption (GHS) and annual sales of cigarettes (TAC) (%)
1972	102 551	130 500	21.4
1974	107 861	137 000	21.3
1976	104 101	130 600	20.3
1978	101 913	125 200	18.6
1980	98 465	121 500	19.0
1982	86 735	102 000	15.0
1984	80 980	99 000	18.2
1986	79 887	95 500	16.3
1988	79 513	93 800 (E)[2]	15.2 (E)[2]

1 See Table 1.5 for further explanation
2 Estimated from a linear regression of percentage difference between the GHS consumption data and the TAC sales data on time

Source: GHS
TAC

Fig. 1.4 Total annual consumption of cigarettes (manufactured and hand-rolled) in numbers, 1972-1988 (Great Britain, *Source*: GHS), total annual sales of manufactured cigarettes in numbers, 1972-1986 (UK, *Source*: TAC), and the estimated annual sales for 1988 (see Table 1.6)

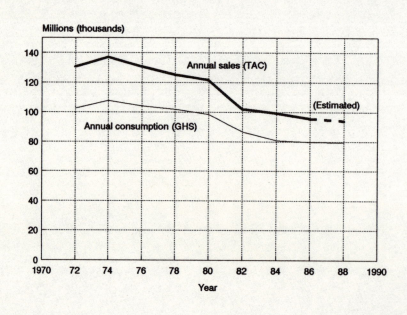

As TAC data have not been provided after 1987 and the GHS does not collect data on the annual weight of tobacco consumed, these data will not be available in the future unless steps are taken to obtain the information. If they are not it will represent an important gap in our knowledge of national smoking habits.

Consumption per person

Cigarettes

Men

Apart from a brief decline after the end of the First World War, manufactured cigarette consumption among men rose steadily from about 1890 until the end of the Second World War in 1945, when it reached a peak of 12 manufactured cigarettes per adult male per day (4420 cigarettes per year). For the next 30 years consumption in terms of number of cigarettes remained fairly stable, varying between 9 and 11 manufactured cigarettes per day (3320 and 4030 cigarettes per year). Since 1974, consumption has decreased steadily to 6.3 manufactured cigarettes per day (2290 cigarettes per year) in 1987. An earlier decline in the amount of cigarettes smoked in terms of weight of tobacco (from 1964) was due to the change from non-filter to filter cigarettes containing less tobacco.

Consumption of hand-rolled cigarettes, always much less than consumption of manufactured cigarettes, increased until 1965 when it reached a maximum of about 1.5 cigarettes per adult male per day (about 570 cigarettes per year). Thereafter it decreased slightly. (As almost all hand-rolled cigarettes are smoked by men, the consumption per adult male can be approximated to twice the adult (male plus female) per person consumption.)

Women

Cigarette smoking among women began at about 1920, and rose rapidly, to reach a maximum of just over 7 manufactured cigarettes per adult female per day (2630 cigarettes per year) in 1974. Since then, there has been a steady decline, although the rate of decline in women has been less than in men. In 1987 manufactured cigarette consumption per adult female was 81 per cent of that among adult males, and 70 per cent if all cigarettes (manufactured plus hand-rolled) are included.

All tobacco products

Men

Annual consumption of all tobacco products rose from 2.6 kg per adult male in 1871 to a maximum of 5.7 kg in 1945, and then fell steadily to 2.4 kg in 1987. In 1871 the tobacco was used for pipe and cigar smoking, as snuff, and for chewing. By 1906, 30 per cent of all tobacco consumed by men was in manufactured cigarettes. This proportion increased steadily to around 80 per cent by 1945, and has remained at this level until 1987.

Women

Consumption of all tobacco products has not been estimated for women, as forms of tobacco other than manufactured cigarettes have never been much used by women.

Consumption per smoker

Cigarettes

Men

According to TAC data, consumption of manufactured cigarettes per adult male smoker rose from 14 per day in 1949 to 19 per day in 1955, and remained at about this level until 1970, when there was a small increase to 22 per day by 1973. From 1972 the consumption of cigarettes per smoker has been estimated by the GHS, but their figures are lower than those of the TAC; for example, in 1986 TAC estimated that the consumption of manufactured cigarettes per adult male smoker was 19 per day, while GHS estimated that the consumption of cigarettes (manufactured and hand-rolled) per smoker was 16 per day. The discrepancy is at least in part due to the fact that the GHS data are not sales-adjusted (i.e., the estimated total number of cigarettes smoked has not been adjusted to agree with the number of cigarettes sold in the same period).

TAC data show that smokers who smoke only hand-rolled cigarettes consume a smaller quantity of tobacco annually than smokers who smoke only manufactured cigarettes.

Women

According to TAC data, consumption of manufactured cigarettes per adult female smoker rose steadily from 7 cigarettes per day in 1949 to a maximum of 17 per day in 1976. In 1986, consumption of manufactured cigarettes per smoker was 15 per day according to TAC data, while that of all cigarettes was 14 per day according to GHS data.

Cigars

Men

TAC data on the annual weight of cigar tobacco consumed per adult male cigar smoker are available from 1975 to 1987. Between these years there have been some fluctuations in consumption per smoker among all smokers of cigars and among smokers of cigars only, but no clear upward or downward trend. These fluctuations may be due to the relatively small number of cigar smokers interviewed.

Pipes

Men

TAC data on the annual weight of pipe tobacco consumed per adult male pipe smoker are available from 1956 to 1987. Among all smokers of pipes there has been little change in the annual weight of pipe tobacco consumed per smoker. Data on pipe-only smokers show greater fluctuations over the same period, but may be less reliable, due to the small number of pipe-only smokers interviewed.

Table 2.1 Annual consumption of tobacco products per person, 1870-1987
Men and women aged 15 and over, United Kingdom

Year	Manufactured cigarettes number/person			Manufactured cigarettes kg/person			Hand-rolled cigarettes number/ person	kg/ person	All tobacco products kg/person	
	Men	Women	Adults	Men	Women	Adults	Adults	Adults	Men	Adults
1871	..	..	..	0.0	..	0.0	..	..	2.6	1.2
1881	..	..	..	0.0	..	0.0	..	..	2.7	1.3
1890-94	..	..	..	0.0	..	0.0	..	..	2.9	1.4
1895-99	..	..	..	0.2	..	0.1	..	..	3.0	1.4
1900-04	..	..	..	0.5	..	0.3	..	..	3.1	1.5
1905	800	..	380	0.8	..	0.4	..	..	3.0	1.5
1906	870	..	420	0.9	..	0.4	..	..	3.0	1.5
1907	940	..	450	1.0	..	0.5	..	..	3.1	1.5
1908	980	..	470	1.0	..	0.5	..	..	3.0	1.5
1909	1 000	..	480	1.0	..	0.5	..	..	2.9	1.4
1910	1 090	..	530	1.1	..	0.5	..	..	2.9	1.5
1911	1 200	..	580	1.2	..	0.6	..	..	3.0	1.5
1912	1 270	..	610	1.3	..	0.6	..	..	3.0	1.5
1913	1 340	..	650	1.3	..	0.6	..	..	3.1	1.5
1914	1 430	..	690	1.4	..	0.7	..	..	3.2	1.5
1915	1 710	..	780	1.7	..	0.8	..	..	3.7	1.7
1916	1 740	..	770	1.7	..	0.8	..	..	3.6	1.6
1917	1 860	..	810	1.9	..	0.8	..	..	3.9	1.7
1918	1 920	..	830	1.9	..	0.8	..	..	4.0	1.7
1919	2 490	..	1 130	2.5	..	1.1	..	..	4.9	2.2
1920	2 290	0	1 080	2.3	0.0	1.1	..	..	4.4	2.1
1921	2 160	13	1 030	2.2	0.0	1.0	..	..	4.2	2.0
1922	2 030	45	980	2.0	0.0	1.0	..	..	3.9	1.9
1923	1 980	45	970	2.0	0.0	1.0	..	..	3.8	1.8
1924	2 070	90	1 020	2.1	0.1	1.0	..	..	3.9	1.9
1925	2 210	90	1 080	2.2	0.1	1.1	..	..	3.9	1.9
1926	2 250	90	1 110	2.3	0.1	1.1	..	..	3.9	1.9
1927	2 390	130	1 180	2.4	0.1	1.2	..	..	4.0	2.0
1928	2 520	130	1 260	2.5	0.1	1.3	..	..	4.1	2.0
1929	2 610	180	1 330	2.6	0.2	1.4	..	..	4.2	2.1
1930	2 760	180	1 380	2.8	0.2	1.4	..	..	4.3	2.1
1931	2 760	230	1 410	2.8	0.2	1.4	26	0.0	4.2	2.1
1932	2 720	230	1 410	2.7	0.2	1.4	57	0.0	4.0	2.0
1933	2 820	270	1 470	2.8	0.3	1.5	84	0.1	4.1	2.1
1934	2 840	270	1 500	2.9	0.3	1.5	116	0.1	4.2	2.1
1935	2 980	320	1 590	3.0	0.3	1.6	112	0.1	4.3	2.2
1936	3 200	360	1 690	3.2	0.4	1.7	111	0.1	4.4	2.3
1937	3 360	400	1 790	3.4	0.4	1.8	107	0.1	4.6	2.4
1938	3 490	450	1 880	3.5	0.5	1.9	106	0.1	4.7	2.4
1939	3 630	500	1 970	3.6	0.5	2.0	109	0.1	4.8	2.5
1940	3 670	600	2 020	3.6	0.6	2.0	..	..	4.7	2.5
1941	3 920	790	2 230	3.9	0.8	2.2	..	..	5.0	2.7
1942	4 020	920	2 340	4.0	0.9	2.3	..	..	5.2	2.9

Year	Manufactured cigarettes number/person			Manufactured cigarettes kg/person			Hand-rolled cigarettes number/ person	kg/ person	All tobacco products kg/person	
	Men	Women	Adults	Men	Women	Adults	Adults	Adults	Men	Adults
1943	3 930	1 040	2 330	3.9	1.0	2.4	..	..	5.1	2.9
1944	4 010	1 110	2 380	4.1	1.1	2.4	..	..	5.3	2.9
1945	4 420	1 250	2 600	4.5	1.3	2.6	..	..	5.7	3.2
1946	4 280	1 120	2 600	4.4	1.1	2.6	132	0.1	5.5	3.2
1947	3 670	1 040	2 270	3.7	1.0	2.3	146	0.1	4.7	2.7
1948	3 520	920	2 170	3.5	0.9	2.1	171	0.1	4.6	2.6
1949	3 320	1 010	2 110	3.3	1.0	2.1	207	0.2	4.3	2.6
1950	3 370	1 080	2 180	3.3	1.0	2.1	192	0.1	4.2	2.6
1951	3 610	1 120	2 300	3.5	1.1	2.2	198	0.1	4.4	2.7
1952	3 640	1 170	2 320	3.5	1.1	2.3	210	0.2	4.5	2.7
1953	3 690	1 210	2 370	3.6	1.2	2.3	206	0.1	4.5	2.7
1954	3 740	1 260	2 430	3.6	1.2	2.4	215	0.1	4.5	2.8
1955	3 830	1 360	2 510	3.7	1.3	2.4	210	0.1	4.6	2.9
1956	3 740	1 430	2 530	3.7	1.4	2.5	208	0.1	4.5	2.9
1957	3 790	1 530	2 590	3.7	1.5	2.5	214	0.1	4.5	2.9
1958	3 840	1 530	2 620	3.8	1.5	2.6	236	0.2	4.6	3.0
1959	3 890	1 570	2 670	3.8	1.5	2.6	247	0.2	4.7	3.0
1960	4 030	1 620	2 760	3.9	1.6	2.7	256	0.2	4.8	3.1
1961	4 010	1 680	2 800	3.9	1.6	2.7	260	0.2	4.7	3.1
1962	3 770	1 710	2 690	3.7	1.6	2.5	276	0.2	4.5	2.9
1963	3 820	1 880	2 800	3.7	1.7	2.6	271	0.2	4.5	3.0
1964	3 780	1 840	2 770	3.5	1.6	2.5	279	0.2	4.4	2.9
1965	3 610	1 870	2 700	3.3	1.6	2.4	283	0.2	4.1	2.8
1966	3 680	2 050	2 820	3.2	1.7	2.4	268	0.2	4.0	2.8
1967	3 760	2 020	2 850	3.2	1.6	2.4	266	0.2	4.0	2.8
1968	3 880	2 030	2 910	3.3	1.6	2.4	271	0.2	4.0	2.8
1969	3 800	2 220	2 980	3.0	1.7	2.4	266	0.2	3.8	2.7
1970	3 920	2 250	3 040	3.0	1.7	2.3	259	0.1	3.8	2.7
1971	3 700	2 170	2 900	2.9	1.6	2.2	235	0.1	3.6	2.5
1972	3 930	2 300	3 080	3.0	1.7	2.3	252	0.1	3.8	2.7
1973	3 980	2 540	3 230	3.1	1.9	2.4	244	0.1	3.8	2.8
1974	3 840	2 630	3 210	2.9	1.9	2.4	236	0.1	3.7	2.8
1975	3 730	2 500	3 090	2.8	1.8	2.3	255	0.1	3.5	2.6
1976	3 530	2 580	3 050	2.6	1.8	2.2	267	0.1	3.3	2.5
1977	3 310	2 540	2 900	2.4	1.8	2.1	256	0.1	3.1	2.4
1978	3 330	2 450	2 850	2.6	2.0	2.3	242	0.1	3.3	2.6
1979	3 300	2 410	2 850	2.6	1.9	2.3	217	0.1	3.3	2.5
1980	3 230	2 330	2 750	2.6	1.9	2.2	213	0.1	3.2	2.5
1981	2 760	2 200	2 470	2.2	1.8	2.0	257	0.1	2.8	2.3
1982	2 540	2 030	2 270	2.1	1.6	1.8	260	0.1	2.6	2.1
1983	2 500	2 020	2 250	2.0	1.7	1.8	248	0.1	2.6	2.1
1984	2 500	1 890	2 190	2.1	1.6	1.8	217	0.1	2.6	2.1
1985	2 380	1 930	2 150	2.0	1.6	1.8	209	0.1	2.4	2.0
1986	2 310	1 880	2 090	1.9	1.6	1.7	197	0.1	2.4	2.0
1987	2 290	1 870	2 070	1.9	1.6	1.7	193	0.1	2.4	1.9

Source: TAC

Fig 2.1 Annual consumption (weight) of all tobacco products and of manufactured cigarettes per adult male, 1890-1987 (5-year averages plotted)
Men aged 15 and over, United Kingdom. *Source*: TAC

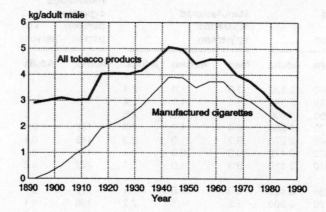

Table 2.2 Weekly and daily consumption of manufactured cigarettes per person, 1910-1987
Men and women aged 15 and over, United Kingdom

Year	Manufactured cigarettes number/ person/week		Manufactured cigarettes number/ person/day	
	Men	Women	Men	Women
1910-1914	24	..	3.5	..
1915-1919	37	..	5.3	..
1920-1924	41	1	5.8	0.1
1925-1929	46	2	6.6	0.3
1930-1934	53	5	7.6	0.6
1935-1939	64	8	9.1	1.1
1940-1944	75	17	10.7	2.4
1945-1949	74	21	10.5	2.9
1950-1954	69	22	9.9	3.2
1955-1959	73	29	10.5	4.1
1960-1964	75	34	10.6	4.8
1965-1969	72	39	10.3	5.6
1970-1974	75	46	10.6	6.5
1975-1979	66	48	9.4	6.8
1980-1984	52	40	7.4	5.7
1985	46	37	6.5	5.3
1986	44	36	6.3	5.2
1987	44	36	6.3	5.1

Source: TAC, derived from Table 2.1

SECTION 2 Consumption of tobacco products per person and per smoker, 1870-1988

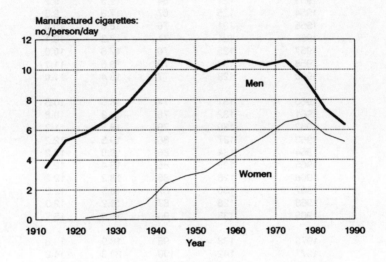

Table 2.3 Weekly and daily consumption of manufactured cigarettes per smoker, 1949-1987[1]
Manufactured cigarette smokers, men and women aged 16 and over, Great Britain: sales-adjusted

Year	Manufactured cigarettes number/ smoker/week		Manufactured cigarettes number/ smoker/day	
	Men	Women	Men	Women
1949	99	48	14.1	6.8
1950	107	56	15.2	7.9
1951	110	57	15.6	8.1
1952	120	60	17.1	8.5
1953	121	64	17.3	9.2
1954	125	67	17.8	9.6
1955	131	70	18.6	10.0
1956	121	71	17.3	10.1
1957	125	70	17.8	10.0
1958	130	78	18.5	11.1
1959	129	77	18.4	11.0
1960	131	74	18.6	10.5
1961	132	76	18.8	10.8
1962	130	79	18.5	11.2
1963	137	86	19.5	12.2
1964	134	86	19.0	12.2
1965	129	85	18.4	12.1
1966	128	86	18.2	12.2
1967	130	87	18.5	12.3
1968	128	87	18.2	12.3
1969	133	96	18.9	13.7
1970	133	95	18.9	13.6
1971	142	100	20.3	14.2
1972	148	105	21.1	14.9
1973	156	113	22.2	16.2
1974	149	115	21.2	16.4
1975	152	111	21.6	15.8
1976	155	120	22.1	17.1
1977	152	119	21.6	17.0
1978	155	118	22.1	16.8
1979	152	116	21.6	16.6
1980	149	115	21.2	16.4
1981	141	113	20.1	16.2
1982	139	112	19.9	15.9
1983	139	112	19.9	15.9
1984	138	108	19.6	15.3
1985	134	110	19.0	15.6
1986	136	111	19.4	15.8
1987	135	108	19.2	15.4

1 Data on consumption of manufactured cigarettes
per smoker was not available before 1949

Source: TAC

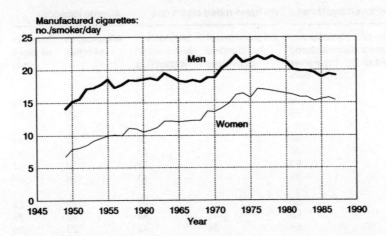

Table 2.4 Weekly and daily consumption of cigarettes (manufactured and hand-rolled) per smoker, 1972-1988
Cigarette smokers, men and women aged 16 and over, Great Britain

Year	Cigarettes number/ smoker/week		Cigarettes number/ smoker/day	
	Men	Women	Men	Women
1972	120	87	17.1	12.4
1974	125	94	17.9	13.4
1976	129	101	18.4	14.4
1978	127	101	18.1	14.4
1980	124	102	17.7	14.6
1982	121	98	17.3	14.0
1984	115	96	16.4	13.7
1986	115	97	16.4	13.9
1988	120	99	17.1	14.1

Source: GHS

Table 2.5 Annual weight[1] of tobacco consumed (hundreds of grams) per adult male smoker: by type of smoker, 1956-1987
Smokers, men aged 16 and over, Great Britain: sales-adjusted except for cigar tobacco

Year	As manufactured cigarettes		As hand-rolled cigarettes		As pipe tobacco		As cigar tobacco	
	All smokers of manufactured cigarettes	Smokers of manufactured cigarettes only	All smokers of hand-rolled cigarettes	Smokers of hand-rolled cigarettes only	All smokers of pipes	Smokers of pipes only	All smokers of cigars	Smokers of cigars only
1956	..	66	..	44	27	29	..	..
1958	..	66	..	44	27	33	..	..
1961	..	66	..	37	27	44	..	..
1963	..	70	..	41	25	37	..	..
1965	..	63	..	37	24	37	..	..
1968	..	59	..	41	24	29	..	..
1971	..	59	..	41	23	29	..	..
1973	..	63	..	41	23	29	..	..
1975	56	56	26	41	23	36	12	22
1976	56	56	27	40	25	36	19	27
1977	56	56	27	39	26	33	14	20
1978	64	63	29	44	27	36	11	17
1979	62	62	28	44	25	30	13	23
1980	61	63	27	40	26	36	12	17
1981	59	61	23	35	27	36	13	19
1982	58	59	23	37	25	33	10	15
1983	58	60	24	36	26	34	14	20
1984	57	58	24	38	32	38	12	18
1985	57	57	21	34	29	43	14	22
1986	56	56	23	34	26	36	12	17
1987	56	56	22	36	23	30	13	20

1 Figures before 1975 have been converted from lb/year or oz/week, and may be less accurate than those for the years 1975-1987

Source: TAC

Percentage of population who smoke 3

Information on the percentages of men and women in the population who smoke is available from 1948 onwards, when the TRC/TAC surveys started. From 1972 data are also available from the GHS.

Cigarettes

Men

According to TAC data, the percentage of men who smoke manufactured cigarettes fell from 65 per cent in 1948 to 34 per cent in 1987. The percentage of men who smoke hand-rolled cigarettes fell slightly from 13 per cent in 1961 to 10 per cent in 1987. (Men who smoke both manufactured and hand-rolled cigarettes are included in both figures.) GHS data indicate a decline in the percentage of men who smoke cigarettes (manufactured and hand-rolled) from 52 per cent in 1972 to 33 per cent in 1988.

Women

According to TAC data, the percentage of women who smoke manufactured cigarettes fluctuated between 36 and 45 per cent during the years between 1948 and 1975. Since 1975, it has decreased steadily to 34 per cent in 1987, the same level as men. TAC surveys indicate that less than 1 per cent of women smoke hand-rolled cigarettes.

The GHS provides data on the percentage of men and women in the population who smoke all types of cigarettes (i.e., manufactured plus hand-rolled). In spite of this, the GHS estimates for the percentage of women who smoke cigarettes are consistently less than those produced by the TAC for women who smoke manufactured cigarettes. Possible reasons for the discrepancy between GHS and TAC data, in addition to the fact that the TAC data are sales-adjusted whereas the GHS data are not, are discussed on page xxxiii.

Cigars

Men

The TAC surveys estimate that the percentage of men who smoke cigars rose from 9 per cent in 1965 to a maximum of 14 per cent in 1973, and then declined to 7 per cent in 1987. In 1965, 27 per cent of men who smoked cigars smoked cigars only. By 1987 this proportion had risen to 45 per cent.

Miniature and small cigars have remained more popular than cigarillos or medium and large cigars. In 1987, less than 0.1 per cent of men smoked cigarillos.

Women

Both the TAC and GHS surveys indicate that very few women smoke cigars.

Pipes

Men

The TAC surveys show that pipe smoking among men decreased from around 17 per cent in 1958 to 5 per cent in 1987.

Women

The TAC and GHS surveys did not question women about pipe smoking.

Table 3.1.1 Numbers of men (millions) with various smoking habits, 1956-1987
Men aged 16 and over, Great Britain: sales-adjusted 1969-1987, except for cigar and pipe tobacco

Smoking habit[1]	1956	1958	1961	1963	1965	1968	1971	1972	1973	1974	1975	1976	1977
Smokers of any tobacco	13.7	13.2	13.6	13.0	13.2	13.5	12.7	13.0	13.0	12.8	12.4	11.8	11.7
Ex-smokers (any tobacco)	2.0	2.5	2.7	3.0	3.0	2.9	3.4	3.0	3.2	3.2	3.7	3.9	3.9
Have never smoked (any tobacco)	2.6	2.7	2.6	3.3	3.4	3.4	3.6	3.8	3.6	3.9	4.1	4.4	4.6
All smokers of manufactured cigarettes	..	10.6	11.1	10.4	10.5	10.8	9.9	10.0	9.8	9.9	9.4	9.0	8.5
Usual brand[2]: plain	..	9.5	9.0	7.2	5.3	3.7	2.3	2.3	2.0	2.0	1.8	1.4	1.3
filter	..	0.8	1.8	2.9	5.0	7.0	7.5	7.6	7.8	7.7	7.5	7.5	7.1
All smokers of hand-rolled cigarettes	..	1.7	2.5	2.5	2.7	2.5	2.2	2.0	2.1	2.4	2.4	2.3	2.1
All smokers of cigars	..	..	..	..	1.8	2.3	2.2	2.5	2.8	2.5	2.6	2.5	2.3
All smokers of cigarillos	..	..	..	..	..	0.3	0.1	0.1	0.1	0.1	0.1	0.1	0.1
All smokers of miniature & small cigars	..	..	..	..	..	1.4	1.3	1.7	1.7	1.7	1.8	1.6	1.6
All smokers of medium & large cigars	..	..	..	..	..	1.0	0.9	1.0	1.1	1.0	1.0	1.0	0.9
All smokers of pipes	..	3.1	2.6	2.8	2.7	2.8	2.6	2.6	2.4	2.3	2.2	1.9	1.9
Smokers of manufactured cigarettes only	9.1	8.6	8.9	8.1	7.2	7.2	6.8	7.1	7.0	6.9	6.4	6.3	6.3
Smokers of hand-rolled cigarettes only	0.8	0.9	1.2	1.2	1.1	0.8	0.8	0.8	0.9	0.9	0.9	0.8	0.9
Smokers of cigars only	..	..	..	..	0.3	0.5	0.6	0.7	0.8	0.7	0.8	0.7	0.9
Smokers of pipes only	1.7	1.6	1.1	1.2	0.8	0.9	1.0	1.0	1.0	0.9	0.8	0.7	0.9
Total population aged 16 and over	18.3	18.4	18.9	19.3	19.6	19.7	19.7	19.8	19.9	20.0	20.1	20.1	20.3

Smoking habit[1]	1978	1979	1980	1981	1982	1983	1984	1985	1986	1987
Smokers of any tobacco	11.1	11.2	11.4	10.5	10.3	10.0	10.1	9.9	9.3	9.5
Ex-smokers (any tobacco)	4.1	3.9	4.1	4.6	5.0	5.1	4.9	5.0	5.4	5.1
Have never smoked (any tobacco)	5.2	5.3	5.2	5.9	5.7	6.1	6.3	6.5	6.9	7.1
All smokers of manufactured cigarettes	8.4	8.5	8.6	7.7	7.5	7.4	7.5	7.4	7.1	7.3
Usual brand[2]: plain	1.1	0.9	0.8	0.6	0.5	0.5	0.3	0.3	0.3	0.3
filter	7.3	7.5	7.8	7.1	7.0	6.8	7.2	7.1	6.9	7.0
Tar yield[2,3]: low	0.6	0.8	1.1	0.8	0.8	0.6	0.8	0.9	0.8	0.8
low/middle	0.4	0.5	0.9	1.2	0.8	3.6	3.3	2.7	2.9	2.9
middle	6.9	7.0	6.4	5.5	5.8	3.0	3.1	3.5	3.1	3.1
middle/high or high	0.2	0.1	0.0	0.0	0.0	..	..	..	0.0	0.0
All smokers of hand-rolled cigarettes	2.1	2.0	2.1	2.4	2.4	2.3	2.1	2.3	2.2	2.2
All smokers of cigars	2.1	2.1	1.9	1.9	1.7	1.7	1.5	1.6	1.5	1.5
All smokers of cigarillos	0.1	0.0	0.1	0.0	0.0	0.0	0.0	0.0	0.0	0.0
All smokers of miniature & small cigars	1.4	1.4	1.1	1.3	1.1	0.9	0.9	1.0	0.9	0.9
All smokers of medium & large cigars	0.8	0.9	0.8	0.9	0.6	0.5	0.4	0.4	0.3	0.4
All smokers of pipes	1.7	1.7	1.7	1.5	1.3	1.2	1.2	1.2	1.1	1.0
Smokers of manufactured cigarettes only	6.2	6.2	6.5	5.6	5.5	5.4	5.7	5.4	5.1	5.4
Smokers of hand-rolled cigarettes only	0.8	0.7	0.9	0.9	1.0	0.9	0.9	0.8	0.7	0.8
Smokers of cigars only	0.8	0.8	0.7	0.7	0.8	0.8	0.8	0.8	0.7	0.6
Smokers of pipes only	0.8	0.7	0.7	0.6	0.6	0.6	0.7	0.6	0.5	0.5
Total population aged 16 and over	20.4	20.5	20.6	20.9	21.1	21.2	21.3	21.4	21.5	21.6

1 Figures for 1956-1963 do not include smokers of cigars only
2 Smokers with no usual brand are excluded from the plain/filter and tar yield categories,
but are included in smokers of manufactured cigarettes
3 1985 data are given according to the tar bands that applied for 1972-1984, namely:

Low	0-10 mg tar/cigarette
Low/middle	11-16 mg tar/cigarette
Middle	17-22 mg tar/cigarette
Middle/high	23-28 mg tar/cigarette
High	29+ mg tar/cigarette

Source: TAC

Table 3.1.2 Numbers of women (millions) with various smoking habits, 1956-1987
Women aged 16 and over, Great Britain: sales-adjusted 1969-1987, except for cigar tobacco

Smoking habit[1]	1956	1958	1961	1963	1965	1968	1971	1972	1973	1974	1975	1976	1977
Smokers of any tobacco (except pipe)	8.4	8.2	9.1	9.2	9.1	9.3	9.1	9.1	9.5	9.7	9.5	9.3	9.2
Ex-smokers (any tobacco except pipe)	1.5	1.3	1.5	1.5	1.7	2.0	2.4	2.3	2.3	2.5	2.7	3.0	3.1
Have never smoked (any tobacco except pipe)	10.5	11.1	10.3	10.5	10.7	10.2	10.1	10.3	9.9	9.7	9.7	9.7	9.8
All smokers of manufactured cigarettes	..	8.2	9.0	9.1	9.1	9.2	9.1	9.0	9.5	9.6	9.4	9.2	9.1
Usual brand[2]: plain	..	6.5	5.6	4.0	2.5	1.3	0.9	0.7	0.7	0.6	0.6	0.5	0.5
filter	..	1.4	3.1	4.9	6.4	7.7	8.1	8.3	8.7	8.9	8.8	8.6	8.5
All smokers of hand-rolled cigarettes	..	0.1	0.2	0.2	0.3	0.3	0.2	0.2	0.2	0.3	0.3	} 0.4	} 0.4
All smokers of cigars	..	..	..	..	0.0	0.1	0.1	0.1	0.1	0.1	0.1		
Smokers of manufactured cigarettes only	8.3	8.1	8.9	9.0	8.9	8.9	8.8	8.8	9.3	9.3	9.1	8.9	8.8
Smokers of hand-rolled cigarettes only	..	0.0	0.1	0.1	0.1	0.1	0.1	0.0	0.0	0.1	0.1	..	..
Smokers of cigars only	..	..	..	..	0.0	0.0	0.0	0.0	0.0	0.0	0.1	..	..
Total population aged 16 and over	20.5	20.6	20.9	21.2	21.5	21.5	21.6	21.8	21.8	21.9	21.9	22.0	22.1

Smoking habit[1]	1978	1979	1980	1981	1982	1983	1984	1985	1986	1987
Smokers of any tobacco (except pipe)	8.9	8.9	8.8	8.4	8.3	8.2	8.0	8.1	7.8	8.0
Ex-smokers (any tobacco except pipe)	3.2	3.3	3.2	3.8	3.8	4.2	4.0	3.9	4.3	4.1
Have never smoked (any tobacco except pipe)	10.2	10.2	10.4	10.6	10.9	10.6	11.1	11.2	11.2	11.3
All smokers of manufactured cigarettes	8.8	8.8	8.7	8.3	8.1	8.1	7.9	8.0	7.7	7.9
Usual brand[2]: plain	0.5	0.3	0.3	0.2	0.2	0.1	0.2	0.1	0.1	0.1
filter	8.3	8.4	8.4	8.0	7.9	8.0	7.3	7.9	7.6	7.8
Tar yield[2,3]: low	1.5	1.7	2.1	1.9	1.7	1.7	1.5	1.8	1.6	1.8
low/middle	0.6	0.7	1.3	1.3	1.1	3.7	3.5	2.7	2.9	3.2
middle	6.4	6.2	5.2	4.9	4.9	2.5	2.4	3.1	2.8	2.5
middle/high or high	0.1	0.1	0.0	0.0	0.0	..	..	..	..	0.0
All smokers of other tobacco (except pipe)	0.4	0.3	0.2	0.4	0.5	0.4	0.5	0.4	0.5	0.4
Smokers of manufactured cigarettes only	8.5	8.6	8.5	8.0	7.8	7.8	7.5	7.7	7.3	7.6
Smokers of other tobacco (except pipe) only	0.1	0.1	0.1	0.1	0.1	0.1	0.1	0.1	0.1	0.1
Total population aged 16 and over	22.2	22.3	22.5	22.8	22.9	23.0	23.1	23.2	23.3	23.4

1 Figures for 1956-1963 do not include smokers of cigars only
2 Smokers with no usual brand are excluded from the plain/filter and tar yield categories,
but are included in smokers of manufactured cigarettes
3 1985 data are given according to the tar bands that applied for 1972-1984, namely:

Low	0-10 mg tar/cigarette
Low/middle	11-16 mg tar/cigarette
Middle	17-22 mg tar/cigarette
Middle/high	23-28 mg tar/cigarette
High	29+ mg tar/cigarette

Source: TAC

SECTION 3   Percentage of population who smoke

Table 3.2.1 Percentage of men with various smoking habits, 1956-1987
Men aged 16 and over, Great Britain: sales-adjusted 1969-1987, except for cigar and pipe tobacco

Smoking habit[1]	1956	1958	1961	1963	1965	1968	1971	1972	1973	1974	1975	1976	1977
Smokers of any tobacco	75.2	72.0	71.9	68.0	67.6	68.6	64.5	65.8	65.6	64.3	61.5	58.8	57.9
Ex-smokers (any tobacco)	11.3	13.4	14.2	15.1	15.3	14.5	17.2	15.1	16.0	16.0	18.2	19.3	19.3
Have never smoked (any tobacco)	13.5	14.6	13.9	16.9	17.1	16.9	18.3	19.1	18.4	19.7	20.3	21.9	22.8
All smokers of manufactured cigarettes	..	58.0	58.6	53.9	53.6	54.9	50.6	50.7	49.3	49.4	46.8	44.8	42.2
Usual brand[2]: plain	..	51.6*	47.5	37.3*	27.0	18.7	11.7	11.6*	10.1*	10.0*	8.7	6.8	5.4
filter	..	4.3*	9.7	15.0*	25.6	35.5	38.2	38.4*	39.2*	38.5*	37.5	37.6	35.4
All smokers of hand-rolled cigarettes	..	9.2*	12.9	13.0*	14.0	12.7	11.0	10.1*	10.6*	12.0*	11.8	11.5	10.7
All smokers of cigars	..	..	..	..	9.0	11.7	11.3	12.6*	14.1*	12.5*	13.1	12.2	11.6
All smokers of cigarillos	..	..	..	..	..	1.7	0.6	0.5*	0.5*	0.5*	0.5	0.3	0.3
All smokers of miniature & small cigars	..	..	..	..	..	7.0	6.6	8.6*	8.5*	8.5*	8.9	8.1	7.8
All smokers of medium & large cigars	..	..	..	..	..	5.1	4.8	5.1*	5.5*	5.0*	5.1	5.1	4.3
All smokers of pipes	..	16.8*	13.6	14.5*	13.9	14.3	13.3	13.1*	12.1*	1.5*	10.9	9.7	9.5
Smokers of manufactured cigarettes only	49.7*	46.7*	47.2	42.0*	36.9	36.9	34.6	35.9*	35.2*	34.5*	31.7	31.4	31.3
Smokers of hand-rolled cigarettes only	4.4*	4.9*	6.4	6.2*	5.4	4.2	3.8	4.0*	4.5*	4.5*	4.6	4.1	4.3
Smokers of cigars only	..	..	..	..	2.4	2.6	3.0	3.5*	4.0*	3.5*	4.1	3.7	4.5
Smokers of pipes only	9.3*	8.7*	5.9	6.2*	4.3	4.7	4.9	5.1*	5.0*	4.5*	3.7	3.6	4.5

Smoking habit[1]	1978	1979	1980	1981	1982	1983	1984	1985	1986	1987
Smokers of any tobacco	54.5	54.8	55.0	50.0	49.2	47.3	47.3	46.4	43.1	43.7
Ex-smokers (any tobacco)	20.1	19.1	19.8	21.8	23.8	23.9	23.0	23.4	25.0	23.4
Have never smoked (any tobacco)	25.4	26.1	25.2	28.2	27.0	28.8	29.7	30.2	31.9	32.9
All smokers of manufactured cigarettes	41.1	41.6	41.7	36.9	35.9	34.8	35.2	34.7	33.2	33.6
Usual brand[2]: plain	5.5	4.5	3.9	2.9	2.4	2.5	1.3	1.3	1.3	1.2
filter	35.5	36.7	37.7	33.9	33.3	32.2	33.8	33.2	31.8	32.3
Tar yield[2,3]: low	3.0	3.9	5.2	4.0	3.7	3.0	3.9	4.1	3.7	3.8
low/middle	1.8	2.3	4.5	5.5	3.9	16.9	15.7	12.8	13.6	13.5
middle	34.0	33.9	31.1	26.4	27.4	14.1	14.4	16.4	14.5	14.6
middle/high or high	0.9	0.7	0.1	0.0	0.0	..	..	..	0.1	0.1
All smokers of hand-rolled cigarettes	10.1	10.0	10.0	11.7	11.5	10.8	10.1	10.7	10.1	10.1
All smokers of cigars	10.2	10.4	9.3	9.0	8.3	8.0	7.0	7.5	6.7	6.7
All smokers of cigarillos	0.3	0.2	0.2	0.2	0.1	0.1	0.0	0.1	0.1	0.0
All smokers of miniature & small cigars	7.0	6.7	5.6	6.0	5.4	4.4	4.1	4.6	4.2	4.3
All smokers of medium & large cigars	3.8	4.4	4.0	4.1	3.1	2.3	1.9	1.9	1.6	1.7
All smokers of pipes	8.1	8.2	8.2	7.3	6.3	5.9	5.5	5.7	5.0	4.7
Smokers of manufactured cigarettes only	30.4	30.4	31.4	26.7	26.0	25.5	27.0	25.1	23.8	24.9
Smokers of hand-rolled cigarettes only	3.9	3.6	4.4	4.3	4.9	4.4	4.4	3.8	3.4	3.6
Smokers of cigars only	3.7	4.1	3.5	3.4	3.9	3.9	3.5	3.8	3.2	3.0
Smokers of pipes only	3.7	4.6	4.6	3.1	2.9	2.7	3.0	2.8	2.4	2.1

1 Figures for 1956-1963 do not include smokers of cigars only
2 Smokers with no usual brand are excluded from the plain/filter and tar yield categories,
but are included in smokers of manufactured cigarettes
3 1985 data are given according to the tar bands that applied for 1972-1984, namely:

Low	0-10 mg tar/cigarette
Low/middle	11-16 mg tar/cigarette
Middle	17-22 mg tar/cigarette
Middle/high	23-28 mg tar/cigarette
High	29+ mg tar/cigarette

* Figures marked with an asterisk have been derived from Table 3.1.1, and are less accurate than the remainder of the table

Source: TAC

Table 3.2.2 Percentage of women with various smoking habits, 1956-1987
Women aged 16 and over, Great Britain: sales-adjusted 1969-1987, except for cigar tobacco

Smoking habit[1]	1956	1958	1961	1963	1965	1968	1971	1972	1973	1974	1975	1976	1977
Smokers of any tobacco (except pipe)	41.6	39.6	43.7	43.0	42.6	43.2	42.3	41.9	43.6	44.2	43.4	42.1	41.4
Ex-smokers (any tobacco except pipe)	7.1	6.7	6.9	7.5	7.8	9.2	11.2	10.7	10.5	11.5	12.5	13.7	14.1
Have never smoked (any tobacco except pipe)	51.3	53.7	49.4	49.5	49.5	47.6	46.5	47.4	45.9	44.3	44.2	44.2	44.4
All smokers of manufactured cigarettes	..	39.5	43.3	42.7	42.3	42.8	41.9	41.5	43.4	43.7	42.8	41.8	41.0
Usual brand[2]: plain	..	31.6*	26.8	18.9*	11.8	6.2	4.0	3.2*	3.2*	2.7*	2.5	2.3	2.4
filter	..	6.8*	14.8	23.1*	29.4	36.0	37.3	38.1*	39.9*	40.6*	39.9	39.2	38.4
All smokers of hand-rolled cigarettes	..	0.5	1.0	0.9*	1.4	1.2	1.0	0.9*	0.9*	1.4*	1.5	}1.8	}1.5
All smokers of cigars	..	..	..	..	0.2	0.5	0.5	0.5*	0.5*	0.5*	0.5		
Smokers of manufactured cigarettes only	40.5*	39.3*	42.7	42.5*	41.1	41.6	40.7	40.4*	42.7*	42.5*	41.5	40.4	39.9
Smokers of other tobacco (except pipe) only	..	..	..	..	..	..	..	..	..	..	0.5	0.2	0.4

Smoking habit[1]	1978	1979	1980	1981	1982	1983	1984	1985	1986	1987
Smokers of any tobacco (except pipe)	39.9	39.8	39.1	36.9	36.1	35.7	34.6	34.8	33.6	34.3
Ex-smokers (any tobacco except pipe)	14.3	14.6	14.4	16.6	16.5	18.3	17.3	17.0	18.6	17.5
Have never smoked (any tobacco except pipe)	45.8	45.6	46.5	46.5	47.5	46.0	48.1	48.2	47.9	48.2
All smokers of manufactured cigarettes	39.5	39.3	38.7	36.3	35.4	35.4	34.0	34.4	33.1	33.8
Usual brand[2]: plain	2.0	1.3	1.1	1.0	0.9	0.6	0.7	0.5	0.3	0.4
filter	37.4	37.6	37.6	35.2	34.4	34.6	31.4	33.9	32.7	33.3
Tar yield[2,3]: low	6.6	7.6	9.3	8.3	7.4	7.4	6.5	7.7	6.8	7.7
low/middle	2.6	3.0	5.6	5.7	5.0	15.9	15.2	11.8	12.6	13.7
middle	28.7	27.8	23.2	21.5	21.4	11.0	10.4	13.5	12.0	10.7
middle/high or high	0.3	0.2	0.0	0.0	0.0	..	..	..	..	..
All smokers of other tobacco (except pipe)	2.0	1.3	1.0	1.7	2.1	1.9	2.3	1.6	2.1	1.8
Smokers of manufactured cigarettes only	38.1	38.5	38.0	35.2	33.9	33.9	32.4	33.2	31.5	32.5
Smokers of other tobacco (except pipe) only	0.3	0.4	0.4	0.6	0.6	0.4	0.6	0.4	0.5	0.5

1 Figures for 1956-1963 do not include smokers of cigars only
2 Smokers with no usual brand are excluded from the plain/filter and tar yield categories, but are included in smokers of manufactured cigarettes
3 1985 data are given according to the tar bands that applied for 1972-1984, namely:

Low	0-10 mg tar/cigarette
Low/middle	11-16 mg tar/cigarette
Middle	17-22 mg tar/cigarette
Middle/high	23-28 mg tar/cigarette
High	29+ mg tar/cigarette

* Figures marked with an asterisk have been derived from Table 3.1.2, and are less accurate than the remainder of the table

Source: TAC

Table 3.3 Percentages of men and women who smoke (i) any form of tobacco (except pipe tobacco, for women), (ii) manufactured cigarettes, 1948-1987
Men and women aged 16 and over, Great Britain: sales-adjusted 1969-1987

Year	Any tobacco[1] Men	Any tobacco[1] except pipe Women	Manufactured cigarettes Men	Manufactured cigarettes Women
1948	82	41	65	41
1949	81	41	63	41
1950	77	38	62	38
1951	78	38	62	38
1952	76	38	59	38
1953	75	37	59	37
1954	75	36	59	36
1955	74	37	58	37
1956	75	42	61	41
1957	75	44	60	44
1958	72	40	58	39
1959	73	42	60	42
1960	74	42	61	42
1961	72	44	59	43
1962	70	43	57	42
1963	68	43	54	43
1964	69	41	54	41
1965	68	43	54	42
1966	68	45	54	45
1967	68	44	54	44
1968	69	43	55	43
1969	68	44	54	44
1970	68	44	55	44
1971	65	42	51	42
1972	66	42	51	42
1973	66	44	49	43
1974	64	44	49	44
1975	62	43	47	43
1976	59	42	45	42
1977	58	41	42	41
1978	55	40	41	40
1979	55	40	42	39
1980	55	39	42	39
1981	50	37	37	36
1982	49	36	36	35
1983	47	36	35	35
1984	47	35	35	34
1985	46	35	35	34
1986	43	34	33	33
1987	44	34	34	34

1 Figures for 1948-1963 do not include smokers of cigars only

Source: TAC

Fig 3.1 Percentages of men who smoke any form of tobacco, and of men and women who smoke manufactured cigarettes, 1948-1987
Men and women aged 16 and over, Great Britain. *Source*: TAC

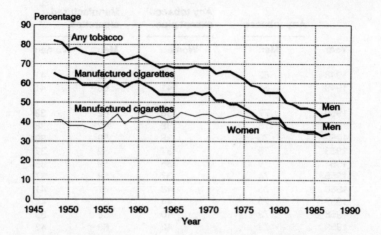

Fig. 3.2 Percentages of men and women who smoke hand-rolled cigarettes, 1961-1987
Men and women aged 16 and over, Great Britain. *Source*: TAC

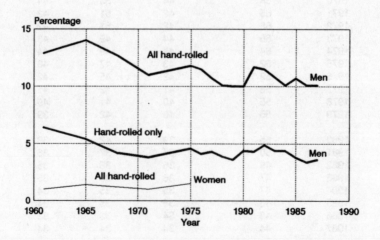

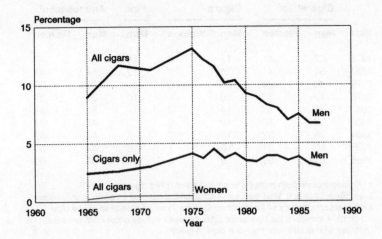

Fig 3.3 Percentages of men and women who smoke cigars, 1965-1987
Men and women aged 16 and over, Great Britain. *Source*: TAC

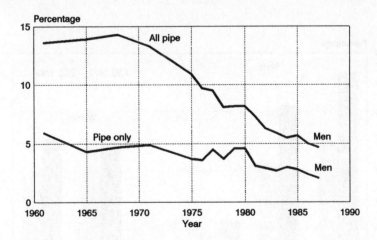

Fig. 3.4 Percentage of men who smoke pipes, 1961-1987
Men aged 16 and over, Great Britain. *Source*: TAC

Table 3.4 Percentages of men and women who smoke: by type of product smoked, 1972-1988
Men and women aged 16 and over, Great Britain

Year	Cigarettes[1]		Cigars		Pipe	Any tobacco[2]	
	Men	Women	Men	Women	Men	Men	Women
1972	52	41	13	0	14	63	41
1974	51	41	34*	3	12	64	41
1976	46	38	31*	3	11	60	39
1978	45	37	16	1	10	55	37
1980	42	37	14	0	..	50	37
1982	38	33	12	0	..	45	34
1984	36	32	10	0	..	43	33
1986	35	31	10	1	6	44	31
1988	33	30	9	0	4	40	30

1 Figures include both manufactured and hand-rolled cigarettes
2 In 1980, 1982 and 1984 men were not asked about pipe smoking, and therefore
the figures for smokers of any tobacco exclude those who smoked only a pipe
* For 1974 and 1976 the figures for cigar smokers include occasional smokers,
i.e. those who smoke less than one cigar a month

Source: GHS

Fig. 3.5 Percentages of men and women who smoke (i) any tobacco, (ii) cigarettes (manufactured and hand-rolled);
percentage of men who smoke cigars; 1972 and 1988
Men and women aged 16 and over, Great Britain. *Source:* GHS

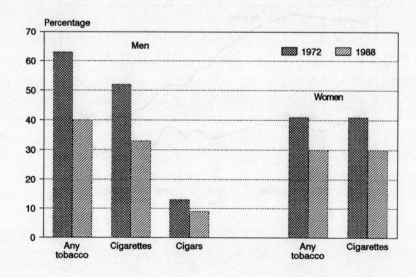

Table 3.5 Percentages of men and women who (i) smoke cigarettes[1]: by number of cigarettes smoked per day; (ii) are ex-smokers of cigarettes; (iii) have never smoked cigarettes; 1972-1988 Men and women aged 16 and over, Great Britain

Year	<20 cigarettes per day	20+ cigarettes per day	All cigarette smokers	Ex-smokers of cigarettes	Never smoked cigarettes
Men					
1972	28	24	52	23	25
1974	25	26	51	23	25
1976	22	24	46	27	27
1978	22	23	45	27	29
1980	21	21	42	28	30
1982	20	18	38	30	32
1984	20	16	36	30	34
1986	20	15	35	32	34
1988	18	15	33	32	35
Women					
1972	30	11	41	10	49
1974	28	13	41	11	49
1976	24	14	38	12	50
1978	23	13	37	14	49
1980	23	13	37	14	49
1982	22	11	33	16	51
1984	22	10	32	17	51
1986	21	10	31	18	51
1988	20	10	30	19	51

1 Figures include both manufactured and hand-rolled cigarettes

Source: GHS

Fig. 3.6 Percentages of men and women who (i) smoke cigarettes: by number of cigarettes smoked per day; (ii) are ex-smokers of cigarettes; (iii) have never smoked cigarettes; 1972 - 1988 Men and women aged 16 and over, Great Britain. *Source*: GHS

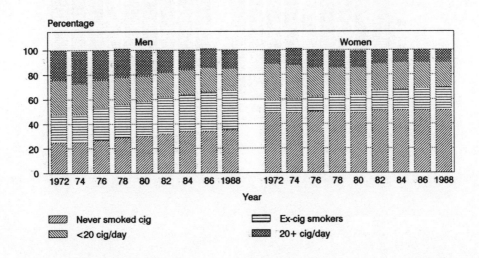

Table 3.6 Percentages of cigarette smokers: by number of cigarettes[1] smoked per day, 1972-1988
Cigarette smokers, men and women aged 16 and over, Great Britain

	Number of cigarettes smoked per day							
Year	<10	10-19	20-29	30+	<10	10-19	20-29	30+
	Men				Women			
1972	19	35	34	12	35	38	23	4
1974	18	31	36	15	31	36	27	6
1976	18	30	36	16	28	35	29	8
1978	18	31	36	15	29	35	28	8
1980	19	31	36	14	27	37	29	7
1982	15	35	37	13	23	41	30	6
1984	20	36	35	10	28	40	27	5
1986	21	36	32	11	28	40	27	5
1988	19	35	34	12	27	40	28	5

1 Figures include both manufactured and hand-rolled cigarettes

Source: GHS

Fig. 3.7 Percentages of cigarette smokers: by number of cigarettes (manufactured and hand-rolled) smoked per day, 1972-1988
Cigarette smokers, men and women aged 16 and over, Great Britain. *Source*: GHS

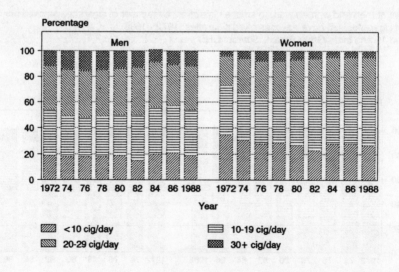

SECTION 3   Percentage of population who smoke

Information on smoking habits at different ages is available from the TAC from 1948, and from the GHS from 1972. The age groups used by the TAC changed in 1976. Before 1976 the TAC used the age groups 16-19, 20-24, 25-34, 35-59, and 60+ years, or alternatively, 16-19, 20-24, 25-34, 35-49, 50-59, 60+ years; from 1976 onwards the age groups 16-24, 25-34, 35-49, 50-64, and 65+ years have been used. In most tables containing TAC data, those for 1975 are presented according to both old and new groupings; the discontinuities caused by these changes are indicated on the relevant graphs by a vertical line.

Percentage of population who smoke: by age

Cigarettes

The TAC data on percentage of smokers of manufactured cigarettes, and percentage of smokers of hand-rolled cigarettes, have been adjusted for under-reporting for the years 1969-1987. The GHS data have not been adjusted in this way.

The TAC data indicate that during the 1950s about 60 per cent of men and 40 per cent of women smoked manufactured cigarettes. However, both the TAC and the GHS data show that, at all ages, the differences in the percentages of men and women who smoke have narrowed since then, so that by 1986, the percentages of men and women in the age range 16-59 (or 16-64) years who smoke cigarettes were about the same, varying from 30 to 42 per cent over the different age groups in the two surveys.

In the TAC surveys the prevalence of cigarette smoking has been less in men and women aged 60 and over (or 65 and over) than in men and women of other ages; in the GHS surveys, it has been least in men and women aged 16-19 years and aged 60 and over.

Men

In 1948, according to the TAC survey, the prevalence of manufactured cigarette smoking among men aged 16-59 was about 70 per cent, while among men aged 60 and over, it was just under 40 per cent.

Manufactured cigarette smoking among men aged 25-59 years decreased slowly between 1948 and 1970, and more rapidly from 1971 until 1987. Seventy-six per cent of men aged 25-34 years smoked manufactured cigarettes in 1948, 60 per cent in 1970, and 38 per cent in 1987. Corresponding figures for men aged 35-59 years were 70 per cent in 1948, 55 per cent in 1970, and approximately 33 per cent in 1987. Smoking in men aged 16-24 fell from just under 70 per cent in 1948 to 54 per cent by 1955, rose to 66 per cent in 1960, and thereafter followed a similar pattern to men aged 25-59, decreasing to 38 per cent in 1984, and then rising slightly to 42 per cent. Smoking among men aged 60 and over rose slightly from 39 per cent in 1948 to 45 per cent by 1956 and fluctuated around this level until 1970, declining thereafter to 21 per cent in 1987 (ages 65 and over).

GHS data on cigarette smoking (manufactured and hand-rolled) show an absolute decline in smoking of about 18 per cent in all age groups between 1972 and 1988. In 1988 the GHS estimated that approximately 36 per cent of men aged 20-59, and 27 per cent of men aged 16-19 or aged 60 and over, smoked cigarettes. The difference from the TAC figures can partly be accounted for by the inclusion of men smoking only hand-rolled cigarettes.

TAC data on hand-rolled cigarette smokers show that in 1987 10 per cent of men smoked hand-rolled cigarettes, and about 40 per cent of these men smoked no other tobacco product. The proportions vary in the different age groups, and in 1987, in the age range 16-24 years, only about one in ten smokers of hand-rolled cigarettes smoked that product only, whereas among those aged 65 and over more than half of those who smoked hand-rolled cigarettes smoked no other product.

Women

The pattern of smoking prevalence among women has been different from that among men. At the end of the Second World War, smoking was more popular with younger than with older women, so that in 1948 the TAC survey estimated that about 50 per cent of women aged 16-34 smoked manufactured cigarettes, compared with 41 per cent of women aged 35-59, and only 23 per cent of women aged 60 and over.

The percentage of young women aged 16-24 who smoked manufactured cigarettes fell from about 48 per cent in 1948 to about 33 per cent in 1955, a fall similar to that experienced by men of the same age. Thereafter the percentage increased to 49 per cent in 1961 and then fluctuated around 50 per cent until 1975. Smoking among women aged 25-34 years remained constant at around 50 per cent from 1948 until 1975. The percentage of women aged 35-59 who smoked manufactured cigarettes rose from 41 per cent in 1948 to 50 per cent in 1961 (as the increasing popularity of smoking among young women which occurred earlier affected this age group) and then remained fairly constant until 1975. Thus, between 1961 and 1975, about half of all women aged under 60 were smokers of cigarettes, about twice the proportion of older women during this period.

The TAC and GHS surveys indicate that cigarette smoking among women started to decline in all age groups from about 1975, approximately five years later than the start of the decline among men. By 1987, TAC estimates indicate that about 38 per cent of women aged 16-64 and 20 per cent of women aged 65 and over were manufactured cigarette smokers. The GHS estimates are very similar to the TAC ones.

Cigars

Men

For cigar smoking, the figures from the GHS and TAC surveys appear somewhat discrepant, with the GHS reporting a higher rate of cigar smoking than the TAC. In 1986, for example, 10 per cent of men aged 16 and over smoked cigars according to the GHS, and 7 per cent according to the TAC. This could be due to the different definitions of a cigar smoker employed by the two surveys. (The TAC defines a cigar smoker as a person smoking at least one cigar a week, whereas the GHS defines cigar smoker as a person smoking at least one cigar a month.) GHS data indicate that cigar smoking is uncommon in men aged 16-19 years, and slightly more popular among those aged 25-59 years than among those aged 60 and over.

Pipes

Men

The TAC surveys indicate that between 1961 and 1987 the percentage of men aged 16 years and over who smoke pipes declined steadily from 14 to 5 per cent, the decline taking place in all age groups. Pipe smoking has consistently been more prevalent among older men (aged 50 years and over) than at other ages and, by 1981, pipes were smoked hardly at all by men aged under 25.

Any tobacco

Men

A greater proportion of older men smoke tobacco in a form other than manufactured cigarettes than do younger men. In 1948, 85 per cent of men aged 60 and over smoked some form of tobacco while only 39 per cent smoked manufactured cigarettes. By 1987 the difference had narrowed; 35 per cent of men aged 65 and over smoked some form of tobacco, compared to 21 per cent who smoked manufactured cigarettes.

The percentage of men aged 16-24 who smoke any tobacco has been only slightly greater than the percentage who smoke manufactured cigarettes, while the difference has averaged about 10 per cent among those aged 25-34, and about 15 per cent among those aged 35-59 throughout the period of the TAC surveys.

Women

The percentage of women smoking any tobacco is approximately equal to the percentage of women smoking manufactured cigarettes, as so few women smoke other forms of tobacco.

Table 4.1.1 Percentage of men who smoke manufactured cigarettes: by age, 1948-1987
Men aged 16 and over, Great Britain: sales-adjusted 1969-1987

Year	16-19	20-24	16-24	25-34	35-59	60+	16+
1948	61	74	68	76	70	39	65
1949	54	73	64	71	68	38	63
1950	51	68	60	70	66	38	62
1951	51	68	60	70	66	42	62
1952	47	62	56	67	64	40	59
1953	47	61	54	67	64	42	59
1954	46	63	55	66	63	42	59
1955	47	59	54	67	62	39	58
1956	52	65	59	67	65	45	61
1957	59	61	60	66	63	45	60
1958	54	63	59	65	63	42	58
1959	60	62	61	65	63	48	60
1960	65	67	66	64	64	46	61
1961	61	67	64	60	61	46	59
1962	61	62	61	59	60	44	57
1963	56	65	61	60	54	42	54
1964	56	61	59	55	57	45	54
1965	50	63	56	56	56	44	54
1966	54	60	57	59	56	44	54
1967	52	61	57	56	56	45	54
1968	57	59	58	57	57	46	55
1969	53	62	59	60	54	44	54
1970	55	58	57	60	55	46	55
1971	53	57	55	55	50	43	51
1972	51	60	56	54	51	42	51
1973	49	62	56	53	49	41	49
1974	48	55	52	55	51	40	49
1975	49	53	51	46	49	41	47

Year			16-24	25-34	35-49	50-64	65+	16+
1975			51	46	47	49	38	47
1976			48	48	46	47	32	45
1977			47	46	43	41	32	42
1978			46	44	43	40	30	41
1979			48	46	43	39	30	42
1980			44	47	43	43	28	42
1981			41	42	39	35	26	37
1982			42	38	37	33	27	36
1983			41	36	37	33	25	35
1984			38	42	35	35	24	35
1985			42	40	36	29	24	35
1986			42	36	35	31	20	33
1987			42	38	35	29	21	34

Source: TAC

Table 4.1.2 Percentage of women who smoke manufactured cigarettes: by age, 1948-1987
Women aged 16 and over, Great Britain: sales-adjusted 1969-1987

Year	16-19	20-24	16-24	25-34	35-59		60+	16+
1948	43	54	49	52	41		23	41
1949	33	53	45	55	43		24	41
1950	36	48	43	53	38		23	38
1951	28	43	37	52	39		21	38
1952	29	45	38	52	40		20	38
1953	26	43	36	49	40		23	37
1954	25	42	35	49	40		21	36
1955	26	39	33	51	41		22	37
1956	33	43	39	52	44		29	41
1957	40	46	44	55	46		28	44
1958	32	45	39	48	45		19	39
1959	33	47	41	55	49		19	42
1960	45	48	46	53	47		22	42
1961	45	51	49	50	50		24	43
1962	46	51	49	49	49		23	42
1963	39	50	45	49	51		24	43
1964	40	49	45	51	48		22	41
1965	40	51	46	50	50		23	42
1966	47	53	50	50	52		26	45
1967	43	52	48	49	51		26	44
1968	46	53	50	47	51		24	43
1969	53	53	53	53	50		25	44
1970	52	54	53	51	50		26	44
1971	48	50	50	49	49		24	42
1972	46	48	47	51	48		25	42
1973	49	54	51	47	52		25	43
1974	47	50	49	52	52		26	44
1975	46	53	50	49	49		27	43

Year			16-24	25-34	35-49	50-64	65+	16+
1975			50	49	50	46	23	43
1976			51	47	48	45	21	42
1977			47	46	47	45	23	41
1978			45	47	47	40	21	40
1979			46	45	44	43	21	39
1980			40	45	44	46	21	39
1981			40	42	43	40	19	36
1982			38	38	41	41	21	35
1983			42	40	39	39	20	35
1984			38	39	37	39	20	34
1985			40	42	38	37	19	34
1986			41	37	40	34	17	33
1987			42	38	37	35	20	34

Source: TAC

Fig. 4.1 Percentages of men and women who smoke manufactured cigarettes: by age, 1948-1987
Men and women aged 16 and over, Great Britain. *Source*: TAC
Where two age groups are given, the first is for years up to and including 1975, and the second for 1976 onwards

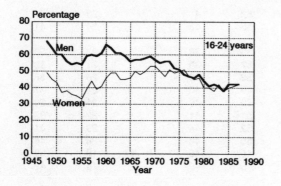

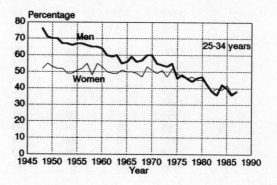

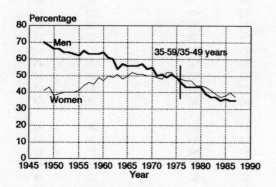

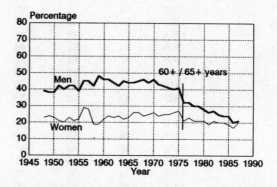

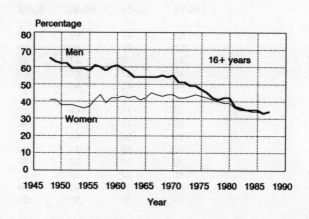

Table 4.2 Percentage of men who smoke hand-rolled cigarettes: by age, 1961-1987
Men aged 16 and over, Great Britain: sales-adjusted 1969-1987

| Year | All smokers of hand-rolled cigarettes | | | | | Smokers of hand-rolled cigarettes only | | | | |
	16-24	25-34	35-59	60+	16+	16-24	25-34	35-59	60+	16+
1961	8	13	15	13	13	1	5	8	9	6
1965	11	14	15	15	14	2	4	6	7	5
1968	10	14	14	12	13	1	3	5	5	4
1971	10	12	12	9	11	1	3	5	5	4
1975	13	11	12	10	12	2	3	5	6	5

Year	16-24	25-34	35-49	50-64	65+	16+	16-24	25-34	35-49	50-64	65+	16+
1975	13	11	12	12	12	12	2	3	5	6	8	5
1978	10	9	10	12	9	10	1	3	4	7	4	4
1981	11	16	11	12	9	12	2	5	4	4	7	4
1982	15	13	11	13	8	12	3	5	4	8	6	5
1983	14	11	11	10	7	11	3	5	4	5	6	4
1984	10	13	12	9	5	10	1	4	7	5	4	4
1985	14	11	12	10	6	11	2	3	5	5	3	4
1986	12	11	12	9	5	10	1	3	4	5	3	3
1987	10	12	12	9	7	10	1	4	5	4	4	4

Source: TAC

Fig. 4.2 Percentage of men who smoke hand-rolled cigarettes: by age, 1987
Men and women aged 16 and over, Great Britain. *Source*: TAC

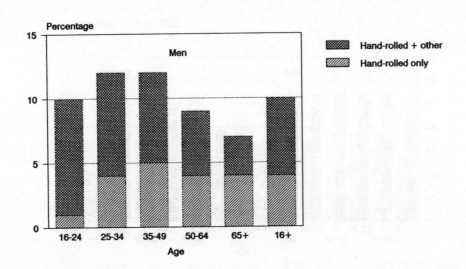

Table 4.3 Percentages of men and women who smoke cigarettes (manufactured and hand-rolled): by age, 1972-1988
Men and women aged 16 and over, Great Britain

Year	16-19	20-24	25-34	35-49	50-59	60+	16+
Men							
1972	43	55	56	55	54	47	52
1974	42	52	56	55	53	44	51
1976	39	47	48	50	49	40	46
1978	35	45	48	48	48	38	45
1980	32	44	47	45	47	36	42
1982	31	41	40	40	42	33	38
1984	29	40	40	39	39	30	36
1986	30	41	37	37	35	29	35
1988	28	37	37	37	33	26	33
Women							
1972	39	48	49	48	47	25	41
1974	38	44	46	49	48	26	41
1976	34	45	43	45	46	24	38
1978	33	43	42	43	42	24	37
1980	32	40	44	43	44	24	37
1982	30	40	37	38	40	23	33
1984	32	36	36	36	39	23	32
1986	30	38	35	34	35	22	31
1988	28	37	35	35	34	21	30

Source: GHS

Fig. 4.3 Percentages of men and women who smoke cigarettes (manufactured and hand-rolled): by age, 1972 and 1988
Men and women aged 16 and over, Great Britain. *Source*: GHS

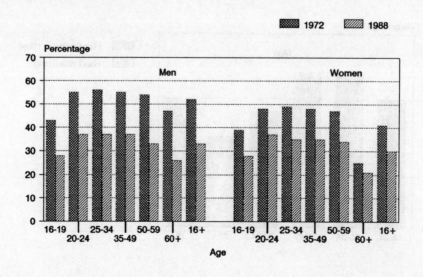

SECTION 4   Smoking habits: by age

Table 4.4 Percentage of men who smoke cigars: by age, 1965-1987
Men aged 16 and over, Great Britain

Year	All smokers of cigars						Smokers of cigars only					
	16-24	25-34	35-59	60+		16+	16-24	25-34	35-59	60+		16+
1965	7	10	10	9		9	1	1	2	2		2
1968	11	14	12	9		12	2	4	3	2		3
1971	9	13	13	8		11	1	4	4	2		3
1975	11	14	15	10		13	3	5	4	3		4
	16-24	25-34	35-49	50-64	65+	16+	16-24	25-34	35-49	50-64	65+	16+
1975	11	14	15	14	8	13	3	5	5	4	3	4
1978	6	12	12	11	9	10	1	4	5	4	4	4
1981	3	9	13	12	6	9	1	3	5	5	3	3
1982	5	10	11	10	5	8	1	5	6	4	3	4
1983	4	9	11	8	6	8	1	6	5	4	3	4
1984	3	8	9	7	7	7	1	1	4	5	4	4
1985	4	10	9	8	6	8	1	5	5	4	3	4
1986	3	7	10	9	4	7	1	3	5	4	2	3
1987	4	6	10	7	5	7	1	3	5	3	3	3

Source: TAC

Fig. 4.4 Percentage of men who smoke cigars: by age, 1987
Men aged 16 and over, Great Britain. *Source*: TAC

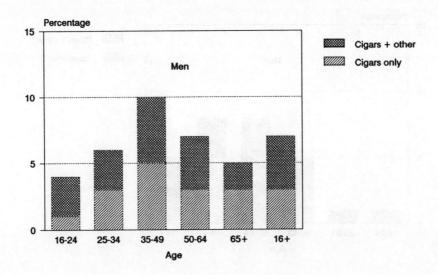

Table 4.5 Percentage of men who smoke cigars: by age, 1972-1988
Men aged 16 and over, Great Britain

Year	16-19[1]	20-24	25-29	30-34	35-49	50-59	60+	16+
1972	5	15	18	18	14	14	8	13
1974[2]	14	38	42	43	39	34	27	34
1976[2]	12	33	38	40	36	30	25	31
1978	7	17	22	23	19	15	11	16
1980	4	13	19	16	18	15	11	14
1982	4	10	12	14	18	14	9	12
1984	3	9	11	13	15	10	8	10
1986	3	11	13	12	13	12	8	10
1988	3	7	8	11	11	12	7	9

1 Data for young people aged 16-17 exclude cigars
2 For 1974 and 1976 the figures include occasional cigar smokers,
that is, those smoking less than one cigar a month

Source: GHS (data for 1984 not previously published)

Fig. 4.5 Percentage of men who smoke pipes: by age, 1987
Men aged 16 and over, Great Britain. *Source*: TAC

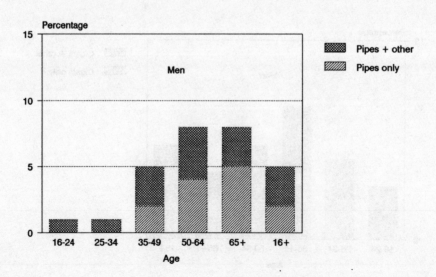

Table 4.6 Percentage of men who smoke pipes: by age, 1961-1987
Men aged 16 and over, Great Britain

Year	All pipe smokers						Pipe only smokers					
	16-24	25-34	35-59	60+		16+	16-24	25-34	35-59	60+		16+
1961	5	9	14	24		14	1	2	5	15		6
1965	6	11	14	22		14	1	2	4	11		4
1968	7	11	15	21		14	1	3	5	10		5
1971	6	12	14	19		13	1	3	5	11		5
1975	4	9	12	16		11	0	2	4	8		4

Year	16-24	25-34	35-49	50-64	65+	16+	16-24	25-34	35-49	50-64	65+	16+
1975	4	9	11	14	16	11	0	2	3	5	9	4
1978	2	4	10	11	14	8	0	2	4	5	8	4
1981	1	6	7	12	11	7	0	1	3	5	8	3
1982	1	4	7	10	10	6	0	1	3	5	6	3
1983	1	3	7	8	11	6	0	1	2	4	7	3
1984	1	3	6	10	9	6	0	1	3	6	6	3
1985	1	3	7	9	9	6	0	1	3	5	6	3
1986	1	2	6	7	9	5	..	1	2	3	7	2
1987	1	1	5	8	8	5	0	0	2	4	5	2

Source: TAC

Table. 4.7 Percentage of men who smoke pipes: by age, 1972-1988
Men aged 16 and over, Great Britain

Year[1]	16-19[2]	20-24	25-29	30-34	35-49	50-59	60+	16+
1972	2	11	13	12	13	17	19	14
1974	2	8	11	14	11	14	17	12
1976	1	5	10	10	12	14	15	11
1978	1	3	7	9	10	11	16	10
1986	0	1	3	4	7	9	11	6
1988	1	1	2	2	4	6	8	4

1 In 1980, 1982 and 1984 men were not asked about pipe smoking
2 Data for young people aged 16-17 exclude pipes

Source: GHS

Table 4.8.1 Percentage of men who smoke any form of tobacco[1]: by age, 1948-1987
Men aged 16 and over, Great Britain: sales-adjusted 1969-1987

Year	16-19	20-24	16-24	25-34	35-59	60+	16+
1948	62	79	71	84	84	85	82
1949	56	78	69	81	84	82	81
1950	52	71	63	79	81	78	77
1951	52	71	64	80	81	81	78
1952	49	67	59	77	80	79	76
1953	48	66	58	76	79	78	75
1954	47	67	58	75	79	80	75
1955	49	63	57	76	78	79	74
1956	55	67	62	74	79	79	75
1957	60	65	63	74	77	79	75
1958	56	66	62	68	77	72	72
1959	62	65	64	73	74	76	73
1960	65	70	68	73	78	69	74
1961	62	71	66	68	75	71	72
1962	63	67	65	67	74	69	70
1963	58	69	64	69	71	64	68
1964	58	66	63	64	73	69	69
1965	52	68	60	67	71	69	68
1966	57	66	61	69	71	69	68
1967	55	68	62	65	73	67	68
1968	58	65	62	67	72	68	69
1969	55	68	63	70	72	66	68
1970	56	65	61	70	71	68	68
1971	55	62	59	67	66	64	65
1972	54	65	60	65	70	63	66
1973	51	69	61	65	68	65	66
1974	48	61	55	66	69	61	64
1975	52	62	57	59	65	61	62

Year	16-24	25-34	35-49	50-64	65+	16+
1975	57	59	62	67	60	62
1976	51	60	62	65	51	59
1977	52	59	61	61	56	58
1978	49	54	58	59	50	55
1979	51	58	58	56	51	55
1980	48	58	58	60	48	55
1981	44	53	53	53	45	50
1982	46	50	52	52	44	49
1983	45	48	50	48	43	47
1984	41	52	51	52	39	47
1985	46	50	51	45	39	46
1986	43	43	48	44	33	43
1987	43	45	50	42	35	44

1 Figures for 1948-1963 do not include smokers of cigars only

Source: TAC

Table 4.8.2 Percentage of women who smoke any form of tobacco[1] (except pipe tobacco): by age, 1956-1987
Women aged 16 and over, Great Britain: sales-adjusted 1969-1987

Year	16-19	20-24	25-29	30-34	35-49	50-59	60+	16+
1956	33	44	47	57	48	37	29	42
1958	32	45	46	51	50	38	19	40

	16-19	20-24	16-24	25-34	35-49	50-59	60+	16+
1961	45	52	49	51	54	42	24	44
1963	40	50	45	49	56	44	24	43
1965	40	51	46	50	54	46	23	43
1968	46	53	50	48	54	48	24	43
1971	49	50	50	49	51	46	24	42
1972	46	48	47	51	51	44	25	42
1973	49	54	52	48	54	51	25	44
1974	47	51	49	52	55	49	27	44
1975	46	53	50	49	51	49	28	43

			16-24	25-34	35-49	50-64	65+	16+
1975			50	49	51	46	24	43
1976			52	48	49	45	21	42
1977			47	47	47	46	23	41
1978			45	48	47	41	22	40
1979			47	45	45	44	22	40
1980			40	46	44	47	21	39
1981			40	43	43	41	20	37
1982			38	38	41	42	22	36
1983			42	41	40	39	20	36
1984			38	40	37	40	20	35
1985			40	42	39	37	19	35
1986			41	38	40	35	17	34
1987			42	39	37	36	21	34

1 Figures for 1956-1963 do not include smokers of cigars only

Source: TAC

Fig. 4.6 Percentages of men who smoke (i) any form of tobacco, (ii) manufactured cigarettes: by age, 1948-1987
Men aged 16 and over, Great Britain. *Source*: TAC
Where two age groups are given, the first is for years up to and including 1975, and the second for 1976 onwards

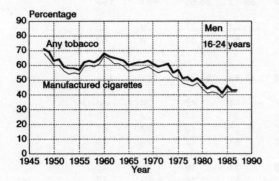

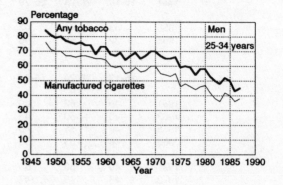

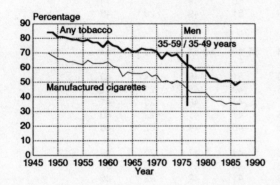

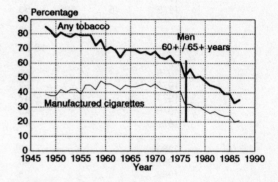

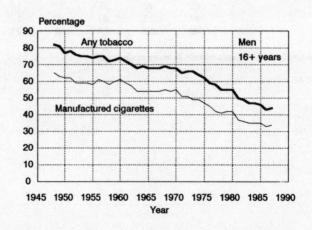

Cigarette consumption: by age

The TAC provides sales-adjusted data on manufactured cigarette consumption on a per person and a per smoker basis, classified according to broad age groups from about 1948 to 1987. From 1966 to 1987 annual consumption of manufactured cigarettes is available from the TAC in five-year age groups; these data are included at the end of this section. The GHS provides data on a consumption per smoker basis for smokers of all cigarettes (i.e. manufactured and hand-rolled) by age from 1972 until 1988. GHS consumption per smoker figures for all cigarettes are lower than the TAC ones for manufactured cigarettes only. This must be partly due to the fact that the GHS data are not sales-adjusted, but could also be partly due to different interviewing and sampling procedures.

The gap in consumption between men and women has narrowed over the period of the surveys. Throughout both the TAC and the GHS surveys consumption per smoker has remained higher in men than in women of the same age. According to the TAC surveys the consumption of manufactured cigarettes per person since 1981 has occasionally been higher in some age groups in women than in men. Both sources report that men and women in the oldest age group consume fewer cigarettes than men or women at younger ages.

Consumption per person at a given age is influenced both by the percentage who smoke and the consumption per smoker at that age.

Consumption per person

Men

Between 1948 and 1960, manufactured cigarette consumption per person rose in young men aged 16-24, while remaining fairly constant at other ages. From around 1960 until 1975 consumption remained reasonably steady at all ages. A decline in consumption per person, which was particularly steep at first, began at all ages around 1975, and has continued until 1987.

Women

Consumption per person rose among women aged under 60 between 1948 and 1976, and declined thereafter.

Consumption per person among women aged 60 and over followed a similar trend to that in younger women, but the changes in consumption have been smaller.

Consumption per smoker

Men

After 1949, manufactured cigarette consumption per manufactured cigarette smoker followed an increasing trend in the age range 16-59 years, with the greatest increases taking place among those aged 16-24. A turning point occurred between 1976 and 1981, the precise year depending upon the age group concerned. The GHS data are confirmatory, showing a small downward trend in cigarette consumption per male cigarette smoker aged under 60 since 1978. Apart from male cigarette smokers aged 16-19, a small increase in cigarette consumption took place in 1988.

Consumption per smoker increased among men aged 60 and over during the early 1950s. Since then there have been fluctuations from year to year, with no clear upward or downward trend.

Cigarette consumption per smoker remains greatest in middle age (35-49 years), and is least in both the young (16-19 years) and the old (65 and over).

Women

Between 1949 and 1976 consumption per smoker increased among women of all ages, with some of the sharpest increases occuring in the early 1970s. Between 1976 and 1987, consumption per smoker has declined most in women aged 16-34 and women aged 50-64, and least in women aged 35-49. The GHS data showed a small increase in cigarette consumption between 1986 and 1988 in the age range 16-59 years.

Table 4.9.1 Weekly consumption of manufactured cigarettes per person: by age, 1946-1987
Men aged 16 and over, Great Britain: sales-adjusted

Year	16-19	20-24	25-29	30-34	35-59		60+	65+	15+
1946	50	88	103	99	100		45	..	82
1947	..	..	..	..	..		..	..	71
1948	38	71	78	78	86		33	..	68
1949	34	66	68	71	76		29	..	64
1950	35	67	78	72	79		31	21	65
1951	38	70	85	83	81		38	27	69
1952	31	69	80	85	85		39	32	70
1953	36	68	80	91	84		42	32	71
1954	33	72	83	88	88		40	29	72
1955	39	68	91	88	90		41	30	74

Year	16-19	20-24	25-29	30-34	35-49	50-59	60+	65+	15+
1956	39	71	82	80	88	87	43	34	72
1957	45	67	81	81	94	79	48	38	73
1958	47	76	70	78	95	84	42	32	74
1959	54	75	79	91	90	88	49	39	75
1960	59	85	81	82	97	89	45	32	78
1961	56	80	80	76	91	85	55	45	77
1962	64	82	80	79	86	84	44	35	73
1963	57	88	87	84	86	77	51	37	73
1964	60	84	76	77	87	77	52	47	73
1965	50	85	76	79	80	74	48	42	69
1966	51	80	83	70	80	71	50	39	71
1967	56	81	83	73	85	72	49	39	72
1968	64	80	73	79	85	75	46	39	75
1969	60	86	87	81	82	77	46	40	73
1970	59	82	86	84	86	74	51	42	75
1971	62	88	80	84	84	70	49	41	71
1972	66	88	88	86	88	72	49	43	76
1973	66	95	93	89	88	75	51	41	77
1974	62	83	82	84	87	76	50	47	74
1975	64	82	72	72	77	83	52	41	72

Year	16-19	20-24	16-24	25-34	35-49	50-64		65+	15+
1975	64	82	73	72	77	81		41	72
1976	62	79	71	79	75	75		34	68
1977	59	76	68	73	70	64		36	64
1978	57	78	67	70	73	63		36	64
1979	55	74	65	75	70	60		37	63
1980	51	63	58	70	73	67		33	62
1981	43	63	51	56	55	50		32	53
1982	44	58	52	54	58	48		33	49
1983	43	54	49	55	56	51		27	48
1984	41	49	45	60	55	49		26	48
1985	47	54	51	54	56	39		26	46
1986	44	53	49	52	52	43		24	45
1987	44	56	51	52	50	42		24	45

Source: TAC

Table 4.9.2 Weekly consumption of manufactured cigarettes per person: by age, 1946-1987
Women aged 16 and over, Great Britain: sales-adjusted

Year	16-19	20-24	25-29	30-34	35-59	60+	15+
1946	17	31	34	36	26	9	22
1947	..	..	..	..	..	..	20
1948	11	24	26	26	20	7	18
1949	11	25	28	28	21	8	19
1950	13	27	27	36	21	11	21
1951	11	22	35	34	26	8	22
1952	13	25	35	34	26	8	23
1953	11	25	30	39	28	10	23
1954	12	26	33	38	30	9	24
1955	13	26	37	37	33	9	26

Year	16-19	20-24	25-29	30-34	35-49	50-59	60+	65+	15+
1956	15	26	34	41	39	27	13	..	28
1957	19	28	40	42	41	28	14	..	29
1958	17	30	36	44	44	30	10	..	29
1959	16	29	38	50	47	32	10	..	30
1960	23	32	33	47	44	30	13	..	31
1961	24	34	40	41	46	34	13	..	32
1962	30	40	39	42	46	36	13	..	33
1963	26	42	44	40	54	37	16	..	36
1964	29	39	46	46	51	35	15	..	35
1965	25	45	47	44	49	41	14	..	36
1966	31	49	48	47	53	38	16	11	39
1967	33	46	45	41	50	44	18	14	39
1968	38	47	46	40	51	42	15	13	39
1969	45	57	60	54	52	44	19	14	43
1970	46	60	51	51	53	46	18	16	43
1971	43	58	51	51	57	46	17	13	42
1972	45	54	60	60	59	44	18	13	44
1973	53	64	60	61	63	56	23	16	49
1974	53	62	63	67	66	57	23	17	51
1975	51	62	63	56	61	50	23	18	48

Year	16-19	20-24	16-24	25-34	35-49	50-64	65+	15+
1975	51	62	57	60	61	46	18	48
1976	59	67	63	60	61	53	18	50
1977	48	62	56	58	61	54	19	49
1978	45	56	51	63	62	45	18	47
1979	43	62	53	59	58	46	18	46
1980	37	52	45	54	55	54	17	45
1981	38	49	42	55	60	44	19	42
1982	33	45	39	44	51	46	17	39
1983	37	50	44	46	50	44	15	39
1984	31	42	38	44	47	40	15	36
1985	38	40	39	47	48	40	16	37
1986	37	45	41	42	52	38	13	37
1987	38	40	39	44	46	39	16	37

Source: TAC

Fig. 4.7 Weekly consumption of manufactured cigarettes per person: by age, 1948-1987
Men and women aged 16 and over, Great Britain. *Source*: TAC
The consumption for men and women aged 25-34 that has been plotted for the years 1948-1974 is equal to the
mean of the consumption for men and women aged 25-29 and 30-34 during those years (see Tables 4.9.1/2)
Where two age groups are given, the first is for years up to and including 1975, and the second for 1976 onwards

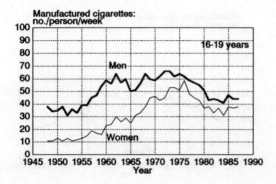

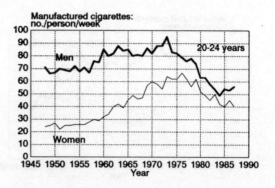

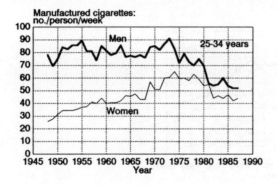

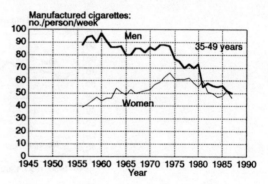

Fig. 4.7 (*continued*)   Weekly consumption of manufactured cigarettes per person: by age, 1948-1987
Men and women aged 16 and over, Great Britain. *Source*: TAC
The consumption for men and women aged 25-34 that has been plotted for the years 1948-1974 is equal to the
mean of the consumption for men and women aged 25-29 and 30-34 during those years (see Tables 4.9.1/2)
Where two age groups are given, the first is for years up to and including 1975, and the second for 1976 onwards

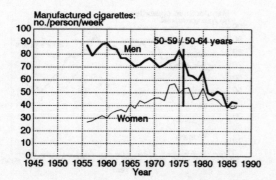

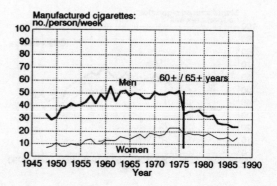

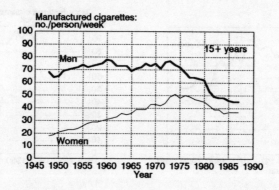

Table 4.10.1 Weekly consumption of manufactured cigarettes per smoker: by age, 1949-1987
Manufactured cigarette smokers, men aged 16 and over, Great Britain: sales-adjusted

Year	16-19	20-24	25-29	30-34	35-59		60-64	60+	65+	16+
1949	62	91	94	103	111		..	75	..	99
1950	68	99	112	104	119		103	..	67	107
1951	72	102	113	116	120		100	..	72	110
1952	65	110	118	125	131		111	..	90	120
1953	77	112	118	136	131		121	..	86	121
1954	72	115	127	132	139		114	..	79	125
1955	83	116	135	131	144		122	..	89	131

Year	16-19	20-24	25-29	30-34	35-49	50-59	60-64	60+	65+	16+
1956	76	110	120	120	134	139	113	..	82	121
1957	77	110	121	124	144	131	123	..	97	125
1958	86	123	116	131	148	142	132	100	82	130
1959	90	120	121	139	144	139	124	..	90	129
1960	91	126	124	131	149	147	128	..	81	131
1961	92	120	127	131	142	148	135	121	111	132
1962	107	130	133	135	142	140	117	106	92	130
1963	100	134	137	140	152	149	..	119	..	137
1964	101	133	136	135	145	145	..	117	..	134
1965	99	130	133	137	143	132	..	110	..	129
1966	96	124	131	122	139	135	131	112	..	128
1967	104	126	140	129	142	137	127	110	..	130
1968	111	131	126	134	142	137	111	100	..	128
1969	110	133	137	135	149	140	113	107	..	133
1970	110	136	137	139	146	139	133	111	..	133
1971	117	149	144	150	153	151	137	118	..	142
1972	127	148	154	160	161	156	139	121	..	148
1973	132	157	168	171	172	160	142	125	..	156
1974	131	151	149	155	170	151	147	125	..	149
1975	132	155	154	158	164	165	162	128	96	152

Year	16-19	20-24	16-24	25-34	35-49	50-64			65+	16+
1975	132	155	143	156	164	163			96	152
1976	134	160	148	167	164	158			107	155
1977	132	152	143	158	162	158			113	152
1978	133	158	145	158	171	158			104	155
1979	123	148	137	163	164	155			121	152
1980	124	138	132	150	170	154			116	149
1981	113	144	133	141	152	138			118	141
1982	109	134	122	143	153	149			119	139
1983	110	129	120	152	151	155			105	139
1984	107	129	119	143	157	140			111	138
1985	114	126	121	135	154	137			108	134
1986	109	125	118	142	147	142			123	136
1987	116	125	122	136	143	143			114	135

Source: TAC

Table 4.10.2   Weekly consumption of manufactured cigarettes per smoker: by age, 1949-1987
Manufactured cigarette smokers, women aged 16 and over, Great Britain: sales-adjusted

Year	16-19	20-24	25-29	30-34	35-59			60+		16+
1949	33	47	48	54	52			33		48
1950	37	55	52	65	62			44		56
1951	37	51	64	62	62			39		57
1952	43	55	67	65	65			38		60
1953	43	58	65	73	71			40		64
1954	47	62	69	76	75			42		67
1955	52	67	77	69	80			41		70

Year	16-19	20-24	25-29	30-34	35-49	50-59	60-64	60+	65+	16+
1956	46	60	71	74	81	71	..	46	..	71
1957	47	59	75	75	80	75	..	50	..	70
1958	52	68	78	86	88	82	..	56	..	78
1959	47	62	80	81	86	86	..	51	..	77
1960	51	67	66	84	86	75	..	57	..	74
1961	54	64	81	80	87	83	..	54	..	76
1962	65	79	84	84	86	83	..	59	..	79
1963	65	84	84	88	97	84	..	68	..	86
1964	69	78	86	95	96	88	..	65	..	86
1965	64	85	92	89	92	90	..	62	..	85
1966	68	87	97	93	96	85	72	59	..	86
1967	76	86	85	87	95	94	76	69	..	87
1968	80	88	93	88	95	88	69	64	..	87
1969	85	102	108	103	97	97	94	77	..	96
1970	89	105	102	96	103	100	82	71	..	95
1971	88	111	103	108	109	100	89	74	..	100
1972	97	113	117	117	117	101	95	76	..	105
1973	108	123	125	123	119	109	99	90	..	113
1974	113	123	123	130	122	118	97	87	..	115
1975	111	119	123	123	122	104	92	85	..	111

Year	16-19	20-24	16-24	25-34	35-49	50-64			65+	16+
1975	111	119	115	123	122	100			72	111
1976	119	126	123	130	127	118			83	120
1977	110	127	119	126	130	119			83	119
1978	106	117	112	132	130	113			81	118
1979	102	125	115	130	130	107			85	116
1980	101	121	113	120	125	117			82	115
1981	98	120	115	119	135	121			87	113
1982	92	111	103	119	127	113			82	112
1983	94	113	105	116	127	114			77	112
1984	85	111	99	114	130	104			80	108
1985	93	107	100	113	124	112			86	110
1986	94	107	102	114	131	110			76	111
1987	89	99	94	115	126	113			79	108

Source: TAC

Fig. 4.8 Weekly consumption of manufactured cigarettes per smoker: by age, 1949-1987
Manufactured cigarette smokers, men and women aged 16 and over, Great Britain. *Source*: TAC
The consumption for men and women aged 25-34 that has been plotted for the years 1948-1974 is equal to the mean of the consumption for men and women aged 25-29 and 30-34 during those years (see Tables 4.10.1/2)
Where two age groups are given, the first is for years up to and including 1975, and the second for 1976 onwards

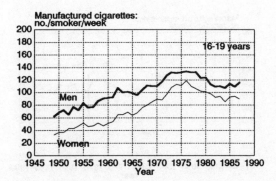

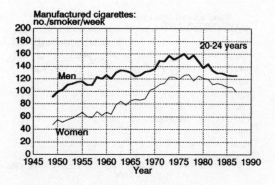

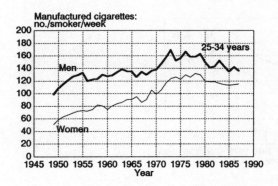

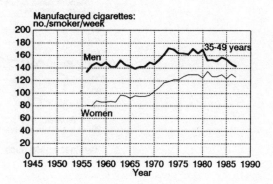

Fig. 4.8 (*continued*)   Weekly consumption of manufactured cigarettes per smoker: by age, 1949-1987
Manufactured cigarette smokers, men and women aged 16 and over, Great Britain. *Source*: TAC
The consumption for men and women aged 25-34 that has been plotted for the years 1948-1974 is equal to the
mean of the consumption for men and women aged 25-29 and 30-34 during those years (see Tables 4.10.1/2)
Where two age groups are given, the first is for years up to and including 1975, and the second for 1976 onwards

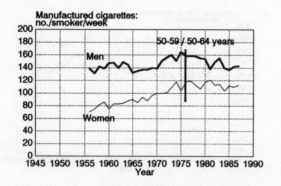

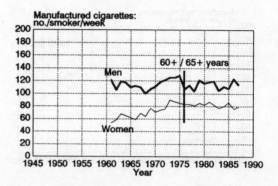

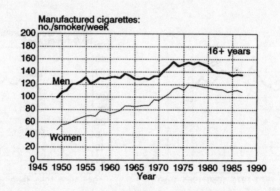

Table 4.11.1 Annual consumption of manufactured cigarettes per person: by age (5-year groups), 1966-1987
Men aged 16 and over, Great Britain: sales-adjusted

Year	16-19	20-24	25-29	30-34	35-39	40-44	45-49	50-54	55-59	60-64	65-69	70-74	75-79	80+	15+
1966	2650	4150	4300	3650	4250	4150	4100	3900	3500	3400	2450	1750	2200	500	3680
1967	2900	4200	4300	3800	4500	4450	4150	3600	3800	3300	2450	2050	1300	1200	3760
1968	3350	4150	3800	4100	4450	4500	4250	4150	3650	2950	2850	2000	1250	700	3880
1969	3100	4450	4500	4200	4200	4900	3850	4400	3650	3000	2700	1800	1300	950	3800
1970	3050	4250	4450	4350	4600	4650	4200	4100	3500	3500	2900	1650	1500	1150	3920
1971	3200	4550	4150	4350	4000	4050	5050	4200	3150	3350	2450	2550	1100	1300	3700
1972	3450	4550	4550	4450	4350	4350	4900	3950	3650	3250	2600	2150	2100	950	3930
1973	3450	4950	4850	4650	4950	4450	4150	4350	3300	3600	2650	1850	1250	1500	3980
1974	3200	4300	4250	4350	4750	4100	4950	4000	3900	2950	3300	2100	1600	1050	3840
1975	3350	4250	3750	3750	4150	4050	3800	4800	3850	3950	2950	1700	1550	700	3730
1976	3200	4100	4150	4050	4000	3650	4050	4350	3550	3700	2250	1650	1100	900	3530
1977	3050	3950	4000	3600	3550	3800	3600	3600	3650	2700	2350	1550	1400	1750	3310
1978	2950	4050	3600	3650	3750	4350	3200	4200	2800	2850	2400	1600	1650	500	3330
1979	2850	3850	3600	4200	3500	3550	3950	3500	2800	3150	2250	1700	2050	1000	3300
1980	2650	3300	3600	3700	4100	3700	3550	4000	3200	3200	1800	1750	1750	950	3230
1981	2250	3250	3350	3050	3400	2900	3100	2850	3000	2050	1650	1850	1000	650	2760
													Age 70+		
1982	2300	3000	2600	3000	3000	2800	3100	3000	2450	2000	2250		1350		2540
1983	2250	2800	2750	2950	2900	3200	2550	2900	2650	2350	1650		1200		2500
1984	2150	2550	3200	3050	2950	2600	3000	2500	3150	2050	1700		1150		2500
1985	2450	2800	3000	2550	3150	2850	2700	2150	2250	1800	1700		1150		2380
1986	2300	2750	2400	2950	2700	2800	2500	2600	2050	2150	1600		1050		2350
1987	2300	2900	2850	2500	2800	2500	2550	2400	2050	2100	1500		1100		2350

Source: TAC

Table 4.11.2 Annual consumption of manufactured cigarettes per person: by age (5-year groups), 1966-1987
Women aged 16 and over, Great Britain: sales-adjusted

Year	16-19	20-24	25-29	30-34	35-39	40-44	45-49	50-54	55-59	60-64	65-69	70-74	75-79	80+	15+
1966	1600	2550	2500	2450	2600	2850	2900	2000	1900	1300	750	750	200	50	2050
1967	1700	2400	2350	2150	2600	2650	2550	2450	2050	1250	1100	600	250	250	2020
1968	1950	2450	2400	2100	2350	2750	2700	2350	2050	1100	950	650	350	150	2030
1969	2350	2950	3100	2800	2550	2950	2650	2400	2100	1650	850	850	350	300	2220
1970	2400	3100	2650	2650	2700	3000	2550	2350	2500	1350	1250	750	400	450	2250
1971	2250	3000	2650	2650	2300	3550	3050	2550	2250	1500	950	700	350	200	2170
1972	2350	2800	3100	3100	3100	3050	3100	2900	1700	1650	1100	550	450	300	2300
1973	2750	3350	3100	3150	2850	3250	3750	2700	3150	1900	1200	850	550	350	2540
1974	2750	3200	3300	3500	3350	3050	3950	3500	2450	2000	1450	850	500	300	2630
1975	2650	3200	3300	2900	3000	3300	3300	2650	2600	2000	1350	850	550	450	2500
1976	3050	3500	3100	3200	3450	2950	3150	3550	2800	1800	1450	800	450	450	2580
1977	2500	3200	3000	3000	3350	3050	3100	3350	2900	2200	1450	1150	350	300	2540
1978	2350	2900	3150	3300	3200	2950	3400	3000	2300	1800	1250	1000	600	250	2450
1979	2250	3200	2700	3400	3000	2800	3150	2650	2600	1850	1110	950	850	450	2410

Year	16-19	20-24	25-29	30-34	35-39	40-44	45-49	50-54	55-59	60-64	65-69	70-74	75-79	80+	15+
1980	1900	2700	2850	2750	3000	2700	2900	3400	2900	2100	1350	900	600	350	2330
1981	1950	2550	2600	2550	2650	2900	3000	2550	2550	1850	1100	900	850	350	2200
													Age 70+		
1982	1700	2350	2150	2500	2750	2900	2350	2800	2500	1900	1350		650		2030
1983	1900	2600	2400	2450	2550	2550	2750	2700	2250	2050	1150		600		2020
1984	1600	2200	2200	2450	2600	2800	2000	2100	2450	1800	1300		600		1890
1985	2000	2100	2550	2300	2200	2600	2700	2100	2300	1950	1500		500		1930
1986	1900	2350	2200	2150	2700	2750	2600	1900	2400	1600	900		500		1900
1987	2000	2100	2150	2450	2350	2400	2450	2150	2050	1950	1450		550		1900

Source: TAC

Table 4.12 Weekly consumption of cigarettes (manufactured and hand-rolled) per smoker: by age, 1972-1988
Cigarette smokers, men and women aged 16 and over, Great Britain

Year	16-19	20-24	25-34	35-49	50-59	60+	16+
Men							
1972	102	123	129	132	124	96	120
1974	110	132	136	138	127	100	125
1976	106	135	138	141	130	108	129
1978	98	122	134	138	137	104	127
1980	99	113	135	140	130	102	124
1982	87	114	121	137	129	109	121
1984	87	107	114	130	126	103	115
1986	86	108	110	133	120	103	115
1988	84	109	120	136	132	102	120
Women							
1972	76	91	97	94	87	60	87
1974	86	99	108	104	91	68	94
1976	89	110	109	112	103	75	101
1978	90	101	113	109	101	79	101
1980	84	102	111	115	105	73	102
1982	76	100	109	108	101	77	98
1984	80	91	105	107	98	80	96
1986	77	85	101	112	99	84	97
1988	79	95	103	113	102	81	99

Source: GHS

Smoking habits: by social class

This section is concerned with current smokers only. Information on ex-smokers and persons who have never smoked, classified according to social class, is given in Section 6.

Details of the TAC classification by social class, and the GHS classification by socio-economic group are given on page xxxi. In the text, little mention is made of trends in smoking habits among men and women in social class VI (TAC data), whose members are described as unoccupied (including for example, persons unemployed for more than two months, married women with unemployed husbands, and divorcees and widows with no occupation). Social class VI is therefore a heterogenous group, and the composition of its members is likely to have changed during the period of the surveys. It cannot appropriately be considered in the social classes I to V 'gradient' described below.

Percentage of population who smoke: by social class

Cigarettes

Men

The TAC first included estimates of smoking and social class in their Annual Consumer Survey in 1958. From 1948 to 1960 the TAC also collected data on the percentages of men and women who smoked manufactured cigarettes by income group. These data are probably less reliable than the data classified by social class; they were based on smaller sample sizes and there were difficulties in assessing the income groups into which the respondents fell. The data do nonetheless indicate a higher prevalence of manufactured-cigarette smoking among men in the higher income groups.

By 1958 the percentage of men who smoked manufactured cigarettes was similar in all social classes. Between 1958 and 1971, this percentage declined from 54 to 37 per cent in social class I, but only from 61 to 59 per cent in social class V. Thereafter the decline affected all social classes so that by 1987 the percentage of men who smoked manufactured cigarettes ranged from 13 per cent in social class I to 46 per cent in social class V. From 1948 to 1987 (the latest year for which TAC provided figures) the social class gradient had therefore reversed, so that a habit once most common among persons of professional occupations had become most common among persons of manual and unskilled occupations.

Data from the GHS surveys show that between 1972 and 1988, as with the TAC data, the decline in cigarette smoking affected all social classes. In the professional group the percentage who smoked cigarettes fell from 33 per cent to 16 per cent, while in the unskilled manual group it fell from 64 to 43 per cent, so that by 1988 more than twice as many unskilled and semi-skilled manual workers were cigarette smokers as in the professional occupations (according to these data).

Data on hand-rolled cigarette smoking classified by social class are available only from 1975 from the TAC; in every survey a greater proportion of men in social classes IIIM, IV, V, and VI smoked hand-rolled cigarettes than men in classes I, II, and IIINM.

Women

TAC data for 1948-1960 show that the percentage of women who smoked manufactured cigarettes was similar in all income groups, apart from a lower rate of smoking in the lowest income group from 1952 onwards. The pattern did not change materially during the 1960s. Between 1971 and 1987 the percentage of women who smoked manufactured cigarettes declined from 34 to 15 per cent in social class I, and from 49 to 40 per cent in social class V.

The GHS data (1972-1988) are again consistent with those from the TAC in showing a decline in the percentage who smoked cigarettes among women of all social classes. The decrease was greatest in the professional socio-economic group, from 33 to 17 per cent, and least in the semi-skilled and unskilled groups, from 42 to 38 per cent.

Both sexes

Data from the TAC for 1987 show that approximately the same percentage of men and women within a given social class were smokers of manufactured cigarettes. GHS data relating to all cigarettes, including hand-rolled, for 1988 indicate a similar pattern.

Cigars

Men

Data on cigar smoking according to social class are available from the TAC from 1975 to 1987. During most of this time cigar smoking remained more popular with professional men than with men from other classes. The percentage of men who smoke cigars declined from 16 per cent in 1975 to 7 per cent in 1987 among men in social classes I and II, and from 10 to 5 per cent among men in social classes IV, V, and VI.

Pipes

Men

Data on pipe smoking according to social class are available from the TAC from 1975 to 1987. During this time pipe smoking remained more popular with professional men than with men from other classes. Between 1975 and 1987 the percentage of men who smoke pipes declined from 15 to 6 per cent among men in social classes I and II, and from 9 to 4 per cent among men in social classes IV, V, and VI.

Any tobacco

Men

TAC data for 1958 showed a small social class gradient across classes I to V, with the percentage of men who smoked any form of tobacco increasing from 65 per cent in social class I to 77 per cent in social class V. A decline in the percentage of smokers of any form of tobacco occurred in all classes except IV and V during the 1960s, and in all classes except class VI between 1971 and 1987. By 1987 the social class gradient had increased, with 23 per cent of men in social class I smoking some form of tobacco, and 57 per cent of class V.

Women

For women, the percentage of smokers of any form of tobacco has always been virtually identical to the percentage of smokers of manufactured cigarettes.

Table 5.1 Percentages of men and women who smoke manufactured cigarettes: by income group, 1948-1960
Men and women aged 16 and over, United Kingdom

| | Income group | | | | | | |
| | Clerical | | | Manual | | | All groups |
Year	A	B	C1	C2	D	E	
Men							
1948	68	69	69	72	64	45	65
1952	66	60	59	63	55	39	59
1953	59	61	57	65	54	42	60
1954	62	62	58	63	49	41	59
1955	59	61	55	63	46	37	58
1956	62	63	61	66	60	43	61
1957	56	66	60	63	60	46	60
1958	57	59	55	62	59	45	58
1959	59	64	57	64	60	46	61
1960	55	61	60	61	64	49	61
Women							
1948	46	41	43	39	42	40	41
1952	37	39	41	37	45	28	38
1953	42	40	41	38	40	26	38
1954	41	40	42	38	38	24	37
1955	41	38	40	41	39	23	38
1956	48	46	43	41	45	35	42
1957	55	42	45	46	48	35	44
1958	43	43	42	44	46	24	40
1959	49	42	45	47	50	25	43
1960	39	42	43	45	46	25	42

The income groups were defined as follows, where the income is the likely annual or weekly income of the head of household in 1962:

A	B	C1	C2	D	E
£2000+ p.a.	£1000- £2000 p.a.	Under £1000 p.a.	£13+ p.wk.	£7-13 p.wk.	Under £7 p.wk.

Source: TAC
Table taken from Todd, G.F. 'Social class variations in cigarette smoking and mortality from associated diseases' (TRC Occasional Paper 2) London: Tobacco Research Council, 1976

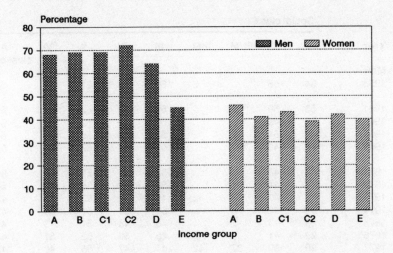

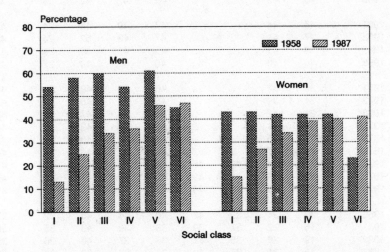

Table 5.2 Percentages of men and women who smoke manufactured cigarettes: by social class, 1958-1987
Men and women aged 16 and over, Great Britain: sales-adjusted 1969-1987

| Year | Social class | | | | | | | | |
	I	II	IIINM	IIIM	III	IV	V	VI	All classes
Men									
1958	54	58	..	..	60	54	61	45	58
1961	53	59	..	..	59	60	62	40	59
1963	43	49	..	..	54	55	62	51	54
1965	44	54	..	..	53	54	59	42	54
1968	44	48	..	..	55	61	62	42	55
1971	37	43	..	..	53	51	59	47	51
1972	30	44	..	..	53	52	58	48	51
1973	39	42	..	..	49	56	63	34	49
1974	37	42	..	..	51	52	61	39	49
1975	29	43	..	..	48	48	57	43	47
1976	29	41	..	..	45	50	52	31	45
1977	25	39	37	42	41	47	56	40	42
1978	20	33	34	45	43	47	51	34	41
1979	29	36	36	44	42	45	48	47	42
1980	29	37	34	45	42	47	49	38	42
1981	22	33	37	37	37	44	40	40	37
1982	19	30	35	37	37	39	45	44	36
1983	18	27	30	37	35	41	43	41	35
1984	23	28	29	37	36	41	43	39	35
1985	20	28	32	36	35	40	40	43	35
1986	21	27	28	32	31	38	47	44	33
1987	13	25	29	36	34	36	46	47	34
Women									
1958	43	43	..	..	42	42	42	23	39
1961	45	44	..	..	47	49	43	24	43
1963	37	41	..	..	47	43	52	24	43
1965	38	41	..	..	45	42	48	24	42
1968	40	40	..	..	46	45	40	27	43
1971	34	37	..	..	46	45	49	24	42
1972	31	39	..	..	45	47	46	29	42
1973	26	42	..	..	47	46	47	26	43
1974	30	41	..	..	47	46	42	27	44
1975	29	38	..	..	45	41	48	39	43
1976	24	37	..	..	45	42	43	32	42
1977	34	34	43	45	44	41	43	32	41
1978	22	36	41	43	42	42	43	32	40
1979	23	35	40	44	42	40	39	39	39
1980	30	34	39	42	40	44	40	32	39
1981	16	32	37	39	38	39	40	35	36
1982	19	29	35	41	38	37	40	36	35
1983	15	31	34	40	37	39	36	36	35
1984	22	27	35	37	36	37	41	34	34
1985	26	28	33	37	35	36	40	40	34
1986	18	27	31	36	34	33	40	43	33
1987	15	27	32	35	34	39	40	41	34

Source: TAC

Fig. 5.3 Percentages of men and women who smoke cigarettes (manufactured and hand-rolled): by socio-economic group, 1972-1988
Men and women aged 16 and over, Great Britain. *Source*: GHS

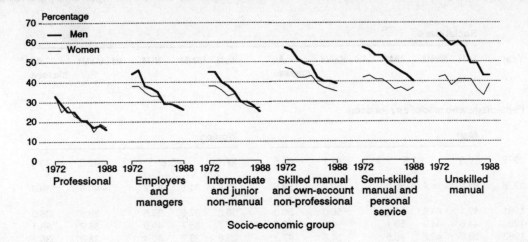

Table 5.3 Percentages of men and women who smoke cigarettes (manufactured and hand-rolled): by socio-economic group, 1972-1988
Men and women aged 16 and over[1],Great Britain

| Year | Socio-economic group | | | | | | |
	Professional	Employers and managers	Intermediate and junior non-manual	Skilled manual and own-account non-professional	Semi-skilled manual and personal service	Unskilled manual	All groups
Men							
1972	33	44	45	57	57	64	52
1974	29	46	45	56	56	61	51
1976	25	38	40	51	53	58	46
1978	25	37	38	49	53	60	45
1980	21	35	35	48	49	57	42
1982	20	29	30	42	47	49	38
1984	17	29	30	40	45	49	36
1986	18	28	28	40	43	43	35
1988	16	26	25	39	40	43	33
Women							
1972	33	38	38	47	42	42	42
1974	25	38	38	46	43	43	41
1976	28	35	36	42	41	38	38
1978	23	33	33	42	41	41	37
1980	21	33	34	43	39	41	37
1982	21	29	30	39	36	41	33
1984	15	29	28	37	37	36	32
1986	19	27	27	36	35	33	31
1988	17	26	27	35	37	39	30

1 Aged 15 and over in 1972

Source: GHS

SECTION 5   Smoking habits: by social class

67

Table 5.4 Percentages of men and women who smoke: by form of tobacco and social class, 1975-1987
Men and women aged 16 and over, Great Britain: sales-adjusted, except for cigar and pipe tobacco

Year	I+II	IIINM	IIIM	IV+V+VI	All classes	I+II	IIINM	IIIM	VI+V+VI	All classes

Social class

Percentage who smoke any tobacco

Year	I+II	IIINM	IIIM	IV+V+VI	All classes	I+II	IIINM	IIIM	VI+V+VI	All classes
	Men					Women				
1975	56.5	61.5		65.2	61.5	37.4	45.8		42.8	43.4
1978	44.9	46.2	58.3	59.5	54.5	33.8	41.6	43.2	40.0	39.9
1981	42.1	48.6	50.8	56.0	50.0	30.0	37.6	39.5	38.8	36.9
1982	44.6	44.9	50.1	52.9	49.2	27.7	35.7	40.9	38.2	36.1
1983	38.9	42.2	48.5	54.6	47.3	28.8	33.7	40.4	38.3	35.7
1984	40.0	39.1	49.8	52.6	47.3	26.6	34.8	37.6	37.4	34.6
1985	39.2	42.8	48.2	51.0	46.4	28.2	32.8	37.6	38.3	34.8
1986	37.2	35.2	42.8	50.6	43.1	26.4	31.2	36.3	37.7	33.6
1987	32.8	37.5	46.0	52.1	43.7	25.7	32.4	35.8	40.4	34.3

Percentage who smoke manufactured cigarettes

Year	I+II	IIINM	IIIM	IV+V+VI	All classes	I+II	IIINM	IIIM	VI+V+VI	All classes
	Men					Women				
1975	40.3	47.6		49.9	46.8	36.5	45.4		42.1	42.8
1978	31.0	33.7	45.0	46.1	41.1	33.2	41.1	43.1	39.6	39.5
1981	30.5	37.2	36.8	42.4	36.9	29.0	37.3	39.1	38.0	36.3
1982	27.6	35.0	36.9	41.2	35.9	27.3	35.0	40.5	37.2	35.4
1983	25.4	29.5	36.6	41.6	34.8	28.4	33.7	40.1	37.9	35.4
1984	27.3	28.6	37.3	40.7	35.2	26.1	34.6	37.0	36.6	34.0
1985	26.3	32.1	35.7	41.1	34.7	27.8	32.6	37.2	37.9	34.4
1986	25.9	27.8	32.2	41.8	33.2	25.5	30.9	35.8	37.4	33.1
1987	23.0	28.8	35.6	41.7	33.6	25.3	32.2	35.2	39.7	33.8

Percentage who smoke manufactured cigarettes only

Year	I+II	IIINM	IIIM	IV+V+VI	All classes	I+II	IIINM	IIIM	VI+V+VI	All classes
	Men					Women				
1975	25.8	32.0		35.4	31.7	35.8	44.2		40.3	41.5
1978	21.4	24.7	33.8	34.8	30.4	32.2	39.9	42.3	37.0	38.1
1981	22.5	27.3	26.2	29.8	26.7	28.2	36.2	38.4	36.6	35.2
1982	20.2	26.6	26.7	29.4	26.0	26.4	34.1	38.9	34.9	33.9
1983	19.0	23.1	26.9	29.5	25.5	27.6	32.6	38.3	35.7	33.9
1984	20.7	23.8	29.6	29.3	27.0	25.3	33.1	35.3	34.6	32.4
1985	20.1	26.1	26.6	26.9	25.1	27.7	31.9	36.1	35.6	33.2
1986	18.2	20.8	23.2	30.1	23.8	24.0	30.4	33.8	35.3	31.5
1987	18.1	22.0	26.6	29.6	24.9	24.4	31.6	33.5	38.0	32.5

Table 5.4 (*continued*) Percentages of men and women who smoke: by form of tobacco and social class, 1975-1987

Men and women aged 16 and over, Great Britain: sales-adjusted, except for cigar and pipe tobacco

Percentage who smoke hand-rolled cigarettes

	Social class									
Year	I+II	IIINM	IIIM	IV+V+VI	All classes	I+II	IIINM	IIIM	VI+V+VI	All classes
	Men					**Women**				
1975	5.5	12.1		15.7	11.8	1.7	4.6		6.6	4.6
1978	5.0	7.4	10.5	14.6	10.1	1.9	3.1	3.5	6.4	3.9
1981	4.2	6.6	14.1	16.2	11.7	1.5	1.4	6.0	5.1	4.3
1982	4.5	8.2	13.4	16.9	11.5	2.2	2.5	5.4	7.1	4.9
1983	5.1	5.6	10.7	17.3	10.8	2.5	1.8	4.3	7.2	4.4
1984	4.0	4.2	10.0	17.1	10.1	1.1	2.2	4.8	7.4	4.4
1985	5.0	6.2	10.7	16.7	10.7	1.8	3.4	4.3	4.9	3.8
1986	3.9	6.2	11.1	15.0	10.1	1.2	1.8	4.1	4.6	3.4
1987	3.8	4.9	10.9	16.2	10.1	1.6	1.0	4.3	5.3	3.6

Percentage who smoke cigars

	Cigars Men					Cigars only Men				
Year	I+II	IIINM	IIIM	IV+V+VI	All classes	I+II	IIINM	IIIM	VI+V+VI	All classes
1975	15.9	13.4		10.4	13.1	5.7	4.1		3.1	4.1
1978	12.6	7.8	11.6	7.4	10.2	5.3	2.5	3.9	2.6	3.7
1981	9.9	11.5	8.7	7.8	9.0	4.4	3.2	3.4	2.6	3.4
1982	11.8	8.0	8.5	5.2	8.3	6.6	3.3	3.8	2.1	3.9
1983	9.7	11.1	8.5	4.8	8.0	4.8	5.1	4.3	2.2	3.9
1984	10.4	6.9	7.2	4.0	7.0	6.2	3.9	3.7	1.0	3.5
1985	10.5	8.2	7.5	5.0	7.5	5.9	4.6	4.0	1.8	3.8
1986	9.6	7.1	6.9	4.2	6.7	4.8	3.0	3.2	1.9	3.2
1987	7.2	7.3	7.7	4.9	6.7	3.5	4.0	3.2	1.9	3.0

Percentage who smoke pipes

	Pipes Men					Pipes only Men				
Year	I+II	IIINM	IIIM	IV+V+VI	All classes	I+II	IIINM	IIIM	VI+V+VI	All classes
1975	15.0	10.2		9.2	10.9	5.9	3.0		3.5	3.7
1978	9.8	9.8	7.9	6.4	8.1	3.8	4.8	3.5	3.5	3.7
1981	9.3	7.7	6.1	7.5	7.3	3.5	3.7	2.8	3.0	3.1
1982	10.8	5.8	5.5	4.1	6.3	5.9	2.7	2.3	1.6	2.9
1983	7.8	6.4	5.1	5.3	5.9	3.8	3.1	2.0	2.7	2.7
1984	7.4	6.4	5.1	4.3	5.5	4.4	3.5	2.9	2.1	3.0
1985	6.2	4.1	5.9	5.7	5.7	3.6	2.5	3.1	2.1	2.8
1986	7.7	4.0	4.6	3.7	5.0	3.9	2.3	2.0	1.9	2.4
1987	5.8	5.0	4.3	4.1	4.7	3.2	2.9	1.5	1.9	2.1

Source: TAC

Fig. 5.4 Percentages of men and women who smoke: by form of tobacco and social class, 1987
Men and women aged 16 and over, Great Britain. *Source*: TAC

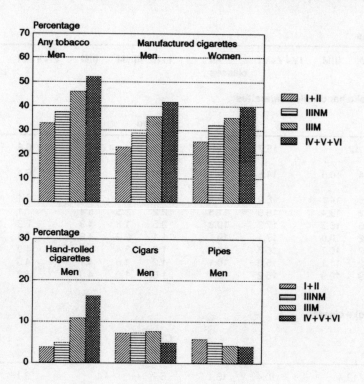

Fig. 5.5 Percentage of men who smoke any form of tobacco: by social class, 1958 and 1987
Men aged 16 and over, Great Britain. *Source*: TAC

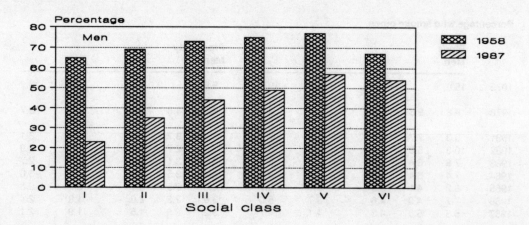

Table 5.5 Percentages of men and women who smoke any form of tobacco (except pipe tobacco, for women): by social class, 1958-1987
Men and women aged 16 and over, Great Britain: sales-adjusted 1969-1987

Year	Social class								All classes
	I	II	IIINM	IIIM	III	IV	V	VI	
Men									
1958	65	69	..	..	73	75	77	67	72
1961	65	68	..	..	72	74	79	63	72
1963	55	61	..	..	68	71	79	60	68
1965	59	67	..	..	66	71	73	63	68
1968	54	64	..	..	67	75	78	51	69
1971	53	58	..	..	65	68	73	50	65
1972	50	60	..	..	68	68	70	58	66
1973	57	60	..	..	66	71	80	41	66
1974	49	61	..	..	65	68	74	40	64
1975	48	58	..	..	62	67	70	53	62
1976	45	57	..	..	59	64	64	34	59
1977	45	54	..	..	57	63	72	50	58
1978	35	47	46	58	56	61	66	45	55
1979	38	52	..	..	55	59	63	51	55
1980	44	49	..	..	56	60	64	47	55
1981	36	44	49	51	50	58	56	51	50
1982	39	46	45	50	49	51	58	52	49
1983	33	40	42	49	47	56	57	50	47
1984	33	42	39	50	48	53	59	48	47
1985	31	41	43	48	47	50	51	52	46
1986	35	38	35	43	41	47	57	52	43
1987	23	35	38	46	44	49	57	54	44
Women									
1958	43	43	..	..	42	42	42	23	40
1961	45	43	..	..	47	50	44	24	44
1963	38	41	..	..	47	44	53	24	43
1965	38	42	..	..	46	43	49	24	43
1968	40	41	..	..	46	45	40	28	43
1971	34	38	..	..	46	46	49	24	42
1972	32	39	..	..	45	47	46	29	42
1973	26	42	..	..	47	47	47	27	44
1974	30	42	..	..	47	47	42	27	44
1975	30	39	..	..	46	42	48	40	43
1976	24	37	..	..	46	42	43	32	42
1977	34	35	..	..	45	42	44	33	41
1978	23	36	42	43	43	42	44	32	40
1979	25	35	..	..	42	40	40	41	40
1980	30	34	..	..	41	44	40	33	39
1981	17	33	38	40	39	40	41	36	37
1982	20	29	36	41	39	37	43	37	36
1983	15	31	34	40	37	39	37	37	36
1984	22	28	35	38	36	37	41	36	35
1985	26	29	33	38	35	36	40	41	35
1986	19	28	31	36	34	33	40	43	34
1987	15	28	32	36	34	39	41	42	34

Source: TAC

Cigarette consumption: by social class

The TAC provides data on the consumption of manufactured cigarettes per person and per manufactured cigarette smoker, classified according to social class, from 1958 to 1987. The GHS provides data on the consumption of cigarettes (manufactured and hand-rolled) per cigarette smoker classified according to socio-economic group from 1972 to 1988. The GHS does not provide data on a per person basis.

Consumption per person

Men

In 1958 the consumption of manufactured cigarettes per person across the social classes was similar, apart from lower consumption in class VI. Manufactured cigarette consumption per person began to fall among men in social class I during the 1960s, as the percentage of men who smoked in this social class began to fall. In most other social classes, consumption per person did not begin to fall until about 1975. By 1987 there was a striking gradient across social classes I to V, with consumption per person among men in social class V five times that of men in social class I, namely, 63 and 13 manufactured cigarettes a week per person respectively.

Women

In 1958, consumption per person among women was similar across the social classes, apart from a low value in social class VI. During the 1960s and 1970s consumption per person remained fairly constant in social class I, at about 30 manufactured cigarettes a week per person, but fell in the early 1980s to half the 1958 value. Consumption per person among women of social classes II to V reached their highest levels during the 1970s (more than 50 manufactured cigarettes a week per person in social classes III, IV, and V), and declined thereafter. In 1987 consumption per person among women in social class I was 14 manufactured cigarettes a week compared with 47 cigarettes a week among women in social class V.

Consumption per smoker

Men

Cigarette consumption per smoker classified by social class has been erratic. Neither TAC nor GHS data indicate a social-class gradient in consumption per smoker among men, although in many years men in social classes I and VI report lower consumption than men from other classes. In social classes I to V the TAC estimated that consumption per smoker reached a maximum of between 150 and 165 manufactured cigarettes a week per smoker during the 1970s. GHS figures, not sales-adjusted, on the consumption of manufactured and hand-rolled cigarettes per smoker, are lower, indicating a maximum consumption of 109 cigarettes a week per smoker among professional men, and between 120 and 139 cigarettes among men of other socio-economic groups. GHS data show that between 1972 and 1988 the average number of cigarettes smoked in 1988 was similar to the number smoked in 1972 for men in all socio-economic groups.

Women

In 1958 consumption per smoker among women was similar across classes II to V, with slightly lower values in social classes I and VI. Consumption per smoker changed very little during the 1960s, but then rose in all classes during the 1970s, reaching a maximum of about 120 manufactured cigarettes a week per smoker according to TAC data, and somewhat less according to GHS data. TAC data indicate a small downward trend in consumption per smoker between the late 1970s and 1987. GHS data also indicate a small downward trend between the late 1970s and 1984, but thereafter indicate an increase in consumption. GHS data show an increase in consumption per smoker for all classes between 1972 and 1988.

GHS data for 1972 to 1988 show that professional women who smoke consume fewer cigarettes than other women smokers, although this pattern is not so clearly displayed by the TAC data.

Both sexes

Throughout the period of the surveys, female smokers of all social classes have consumed fewer cigarettes per smoker than male cigarette smokers of the same class.

Table 5.6 Weekly consumption of manufactured cigarettes per person: by social class, 1958-1987
Men and women aged 16 and over, Great Britain: sales-adjusted

	Social class								
Year	I	II	IIINM	IIIM	III	IV	V	VI	All classes (ages 16+)
Men									
1958	76	76	..	..	82	70	78	44	76
1961	65	83	..	..	76	78	84	43	77
1963	42	67	..	..	75	72	91	56	74
1965	56	76	..	..	69	65	76	41	69
1968	46	62			71	75	81	38	70
1971	50	62	..	..	77	68	83	52	72
1972	36	66	..	..	79	75	91	64	75
1973	51	69	..	..	78	82	103	32	77
1974	44	66	..	..	76	76	99	34	74
1975	36	70	..	..	73	71	85	51	72
1976	39	62	..	..	70	78	84	35	68
1977	37	56	55	66	64	71	83	54	64
1978	25	51	45	73	67	73	75	48	64
1979	43	56	51	69	65	68	72	54	63
1980	36	53	48	69	65	69	76	42	62
1981	30	49	51	53	53	63	49	50	52
1982	28	41	47	53	52	56	56	53	50
1983	20	38	41	52	50	58	63	51	48
1984	30	42	37	53	49	55	60	45	48
1985	29	38	40	48	47	49	61	54	46
1986	26	38	41	44	44	48	65	55	45
1987	13	35	36	49	46	50	63	59	45
Women									
1958	30	36	..	..	34	34	32	16	31
1961	32	34	..	..	36	38	32	14	32
1963	34	36	..	..	40	40	48	16	36
1965	28	34	..	..	39	38	46	15	36
1968	28	34	..	..	40	41	33	19	37
1971	28	38	..	..	47	45	56	16	42
1972	32	39	..	..	50	51	48	24	44
1973	22	44	..	..	57	49	58	24	49
1974	29	44	..	..	55	55	50	22	50
1975	26	40	..	..	52	45	52	38	47
1976	27	42	..	..	55	52	53	34	50
1977	37	40	53	57	55	46	51	35	49
1978	26	42	49	50	50	52	51	36	47
1979	27	40	47	50	48	48	51	34	46
1980	25	38	45	50	48	52	42	36	44
1981	22	35	42	44	43	43	51	39	41
1982	15	32	38	46	42	43	43	39	39
1983	15	31	37	46	41	47	41	40	39
1984	17	29	38	42	40	38	48	34	37
1985	23	27	35	42	38	42	43	46	38
1986	13	29	35	40	38	38	48	47	37
1987	14	31	32	38	36	45	47	41	37

Source: TAC

Fig. 5.6 Weekly consumption of manufactured cigarettes per person: by social class, 1958 and 1987
Men and women aged 16 and over, Great Britain. *Source*: TAC

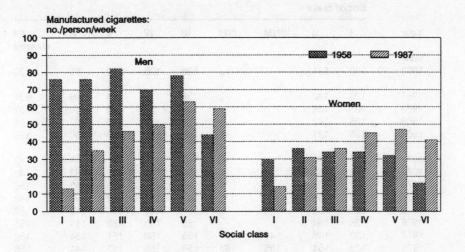

Fig. 5.7 Weekly consumption of manufactured cigarettes per smoker: by social class, 1958 and 1987
Manufactured cigarette smokers, men and women aged 16 and over, Great Britain. *Source*: TAC

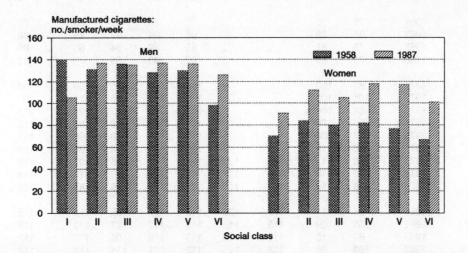

Table 5.7 Weekly consumption of manufactured cigarettes per smoker: by social class, 1958-1987
Manufactured cigarette smokers, men and women aged 16 and over
Great Britain: sales-adjusted

| Year | Social class | | | | | | | | All classes |
	I	II	IIINM	IIIM	III	IV	V	VI	
Men									
1958	140	131	..	..	136	128	130	98	130
1961	123	142	..	..	128	130	134	106	131
1963	101	136	..	..	139	132	148	110	137
1965	126	142	..	..	129	122	130	97	129
1968	105	131	..	..	130	124	129	90	128
1971	137	143	..	..	145	133	141	111	142
1972	120	148	..	..	150	145	157	133	148
1973	132	163	..	..	158	147	165	95	156
1974	118	159	..	..	149	148	162	88	149
1975	124	163	..	..	154	147	147	119	152
1976	135	154	..	..	155	155	160	114	155
1977	150	146	149	156	155	152	151	134	152
1978	123	154	135	163	158	156	147	141	155
1979	146	156	142	155	153	152	151	117	152
1980	126	146	141	156	153	148	155	112	149
1981	138	149	137	145	143	143	123	125	141
1982	151	139	136	143	141	144	124	121	139
1983	115	141	140	142	142	141	149	123	139
1984	126	150	126	141	138	136	137	116	138
1985	147	141	126	136	134	123	151	125	134
1986	124	143	149	138	140	125	140	124	136
1987	105	137	123	137	135	137	136	126	134
Women									
1958	70	84	..	..	80	82	77	67	79
1961	72	79	..	..	77	78	76	58	76
1963	88	88	..	..	85	94	92	66	86
1965	75	81	..	..	85	89	94	63	85
1968	71	85	..	..	87	90	83	70	86
1971	83	102	..	..	102	99	115	68	100
1972	105	100	..	..	110	109	105	81	105
1973	84	106	..	..	119	106	122	91	113
1974	95	106	..	..	119	118	120	83	115
1975	87	106	..	..	115	109	110	98	111
1976	116	115	..	..	122	122	124	106	120
1977	108	117	123	125	124	111	118	107	119
1978	116	116	120	117	118	123	119	113	118
1979	118	114	117	115	116	122	129	89	116
1980	84	111	117	120	118	117	105	112	115
1981	135	109	113	113	113	112	127	112	113
1982	80	110	112	113	113	116	106	110	112
1983	108	99	108	115	112	121	115	112	112
1984	82	108	110	115	113	102	118	97	108
1985	88	94	107	113	111	118	111	115	110
1986	70	107	111	113	112	113	120	111	111
1987	91	112	99	110	105	118	117	101	108

Source: TAC

Table 5.8 Weekly consumption of cigarettes (manufactured and hand-rolled) per smoker: by socio-economic group, 1972-1988
Cigarette smokers, men and women aged 16 and over[1], Great Britain

Year	Socio-economic group						
	Professional	Employers and managers	Intermediate and junior non-manual	Skilled manual and own-account non-professional	Semi-skilled manual and personal service	Unskilled manual	All groups
Men							
1972	102	126	114	124	119	111	120
1974	107	134	118	130	120	117	125
1976	103	132	124	133	128	118	129
1978	100	128	120	131	126	120	127
1980	98	125	120	130	122	118	124
1982	108	139	109	126	118	120	121
1984	108	121	108	121	108	114	115
1986	85	130	103	118	114	110	115
1988	109	132	113	122	117	111	120
Women							
1972	75	86	81	93	85	87	87
1974	82	97	89	100	92	91	94
1976	81	101	98	107	102	96	101
1978	72	94	97	107	103	102	101
1980	86	96	95	110	103	97	102
1982	73	97	92	106	98	93	98
1984	78	93	93	101	99	96	96
1986	82	101	91	99	101	92	97
1988	90	101	88	104	102	104	99

1 Aged 15 and over in 1972

Source: GHS

Fig. 5.8   Weekly consumption of cigarettes (manufactured and hand-rolled) per smoker: by socio-economic group, 1972-1988
Cigarette smokers, men and women aged 16 and over, Great Britain. *Source*: GHS

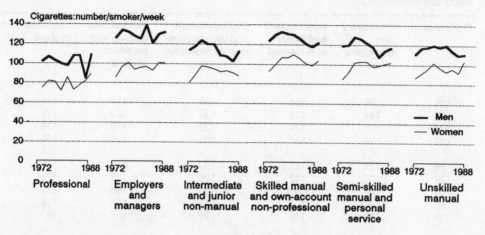

The TAC provides data on ex-smokers of any form of tobacco and on persons who have never smoked any form of tobacco, classified according to age from 1956-1987, and according to social class from 1975-1987. From 1969 onwards these data have been sales-adjusted to correspond with the sales-adjustment that was applied to the percentage of smokers.

Data on ex-smokers of cigarettes are not available from the TAC, but are published by the GHS for the period 1972-1988. The GHS provides data on ex-smokers of cigarettes, and on persons who have never smoked cigarettes (manufactured or hand-rolled), classified by age, and by socio-economic group.

TAC data are also given on the percentage of ex-smokers classified according to age, and to time since giving up smoking, and on cigarette consumption among ex-smokers immediately before stopping smoking. GHS data on percentages of ex-cigarette smokers classified according to age, and to time since giving up smoking, are presented for 1988 (unpublished data).

The TAC data indicate that the percentage of men who are ex-smokers of any form of tobacco rose from 11 per cent to 25 per cent between 1956 and 1986. Over the same period, the percentage of women who are ex-smokers rose from 7 per cent to 19 per cent. The percentages fell slightly in 1987. The GHS data indicate that in 1986 32 per cent of men and 18 per cent of women were ex-smokers of cigarettes.

The TAC data indicate that the percentage of men who have never smoked any form of tobacco rose from 14 per cent to 33 per cent between 1956 and 1987. During the same period, the percentage of women who have never smoked fluctuated between 54 per cent and 44 per cent, and stood at 48 per cent in 1987.

Similar trends are shown by the GHS data. Between 1972 and 1988 the GHS data indicate that the percentage of men who have never smoked cigarettes rose from 25 per cent to 35 per cent while the percentage of women who have never smoked cigarettes remained very close to 50 per cent.

Men and women

The TAC data indicate that between 1956 and 1987 the percentages of ex-smokers increased in all age groups, with the largest increases occurring in the older age groups. In 1987, 45 per cent of men and 26 per cent of women aged 65 years and over were ex-smokers of any form of tobacco.

GHS figures for ex-regular cigarette smokers for 1972-1988 are similar to, though slightly higher than, the TAC figures, as would be expected, since the TAC data relate to ex-smokers of any form of tobacco, rather than to ex-smokers of cigarettes.

Persons who have never smoked: by age

Men

The almost universal adoption of the smoking habit by men during the first quarter of this century is illustrated by the fact that in 1956 the percentage of men aged 50 and over who had never smoked any form of tobacco was estimated by the TAC survey to be as low as 7 per cent.

Between 1956 and 1987 the percentage of men who have never smoked any form of tobacco rose slowly at first, and, in most age groups, more steeply from about 1972 onwards, so that by 1987 the percentages of men aged 25 years and over who had never smoked any form of tobacco had more than doubled, compared with the 1956 figures. In 1987, of men aged 16-24, 25-34, 35-49, and 50 years and over, 51, 43, 30, and approximately 20 per cent, respectively, had never smoked any form of tobacco.

GHS data for 1972-1988 report that the largest increase in men who have never smoked cigarettes occurred in the 20-34 age range. Between 1972 and 1988 the percentage who had never smoked cigarettes rose from 36 to 53 per cent among men aged 20-24, and from 27 to 46 per cent among men aged 25-34.

Women

In 1956 TAC estimated that about 40 per cent of women aged 25-49 years, and about 60 per cent of women of other ages, had never smoked. Between 1956 and 1971 the percentage of women aged 16-24 years who have never smoked fell from about 60 per cent to 43 per cent, as more young women took up smoking. The percentage of women aged 50-59 years who have never smoked also fell, from 56 to 39 per cent. During this period the percentage of women aged 25-49 years and 60 years and over who had never smoked remained stable at around 40 per cent and 66 per cent respectively.

From about 1972 both TAC and GHS data show that the percentage of women who have never smoked increased among women aged under 50 years, and decreased among women aged 60 years and over. TAC data for 1987 indicate that 51 per cent of women aged 16-24 years, and 53 per cent of women aged 65 years and over, had never smoked; for women aged 25-49 years and 50-64 years, the figures were 47 and 44 per cent respectively.

Ex-smokers: by social class

GHS data are available on ex-smokers of cigarettes classified according to socio-economic group for the years 1972-1988. The TAC data on ex-smokers of any form of tobacco are available for grouped social classes (I+II, IIINM, IIIM, IV+V+VI) for the years 1975-1987. The GHS and TAC data display similar trends.

Men

GHS data indicate that, in 1972, the proportion of men who were ex-smokers of cigarettes ranged from 17 per cent among unskilled manual workers to 30 per cent among employers and managers. Between 1972 and 1988 small increases in the percentage of ex-smokers occurred in all socio-economic groups, so that by 1988, the percentage of ex-smokers of cigarettes ranged from 24 per cent among manual workers to 39 per cent among employers and managers.

Women

GHS data indicate that in 1972 the proportion of women who were ex-smokers of cigarettes ranged from 8 per cent among unskilled manual workers to 14 per cent among professional women. Between 1972 and 1988 small increases in the percentage of ex-smokers occurred in all social-economic groups, so that by 1988 the percentage of ex-smokers ranged from 16 per cent among intermediate and junior non-manual workers to 23 per cent among professionals, and employers and managers.

Persons who have never smoked: by social class

Similar GHS and TAC data are available on persons who have never smoked, classified by social class, as data on ex-smokers, classified by social class. Again both sources yield similar results.

Men

GHS data indicate that in 1972 the proportion of men who have never smoked cigarettes ranged from 19 per cent among unskilled manual workers to 39 per cent among professional men. Between 1972 and 1988 increases in the percentage who have never smoked occurred among men of all socio-economic groups. In 1988, 49 per cent of professional men, compared with about 30 per cent of skilled and semi-skilled manual workers, had never smoked cigarettes.

Women

GHS data indicate that between 1972 and 1988 the proportion of professional women who have never smoked cigarettes rose from 53 to 60 per cent; the proportion of unskilled manual women who have never smoked declined from 51 to 43 per cent. During the same period there was little change in the percentages of women from other socio-economic groups who have never smoked.

Ex-smokers: by age at time of survey

TAC data show that the percentage of male ex-smokers of any tobacco who were aged 30-59 years at the time of the survey fell from 63 to 52 per cent between 1961 and 1975, while for female ex-smokers of any tobacco those who were aged 35-49 years fell from 33 to 20 per cent. Corresponding rises in the percentage of ex-smokers of other ages occurred, particularly in men and women aged 60 and over.

Ex-smokers: by time since giving up

TAC data indicate that in 1987 about 8 per cent of men and women ex-smokers of any form of tobacco had given up less than a year ago, about 27 per cent had given up 1-5 years ago, and about 19 per cent had given up 6-10 years ago; over 45 per cent of male and female ex-smokers had given up smoking (any tobacco) 11 or more years ago. GHS data in 1988 show similar results.

Cigarette consumption of ex-smokers of manufactured cigarettes before giving up smoking

Information on the mean weekly consumption of manufactured cigarettes by ex-smokers are available only for 1965-1975. Men who were formerly manufactured cigarette smokers had had higher mean weekly consumption immediately before giving up than continuing manufactured cigarette smokers, while for women the reverse was generally true. Among men, the older ex-smokers smoked more than the younger ex-smokers immediately before giving up; male ex-smokers aged 60 years and over reported a particularly high consumption of manufactured cigarettes, compared with continuing smokers in the same age group.

Table 6.1.1 Percentage of men who are ex-smokers of any form of tobacco: by age, 1956-1987
Men aged 16 and over, Great Britain: sales-adjusted 1969-1987

Year	16-19	20-24	25-29	30-34	35-49	50-59	60+	16+
1956	3	6	9	12	11	14	14	11
1958	3	6	11	13	14	15	21	13
1961	3	5	10	15	14	18	21	14
1963	3	5	11	12	16	18	25	15
1965	4	9	11	11	16	19	23	15
1968	4	7	10	10	14	18	24	15
1971	5	8	14	13	17	23	26	17
1972	4	7	10	12	14	19	25	15
1973	5	6	10	13	16	21	25	16
1974	4	5	10	13	15	20	28	16
1975	5	9	15	17	19	21	26	18

Year		16-24	25-34	35-49	50-64	65+	16+
1975		7	16	19	22	27	18
1976		7	13	18	24	37	19
1977		5	14	19	27	32	19
1978		7	15	20	25	36	20
1979		7	12	19	27	32	19
1980		7	13	19	25	37	20
1981		7	13	21	31	39	22
1982		8	16	22	33	44	24
1983		8	15	23	31	46	24
1984		7	15	22	29	46	23
1985		7	14	21	34	43	23
1986		7	15	21	34	49	25
1987		6	12	21	36	45	23

Source: TAC

Table 6.1.2 Percentage of women who are ex-smokers of any form of tobacco (except pipe tobacco): by age, 1956-1987
Women aged 16 and over, Great Britain: sales-adjusted 1969-1987

Year	16-19	20-24	25-29	30-34	35-49	50-59	60+	16+
1956	1	3	7	9	9	7	5	7
1958	1	4	6	8	9	7	6	7
1961	1	3	7	6	7	8	8	7
1963	3	5	7	9	9	6	8	8
1965	2	6	5	6	9	9	9	8
1968	4	7	8	9	10	12	10	9
1971	5	9	10	10	12	14	12	11
1972	4	7	11	10	10	13	12	11
1973	6	7	9	9	9	17	11	11
1974	4	8	10	12	9	15	15	12
1975	6	7	14	14	11	15	14	13

Table 6.1.2 (*continued*) Percentage of women who are ex-smokers of any form of tobacco (except pipe tobacco): by age, 1956-1987
Women aged 16 and over, Great Britain: sales-adjusted 1969-1987

Year	16-24	25-34	35-49	50-64	65+	16+
1975	6	14	11	15	14	13
1976	6	11	12	18	18	14
1977	8	13	13	18	16	14
1978	7	12	12	19	20	14
1979	7	11	14	18	19	15
1980	5	12	14	17	21	14
1981	8	15	16	21	22	17
1982	8	15	16	22	20	17
1983	7	15	18	23	25	18
1984	8	14	16	20	26	17
1985	7	12	17	21	25	17
1986	7	14	19	24	26	19
1987	7	13	18	21	26	18

Source: TAC

Table 6.2.1 Percentage of men who have never smoked any form of tobacco: by age, 1956-1987
Men aged 16 and over, Great Britain: sales-adjusted 1969-1987

Year	16-19	20-24	25-29	30-34	35-49	50-59	60+	16+
1956	42	27	17	13	10	7	7	14
1958	41	28	22	17	9	8	7	15
1961	35	24	21	17	9	8	8	14
1963	39	26	20	20	13	11	11	17
1965	44	23	24	21	14	10	8	17
1968	38	28	24	22	14	9	8	17
1971	40	30	20	19	16	12	10	18
1972	42	28	25	22	14	14	12	19
1973	42	26	26	20	16	10	9	18
1974	47	34	24	21	17	11	11	20
1975	43	29	27	23	19	10	12	20

Year	16-24	25-34	35-49	50-64	65+	16+
1975	36	25	19	11	13	20
1976	41	27	20	12	11	22
1977	43	28	20	13	12	23
1978	45	31	22	16	14	25
1979	43	30	23	18	17	26
1980	45	30	23	15	14	25
1981	49	34	25	16	16	28
1982	46	34	26	15	13	27
1983	47	37	27	20	11	29
1984	53	34	27	19	15	30
1985	47	37	28	21	18	30
1986	50	42	28	22	18	32
1987	51	43	30	22	19	33

Source: TAC

SECTION 6   Ex-smokers and persons who have never smoked

Fig. 6.1 Percentages of men and women who are ex-smokers of any form of tobacco: by age, 1956-1987
Men and women aged 16 and over, Great Britain. *Source*: TAC
The consumption for men and women aged 16-24 and 25-34 that has been plotted for the years 1956-1974 is
equal to the mean of the consumption for men and women aged 16-19 and 20-24, and 25-29 and 30-34 respectively
during those years (see Tables 6.1.1/2)
Where two age groups are given, the first is for years up to and including 1975, and the second for 1976 onwards

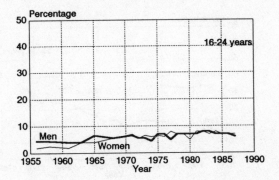

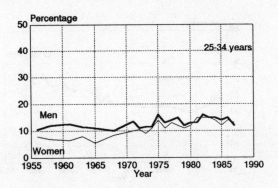

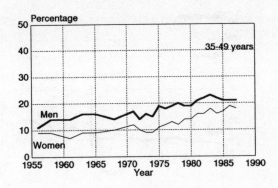

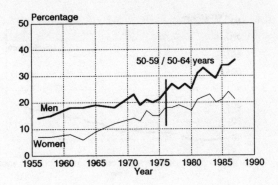

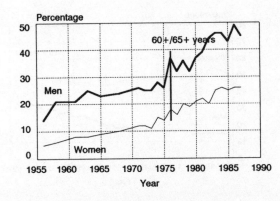

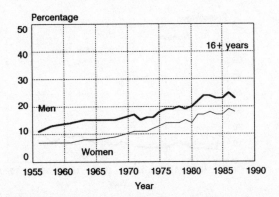

Fig. 6.2 Percentages of men and women who have never smoked any form of tobacco: by age, 1956-1987
Men and women aged 16 and over, Great Britain. *Source*: TAC
The consumption for men and women aged 16-24 and 25-34 that has been plotted for the years 1956-1974 is
equal to the mean of the consumption for men and women aged 16-19 and 20-24, and 25-29 and 30-34 respectively
during those years (see Tables 6.2.1/2)
Where two age groups are given, the first is for years up to and including 1975, and the second for 1976 onwards

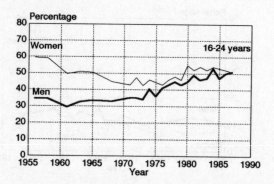

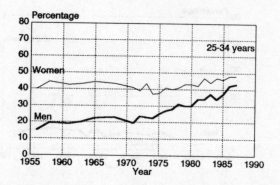

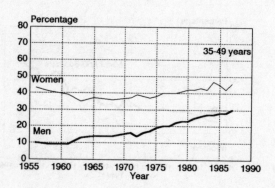

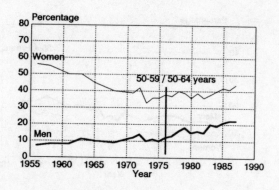

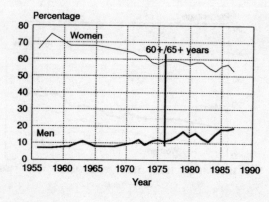

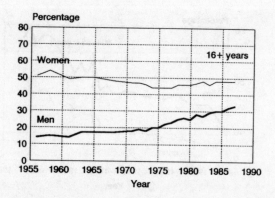

SECTION 6   Ex-smokers and persons who have never smoked

Table 6.2.2 Percentage of women who have never smoked any form of tobacco (except pipe tobacco): by age, 1956-1987
Women aged 16 and over, Great Britain: sales-adjusted 1969-1987

Year	16-19	20-24	25-29	30-34	35-49	50-59	60+	16+
1956	66	53	46	34	43	56	66	51
1958	67	51	48	41	41	55	75	54
1961	54	45	42	43	39	50	68	49
1963	57	45	41	45	35	50	68	50
1965	58	43	44	45	37	45	68	50
1968	50	40	43	44	36	40	66	48
1971	46	40	39	43	37	39	64	47
1972	50	45	38	40	39	42	62	47
1973	45	40	45	42	38	33	62	46
1974	50	42	38	36	37	36	58	44
1975	48	41	36	39	38	36	57	44

Year		16-24	25-34	35-49	50-64	65+	16+
1975		44	37	38	38	62	44
1976		43	41	40	38	59	44
1977		46	40	40	37	59	44
1978		48	41	40	40	59	46
1979		46	43	41	39	58	46
1980		55	43	42	36	57	46
1981		52	42	42	39	58	47
1982		54	47	43	36	58	48
1983		52	44	42	38	55	46
1984		54	47	47	40	53	48
1985		53	46	45	42	56	48
1986		52	48	42	41	57	48
1987		51	48	46	44	53	48

Source: TAC

Table 6.3 Percentages of men and women who are ex-smokers of cigarettes (manufactured and hand-rolled): by age, 1972-1988
Men and women aged 16 and over[1], Great Britain

Year	16-19	20-24	25-34	35-49	50-59	60+	16+
Men							
1972	4	9	17	23	30	35	23
1974	3	9	18	21	30	37	23
1976	5	11	20	27	33	43	27
1978	4	9	18	26	35	43	27
1980	5	8	18	27	35	45	28
1982	4	9	20	32	38	47	30
1984	5	8	20	31	37	48	30
1986	5	11	20	33	38	52	32
1988	4	10	17	31	41	53	32

Table 6.3 (*continued*) Percentages of men and women who are ex-smokers of cigarettes (manufactured and hand-rolled): by age, 1972-1988
Men and women aged 16 and over[1], Great Britain

Year	16-19	20-24	25-34	35-49	50-59	60+	16+
Women							
1972	3	8	10	10	11	9	9
1974	4	9	12	10	13	11	11
1976	5	10	13	12	15	14	12
1978	5	8	14	13	18	16	14
1980	4	9	13	13	17	19	14
1982	6	9	15	15	19	20	16
1984	6	9	16	17	18	22	17
1986	7	9	16	20	18	23	18
1988	5	8	16	21	19	25	19

1 Aged 15 and over in 1972

Source: GHS

Table 6.4 Percentages of men and women who have never smoked cigarettes (manufactured and hand-rolled): by age, 1972-1988
Men and women aged 16 and over[1], Great Britain

Year	16-19	20-24	25-34	35-49	50-59	60+	16+
Men							
1972	58	36	27	22	16	18	25
1974	56	38	26	24	16	18	25
1976	56	42	32	23	18	18	27
1978	61	46	33	26	17	18	29
1980	62	48	34	27	18	19	30
1982	65	50	39	28	20	20	32
1984	66	52	39	30	24	22	34
1986	65	47	43	30	26	19	34
1988	69	53	46	32	26	22	35
Women							
1972	61	44	41	41	41	66	50
1974	58	47	42	41	38	63	49
1976	61	45	45	43	39	62	50
1978	62	49	44	44	39	60	49
1980	63	51	43	44	39	57	49
1982	64	51	48	47	41	57	51
1984	62	55	48	47	43	55	51
1986	62	54	48	46	47	55	51
1988	67	55	50	44	48	53	51

1 Aged 15 and over in 1972

Source: GHS

Fig. 6.3 Percentages of men and women who (i) smoke, (ii) are ex-smokers, or (iii) have never smoked cigarettes (manufactured and hand-rolled): by age, 1972 and 1988
Men and women aged 16 and over (aged 15 and over in 1972), Great Britain. *Source*: GHS

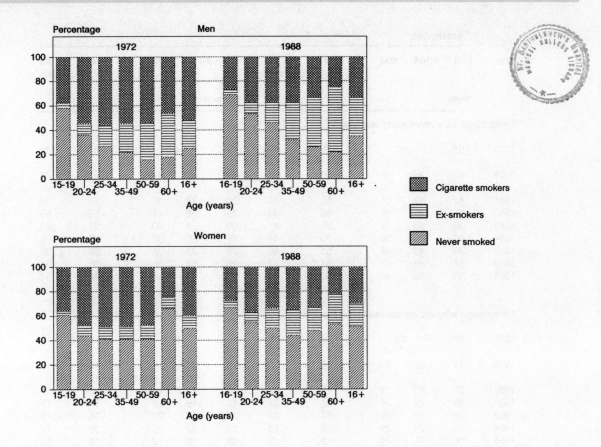

Fig. 6.4 Percentages of men and women who (i) smoke, (ii) are ex-smokers, or (iii) have never smoked any form of tobacco (except pipe tobacco, for women): by social class, 1987
Men and women aged 16 and over, Great Britain. *Source*: TAC

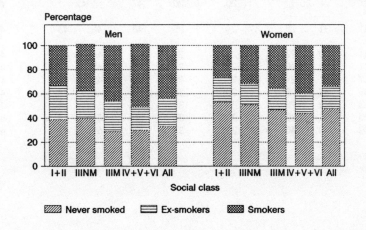

Table 6.5 Percentages of men and women who (i) smoke, (ii) are ex-smokers, or (iii) have never smoked any form of tobacco (except pipe tobacco, for women): by social class, 1975-1987
Men and women aged 16 and over, Great Britain: sales-adjusted

Year	| Men					| Women				
Social class	I+II	IIINM	IIIM	IV+V+VI	All classes	I+II	IIINM	IIIM	IV+V+VI	All classes
Percentage who smoke any tobacco										
1975	57	62 (IIINM–IIIM)		65	62	37	46 (IIINM–IIIM)		43	43
1978	45	46	58	60	55	34	42	43	40	40
1981	42	49	51	56	50	30	38	40	39	37
1982	45	45	50	53	49	28	36	41	38	36
1983	39	42	49	55	47	29	34	40	38	36
1984	40	39	50	53	47	27	35	38	37	35
1985	39	43	48	51	46	28	33	38	38	35
1986	37	35	43	51	43	26	31	36	38	34
1987	33	38	46	52	44	26	32	36	40	34
Percentage who are ex-smokers (any tobacco)										
1975	22	18 (IIINM–IIIM)		15	18	16	12 (IIINM–IIIM)		11	13
1978	24	23	20	16	20	18	14	14	12	14
1981	27	22	23	17	22	20	14	18	15	17
1982	29	22	24	20	24	19	16	16	15	17
1983	29	27	25	17	24	22	17	20	15	18
1984	25	26	24	18	23	19	17	18	16	17
1985	28	24	24	19	23	18	16	19	16	17
1986	28	28	27	20	25	21	18	20	16	19
1987	28	23	25	19	23	21	17	17	16	18
Percentage who have never smoked (any tobacco)										
1975	21	20 (IIINM–IIIM)		20	20	47	42 (IIINM–IIIM)		47	44
1978	31	31	22	24	25	48	45	43	48	46
1981	31	30	27	27	28	50	49	43	46	47
1982	27	33	26	27	27	53	48	43	47	48
1983	32	31	27	28	29	49	49	40	47	46
1984	35	35	26	29	30	54	48	44	47	48
1985	33	33	28	31	30	54	51	44	46	48
1986	35	37	30	30	32	53	51	44	46	48
1987	39	29	40	30	33	53	51	47	44	48

Source: TAC

Fig. 6.5 Percentages of men and women who are ex-smokers of cigarettes (manufactured and hand-rolled): by socio-economic group, 1972-1988
Men and women aged 16 and over, Great Britain. *Source*: GHS

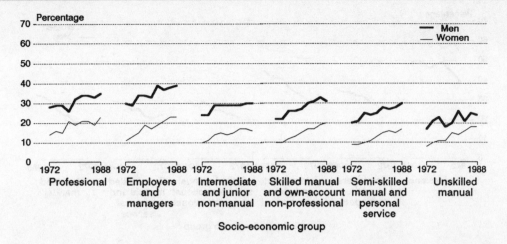

Table 6.6 Percentages of men and women who are ex-smokers of cigarettes (manufactured and hand-rolled): by socio-economic group, 1972-1988
Men and women aged 16 and over[1], Great Britain

| Year | Socio-economic group | | | | | | |
	Professional	Employers and managers	Intermediate and junior non-manual	Skilled and own-account non-professional	Semi-skilled manual and personal service	Unskilled manual	All groups
Men							
1972	28	30	24	22	20	17	23
1974	29	29	24	22	21	21	23
1976	29	34	29	26	25	23	27
1978	26	34	29	26	24	18	27
1980	32	33	29	27	25	20	28
1982	34	39	29	30	28	26	30
1984	34	37	29	31	27	21	30
1986	33	38	30	33	28	25	32
1988	35	39	30	31	30	24	32
Women							
1972	14	11	10	10	9	8	10
1974	16	13	11	10	9	10	11
1976	15	15	14	12	10	11	12
1978	21	19	15	13	11	11	14
1980	19	17	14	15	13	15	14
1982	21	19	15	17	15	14	16
1984	21	21	17	17	16	16	17
1986	19	23	17	19	15	18	18
1988	23	23	16	20	17	18	19

1 Aged 15 and over in 1972

Source: GHS

Fig. 6.6 Percentages of men and women who have never smoked cigarettes (manufactured and hand-rolled): by socio-economic group, 1972-1988
Men and women aged 16 and over, Great Britain. *Source*: GHS

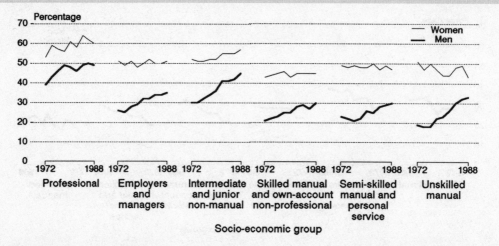

Table 6.7 Percentages of men and women who have never smoked cigarettes (manufactured and hand-rolled): by socio-economic group, 1972-1988
Men and women aged 16 and over[1], Great Britain

| Year | Socio-economic group | | | | | | |
	Professional	Employers and managers	Intermediate and junior non-manual	Skilled manual and own-account non-professional	Semi-skilled manual and personal service	Unskilled manual	All groups
Men							
1972	39	26	30	21	23	19	25
1974	43	25	30	22	22	18	25
1976	46	28	32	23	21	18	27
1978	49	29	34	25	22	22	29
1980	48	32	36	25	26	23	30
1982	46	32	41	28	25	26	32
1984	49	34	41	29	28	30	34
1986	50	34	42	27	29	32	34
1988	49	35	45	30	30	33	35
Women							
1972	53	51	52	43	49	51	50
1974	59	49	51	44	48	47	49
1976	57	51	51	45	49	50	50
1978	56	48	52	46	48	47	49
1980	61	50	52	43	48	44	49
1982	58	52	55	45	50	44	51
1984	64	50	55	45	47	48	51
1986	62	50	55	45	49	49	51
1988	60	51	57	45	47	43	51

1 Aged 15 and over in 1972

Source: GHS

Table 6.8 Percentages of ex-smokers: by age, 1961-1975
Ex-smokers of any form of tobacco (except pipe tobacco, for women),
men and women aged 16 and over, Great Britain

Age	1961	1965	1968	1971	1972	1973	1974	1975
Men								
16-19	2	2	2	2	2	2	2	2
20-24	3	5	5	5	5	4	3	5
25-29	6	6	6	7	7	7	6	9
30-34	11	7	6	6	7	7	7	8
35-49	30	27	25	25	23	25	23	25
50-59	22	21	21	22	20	21	19	19
60+	27	31	35	32	36	34	40	32
All ages	100	100	100	100	100	100	100	100
Women								
16-19	1	2	3	3	3	4	2	4
20-24	4	6	8	8	6	6	6	5
25-29	8	5	7	8	10	9	9	10
30-34	8	6	7	6	7	6	8	9
35-49	33	30	25	24	21	19	18	20
50-59	17	20	20	20	20	25	20	19
60+	29	31	30	30	33	31	38	34
All ages	100	100	100	100	100	100	100	100

Source: TAC

Table 6.9 Percentages of ex-smokers: by time since giving up, 1975-1987
Ex-smokers of any form of tobacco (except pipe tobacco, for women),
men and women aged 16 and over, Great Britain

	Number of years since giving up					All ex-smokers
	< 1	1-5	6-10	11-20	21+	
Men						
1975	13	32	17	17	21	100
1976	11	35	16	18	20	100
1977	11	34	17	20	19	100
1978	7	30	22	17	24	100
1979	6	28	21	19	26	100
1980	9	28	20	22	22	100
1981	12	27	16	21	25	100
1982	9	30	18	21	22	100
1983	8	30	16	20	25	100
1984	9	28	16	24	23	100
1985	7	28	19	20	27	100
1986	9	24	20	23	25	100
1987	7	25	16	26	27	100

Table 6.9 (*continued*) Percentages of ex-smokers: by time since giving up, 1975-1987
Ex-smokers of any form of tobacco (except pipe tobacco, for women),
men and women aged 16 and over, Great Britain

	Number of years since giving up					All ex-smokers
	< 1	1-5	6-10	11-20	21+	
Women						
1975	17	38	16	10	19	100
1976	13	36	20	13	19	100
1977	13	39	19	16	13	100
1978	8	39	19	14	20	100
1979	11	38	18	15	19	100
1980	10	32	21	19	19	100
1981	13	34	18	16	19	100
1982	10	32	21	20	17	100
1983	8	33	21	19	20	100
1984	12	32	17	21	18	100
1985	10	31	16	21	21	100
1986	11	31	16	22	20	100
1987	8	29	22	21	20	100

Source: TAC

Table 6.10 Percentages of ex-cigarette smokers: by age, and by time since giving up, 1988
Ex-regular cigarette smokers, men and women aged 16 and over, Great Britain

	Time since giving up					
	<6 months	6-12 months	1-2 years	2-5 years	5-10 years	>10 years
Men						
16-19[1]	33	33	0	22	11	0
20-24	22	14	20	27	17	0
25-34	8	7	12	27	29	16
35-49	4	3	4	17	22	51
50-59	3	2	3	11	16	65
60+	1	1	2	9	15	72
All ages	4	3	4	14	18	58
Women						
16-19[1]	45	15	10	30	0	0
20-24	13	15	25	27	18	2
25-34	12	7	9	24	31	17
35-49	4	3	5	13	22	53
50-59	4	4	6	13	18	54
60+	3	2	3	12	17	63
All ages	6	4	6	15	20	49

1 The figures shown for this age group are based on a very small number of respondents

Source: GHS (data not previously published)

SECTION 6   Ex-smokers and persons who have never smoked

Table 6.11 Weekly consumption (number) of manufactured cigarettes among ex-smokers immediately before stopping smoking: by age, 1965-1975
Ex-smokers of manufactured cigarettes, men and women aged 16 and over, Great Britain

Age	1965	1968	1971	1972	1973	1974	1975
Men							
16-19	68	70	94	101	109	100	101
20-24	116	114	127	120	147	138	147
25-29	154	124	146	145	156	139	149
30-34	159	128	164	159	162	151	159
35-49	174	141	163	165	172	160	170
50-59	170	157	176	168	180	173	171
60+	167	158	171	161	165	153	166
16+	164	145	164	159	168	156	164
Weekly consumption of current smokers	129	128	142	148	156	149	152
Women							
16-19	68	48	70	72	84	71	59
20-24	92	70	83	82	100	102	106
25-29	92	74	94	92	97	91	96
30-34	93	66	82	91	95	91	102
35-49	88	78	96	92	110	100	107
50-59	91	90	90	85	106	111	98
60+	77	91	76	76	93	85	93
16+	86	83	86	84	100	95	97
Weekly consumption of current smokers	85	87	100	105	113	115	111

Source: TAC

Table 6.12 Distribution of number of manufactured cigarettes smoked by ex-smokers immediately before stopping smoking, and by current smokers, 1965-1975
Ex- and current manufactured cigarette smokers, men and women aged 16 and over, Great Britain

Manufactured cigarettes/day	1965	1968	1971	1972	1973	1974	1975
Men	**Percentage of ex-cigarette smokers**						
< 5	4	6	5	5	3	4	4
5-10	25	28	22	22	23	23	20
11-20	39	39	42	40	43	41	40
21-29	5	5	4	7	4	6	6
30+	27	22	28	26	27	26	30
	Percentage of current cigarette smokers						
< 5	9	9	8	8	8	8	9
5-10	23	18	18	16	15	15	14
11-20	39	41	39	39	37	36	36
21-29	14	15	13	13	15	15	13
30+	16	17	22	23	26	25	28
Women	**Percentage of ex-cigarette smokers**						
< 5	20	15	19	21	18	16	15
5-10	47	54	48	47	40	43	39
11-20	23	22	24	23	29	26	32
21-29	} 10	} 9	2	4	4	4	4
30+			8	6	10	11	9
	Percentage of current cigarette smokers						
< 5	21	18	16	15	14	13	14
5-10	35	34	28	28	23	21	22
11-20	34	37	38	40	42	43	42
21-29	} 10	} 11	8	9	11	11	9
30+			8	8	10	12	12

Source: TAC

SECTION 6   Ex-smokers and persons who have never smoked

Age at starting to smoke

7

Data on age at starting to smoke are available from surveys commissioned by the TAC between 1965 and 1987. Data are available for men and women for all ages combined; they are also stratified according to age at the time of the survey. In the tabulations the data relate to all persons who have ever smoked any form of tobacco, and therefore include ex-smokers as well as current smokers at the time of the survey.

GHS data on age at starting to smoke, stratified according to age at the time of the survey, is presented for 1988 (unpublished data).

In surveys of smoking among children, the definition of smoking used for children is not usually the same as that used for adults. For example, for an adult, a current smoker is often defined as a person smoking one cigarette or more per day, while for a child it is usually taken to be smoking one cigarette or more per week. Data displayed in the tables in this section were estimated from adults, and so the adult definition of smoking was used even though often the information at the time of starting to smoke relates to habits in childhood.

Men

Between 1965 and 1987 the proportion of adult men who started to smoke before the age of 16 years has remained at around 30 per cent. Between 1965 and 1987 the proportion of men who started to smoke between the ages of 16 and 19 years decreased from 37 to 24 per cent, between 20-24 years it decreased from 10 to 7 per cent, while the proportion who started to smoke at age 25 years and over remained approximately the same at about 3 per cent.

Examination of the data stratified according to age at the time of the survey reveals that much of the decline in the proportion of men taking up smoking has occurred among those in the younger age groups, particularly those aged under 35 years at the time of the survey.

The decline in the proportion of men taking up smoking, especially evident among young adults, has meant that the proportion of young men who have never smoked has increased; for example, between 1965 and 1987, the proportion of men aged 20-24 years who had never smoked for as long as one year increased nearly twofold from 26 to 47 per cent.

Women

The proportion of adult women who started to smoke before the age of 16 years rose from 6 to 14 per cent between 1965 and 1987. There was little change in the proportion of women who started to smoke at 16 years and over; in 1987 the proportion of women who started to smoke at 16-19 years, 20-24 years, and 25 years and over, were respectively, 21, 7, and 6 per cent.

The data, when classified according to age at the time of the survey, show that young women who took up smoking did so at an earlier age when asked in 1987 than in 1965. Over this period, the percentage of women aged 20-24 years who started to smoke under the age of 16 years rose from 9 to 21 per cent, while the proportion who started to smoke at ages 16-19 years declined from 37 to 23 per cent. Among women aged 25 and over, there were similar but smaller increases between 1965 and 1987 in the percentage who started to smoke under the age of 16 years.

In contrast to men, a higher percentage of older women surveyed started to smoke later in life than did younger women. For example, in 1987 among women aged 65 and over, 13 per cent started to smoke at the age of 25 years or more, while among women aged 35-49 years only 3 per cent did so. GHS data in 1988 also show that a higher percentage of older women started to smoke later in life than did younger women.

Table 7.1 Percentages of men and women starting to smoke (any tobacco) at different ages, 1965-1987
Men and women aged 16 and over, Great Britain

Recalled age at starting to smoke	Year of survey												
	1965	1968	1971	1973	1975	1978	1981	1982	1983	1984	1985	1986	1987
Men													
13 and less	} 28	} 30	} 30	} 30	9	9	10	9	10	9	10	10	10
14-15					20	19	18	18	18	19	19	17	17
16-17	23	22	21	21	20	18	18	18	17	16	16	16	15
18-19	14	14	12	13	12	11	10	10	10	9	10	9	9
20-24	10	10	10	10	8	8	7	8	8	7	7	6	7
25-29	2	2	2	2	2	2	2	2	1	2	2	2	2
30+	1	2	1	2	1	1	1	1	1	1	1	1	1
Don't know	2	3	3	2	4	5	5	5	4	6	5	5	6
Never smoked for as long as a year	19	19	21	20	22	27	30	29	31	31	31	34	34
	100	100	100	100	100	100	100	100	100	100	100	100	100
Women													
13 and less	} 6	} 8	} 10	} 11	3	3	3	3	3	3	4	3	4
14-15					9	9	9	10	11	10	11	10	10
16-17	10	12	12	12	12	12	13	13	12	13	13	13	13
18-19	9	10	9	9	9	9	9	9	10	7	8	9	8
20-24	9	8	9	9	9	9	8	8	7	7	7	7	7
25-29	3	3	3	3	3	2	2	3	3	3	2	2	2
30+	8	8	7	6	7	5	5	4	4	5	4	4	4
Don't know	1	1	2	1	2	3	3	2	2	3	2	2	2
Never smoked for as long as a year	54	51	50	48	47	49	48	49	48	50	49	50	50
	100	100	100	100	100	100	100	100	100	100	100	100	100

Source: TAC

Fig. 7.1 Percentages of men and women starting to smoke (any tobacco) at different ages, 1987
Men and women aged 16 and over, Great Britain. *Source*: TAC

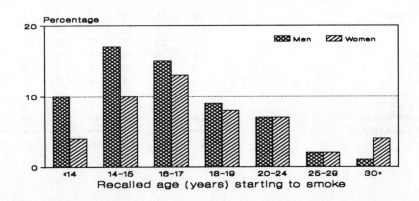

Table 7.2.1 Percentage of men starting to smoke (any tobacco) at different ages: by age at time of survey, 1965-1987
Men aged 16 and over, Great Britain

Age at time of survey	Recalled age at starting to smoke	Year of survey												
		1965	1968	1971	1973	1975	1978	1981	1982	1983	1984	1985	1986	1987
16-19	13 and less	} 32	} 38	} 37	} 33	14	11	12	14	14	12	15	13	12
	14-15					22	20	16	17	16	16	18	19	18
	16-17	15	14	14	14	12	10	9	10	10	10	10	10	8
	18-19	1	2	1	1	1	1	0	1	0	1	1	1	1
	Don't know	0	1	0	0	2	1	2	2	1	3	2	2	1
	Never smoked for as long as a year	52	45	47	51	51	58	61	56	58	59	55	57	61
		100	100	100	100	100	100	100	100	100	100	100	100	100
20-24	13 and less	} 29	} 29	} 31	} 34	9	10	9	10	12	9	11	11	10
	14-15					21	19	15	18	15	14	19	16	17
	16-17	32	27	21	25	25	19	19	17	17	14	16	16	17
	18-19	10	8	11	11	7	6	5	6	6	5	6	5	6
	20-24	2	3	2	2	2	2	2	2	2	2	2	2	1
	Don't know	1	1	2	0	2	1	3	2	2	4	1	2	3
	Never smoked for as long as a year	26	31	34	28	33	42	47	45	46	52	46	50	47
		100	100	100	100	100	100	100	100	100	100	100	100	100
25-34	13 and less	} 23	} 24	} 29	} 29	} 28	..	..	..	..	..	..	..	..
	14-15													
	16-17	24	23	24	23	23	..	..	..	..	..	..	..	..
	18-19	17	16	13	13	12	..	..	..	..	..	..	..	..
	20-24	9	10	8	7	7	..	..	..	..	..	..	..	..
	25-29	2	1	1	1	1	..	..	..	..	..	..	..	..
	30-34	0	0	0	0	0	..	..	..	..	..	..	..	..
	Don't know	1	1	2	1	3	..	..	..	..	..	..	..	..
	Never smoked for as long as a year	25	24	22	25	27	..	..	..	..	..	..	..	..
		100	100	100	100	100								
25-29	13 and less	..	..	..	..	10	10	8	7	7	9	10	8	9
	14-15	..	..	..	..	21	17	19	17	16	21	18	13	16
	16-17	..	..	..	..	23	20	21	17	19	17	17	16	15
	18-19	..	..	..	..	9	9	7	11	9	7	7	9	6
	20-24	..	..	..	..	5	4	5	4	4	3	4	3	5
	25-29	..	..	..	..	1	1	1	0	1	1	1	0	1
	Don't know	..	..	..	..	2	3	5	2	3	3	3	3	3
	Never smoked for as long as a year	..	..	..	..	29	35	34	41	42	39	40	48	46
						100	100	100	100	100	100	100	100	100

Table 7.2.1 (*continued*) Percentage of men starting to smoke (any tobacco) at different ages: by age at time of survey, 1965-1987
Men aged 16 and over, Great Britain

Age at time of survey	Recalled age at starting to smoke	Year of survey												
		1965	1968	1971	1973	1975	1978	1981	1982	1983	1984	1985	1986	1987
30-34	13 and less	..	..	..	..	..	..	9	9	7	8	9	8	12
	14-15	..	..	..	..	..	..	17	16	19	24	16	16	14
	16-17	..	..	..	..	..	..	19	22	17	18	18	18	13
	18-19	..	..	..	..	..	..	8	9	11	11	11	8	9
	20-24	..	..	..	..	..	..	6	6	6	4	6	5	4
	25-29	..	..	..	..	..	..	2	2	2	1	2	1	2
	30+	..	..	..	..	..	..	0	0	1	0	0	0	0
	Don't know	..	..	..	..	..	..	4	5	3	4	3	5	5
	Never smoked for as long as a year	..	..	..	..	..	..	36	30	36	30	35	39	42
								100	100	100	100	100	100	100
35-59 (1965-75) **35-49** (1981+)	13 and less	} 27	} 28	} 27	} 27	} 28	..	9	7	9	7	8	7	9
	14-15						..	17	18	17	18	18	17	16
	16-17	23	22	20	21	20	..	22	20	18	16	17	17	18
	18-19	15	17	15	18	16	..	13	11	11	10	11	11	10
	20-24	13	12	14	14	11	..	7	8	10	10	8	8	8
	25-29	3	3	3	3	2	..	1	2	2	2	2	2	2
	30+	2	2	2	1	0	..	1	1	1	1	1	2	1
	Don't know	2	2	3	1	4	..	4	6	4	8	6	8	6
	Never smoked for as long as a year	14	13	17	15	16	..	27	28	29	28	28	29	31
		100	100	100	100	100		100	100	100	100	100	100	100
50-64	13 and less	..	..	..	..	..	..	12	10	11	10	11	10	10
	14-15	..	..	..	..	..	..	22	19	20	19	19	22	18
	16-17	..	..	..	..	..	..	15	19	17	16	15	15	15
	18-19	..	..	..	..	..	..	13	13	14	14	13	13	13
	20-24	..	..	..	..	..	..	11	13	9	11	9	8	9
	25-29	..	..	..	..	..	..	3	2	1	2	1	2	3
	30+	..	..	..	..	..	..	1	2	2	1	2	1	2
	Don't know	..	..	..	..	..	..	7	7	6	8	8	6	8
	Never smoked for as long as a year	..	..	..	..	..	..	16	16	21	19	21	22	22
								100	100	100	100	100	100	100
60+ (1965-75) **65+** (1981+)	13 and less	} 31	} 34	} 33	} 33	} 31	..	10	9	11	10	11	11	10
	14-15						..	18	20	19	19	20	17	19
	16-17	22	22	24	22	20	..	16	19	20	18	14	19	15
	18-19	13	11	11	11	12	..	12	12	13	9	10	10	11
	20-24	12	12	11	13	10	..	12	12	13	11	13	11	12
	25-29	3	3	2	3	3	..	3	4	3	3	5	4	2
	30+	3	3	2	4	3	..	2	3	2	4	2	3	1
	Don't know	5	6	6	4	7	..	10	9	8	9	7	8	11
	Never smoked for as long as a year	10	9	11	10	12	..	17	13	12	16	18	18	20
		100	100	100	100	100		100	100	100	100	100	100	100

Source: TAC

Age at time of survey	Recalled age at starting to smoke	Year of survey												
		1965	1968	1971	1973	1975	1978	1981	1982	1983	1984	1985	1986	1987
16-19	13 and less	} 14	} 23	} 26	} 29	9	7	9	8	8	10	10	10	11
	14-15					19	16	15	13	18	18	19	17	19
	16-17	15	16	18	15	14	12	13	11	12	8	12	10	12
	18-19	3	2	2	1	1	2	1	1	1	1	1	1	1
	Don't know	1	0	0	0	1	2	1	1	1	3	2	1	1
	Never smoked for as long as a year	68	59	55	55	55	61	61	67	60	61	57	61	57
		100	100	100	100	100	100	100	100	100	100	100	100	100
20-24	13 and less	} 9	} 15	} 17	} 19	5	6	6	6	8	5	7	5	7
	14-15					15	14	15	13	15	12	13	13	14
	16-17	21	24	22	22	23	17	19	18	16	17	15	20	15
	18-19	16	13	15	13	9	10	7	9	7	6	7	6	8
	20-24	5	3	3	3	3	3	1	2	2	1	2	1	2
	Don't know	0	1	0	0	1	2	2	2	1	3	2	1	1
	Never smoked for as long as a year	48	45	44	43	44	48	51	50	51	54	55	54	53
		100	100	100	100	100	100	100	100	100	100	100	100	100
25-34	13 and less	} 8	} 8	} 11	} 11	} 15	..	..	..	..	..	..	..	..
	14-15						..	..	..	..	..	..	..	..
	16-17	15	16	18	19	20	..	..	..	..	..	..	..	..
	18-19	14	16	13	14	14	..	..	..	..	..	..	..	..
	20-24	11	9	9	8	8	..	..	..	..	..	..	..	..
	25-29	3	2	2	1	1	..	..	..	..	..	..	..	..
	30-34	0	0	0	0	0	..	..	..	..	..	..	..	..
	Don't know	0	0	1	0	1	..	..	..	..	..	..	..	..
	Never smoked for as long as a year	48	47	45	45	40	..	..	..	..	..	..	..	..
		100	100	100	100	100								
25-29	13 and less	..	..	..	..	4	6	5	3	4	4	5	4	8
	14-15	..	..	..	..	12	13	16	12	17	13	16	14	11
	16-17	..	..	..	..	22	18	20	20	19	19	17	17	16
	18-19	..	..	..	..	14	10	10	8	8	7	12	6	9
	20-24	..	..	..	..	7	5	4	3	3	3	3	3	4
	25-29	..	..	..	..	1	1	0	0	0	0	0	0	1
	Don't know	..	..	..	..	0	2	2	1	1	2	1	1	1
	Never smoked for as long as a year	..	..	..	..	40	46	44	52	48	52	46	56	51
						100	100	100	100	100	100	100	100	100

Table 7.2.2 (*continued*) Percentage of women starting to smoke (any tobacco) at different ages: by age at time of survey, 1965-1987
Women aged 16 and over, Great Britain

Age at time of survey	Recalled age at starting to smoke	Year of survey												
		1965	1968	1971	1973	1975	1978	1981	1982	1983	1984	1985	1986	1987
30-34	13 and less	..	..	..	..	..	..	4	1	4	3	4	4	5
	14-15	..	..	..	..	..	..	12	12	11	12	14	11	14
	16-17	..	..	..	..	..	..	19	15	18	19	16	18	16
	18-19	..	..	..	..	..	..	11	15	12	9	9	14	9
	20-24	..	..	..	..	..	..	7	7	6	8	6	6	5
	25-29	..	..	..	..	..	..	1	2	2	3	1	1	2
	30+	..	..	..	..	..	..	1	0	0	0	0	0	0
	Don't know	..	..	..	..	..	..	2	1	2	2	2	3	1
	Never smoked for as long as a year	..	..	..	..	..	..	44	46	45	44	48	44	49
								100	100	100	100	100	100	100
35-59 (1965-75) **35-49** (1981+)	13 and less	} 6	} 7	} 9	} 10	} 11	..	2	2	2	2	4	3	3
	14-15						..	8	10	10	10	9	11	10
	16-17	10	12	12	13	12	..	15	14	17	14	15	17	16
	18-19	12	13	12	13	13	..	12	12	12	9	12	11	10
	20-24	14	13	13	15	14	..	10	10	9	9	8	9	9
	25-29	6	5	5	5	4	..	3	3	3	2	3	2	2
	30+	9	9	6	6	6	..	3	2	2	2	3	2	1
	Don't know	1	1	2	1	2	..	3	3	1	4	2	2	2
	Never smoked for as long as a year	44	41	41	37	39	..	43	45	44	48	46	43	47
		100	100	100	100	100		100	100	100	100	100	100	100
50-64	13 and less	..	..	..	..	..	..	2	2	2	2	3	2	3
	14-15	..	..	..	..	..	..	8	10	11	10	10	11	9
	16-17	..	..	..	..	..	..	11	15	9	13	13	10	13
	18-19	..	..	..	..	..	..	11	13	13	9	11	12	8
	20-24	..	..	..	..	..	..	15	12	11	11	11	11	11
	25-29	..	..	..	..	..	..	4	4	4	3	2	3	3
	30+	..	..	..	..	..	..	7	5	7	6	6	6	6
	Don't know	..	..	..	..	..	..	3	3	3	3	1	3	2
	Never smoked for as long as a year	..	..	..	..	..	..	40	38	40	42	42	43	45
								100	100	100	100	100	100	100
60+ (1965-75) **65+** (1981+)	13 and less	} 1	} 2	} 3	} 3	} 3	..	1	0	1	1	1	1	1
	14-15						..	3	5	6	5	5	6	6
	16-17	2	3	4	3	4	..	6	6	4	6	7	4	7
	18-19	2	3	3	4	4	..	7	5	7	4	4	6	7
	20-24	3	5	6	6	8	..	6	9	8	8	10	9	9
	25-29	2	3	2	3	4	..	4	4	5	5	5	4	3
	30+	16	15	14	14	15	..	12	11	11	14	10	9	10
	Don't know	2	1	2	1	3	..	3	3	3	3	2	3	2
	Never smoked for as long as a year	72	69	66	65	59	..	59	59	56	55	57	58	54
		100	100	100	100	100		100	100	100	100	100	100	100

Source: TAC

Table 7.3 Percentages of men and women starting to smoke at different ages: by age at time of survey, 1988
Current and ex-cigarette smokers, men and women aged 16 and over, Great Britain

Age at time of survey	Age started to smoke					
	<16	16-17	18-19	20-24	25-29	30+
Men						
16-19	67	31	2	0	0	0
20-24	43	37	16	3	0	0
25-34	41	32	16	10	2	0
35-49	39	30	16	12	2	1
50-59	38	22	22	15	2	2
60+	36	23	19	16	4	3
All ages	39	27	18	12	2	2
Women						
16-19	64	33	3	0	0	0
20-24	40	41	13	5	0	0
25-34	33	34	21	10	2	1
35-49	23	30	22	17	4	4
50-59	21	24	18	22	6	9
60+	14	18	18	22	9	19
All ages	25	28	19	16	5	7

Source: GHS (data not previously published)

Manufactured cigarettes: trends in type and yields, market shares

8

Plain/filter cigarettes

The first major change to occur in the type of manufactured cigarettes was the switch from plain to filter cigarettes, which began in the 1950s, gathered momentum in the 1960s, and has continued to the present. The original filter cigarettes were unventilated (without perforations in the tip), and these still account for the majority of the filter market. During the 1970s, ventilated filters (with perforations in the tip) were introduced. The subsequent rise in the market share of ventilated filter cigarettes was due both to the introduction of new ventilated brands, and to the change of some existing brands from unventilated to ventilated filters. By 1988 the market shares of unventilated filter, ventilated filter, and plain cigarettes were estimated to be 52, 46, and 2 per cent respectively.

Percentage market share of manufactured cigarettes

The percentage market share of brands of manufactured cigarettes sold in the United Kingdom are available from two sources: Maxwell's international estimates, published annually in the journal *World Tobacco*, and the estimates of brand shares of the UK cigarette market, published annually in the journal *Tobacco*. Only the main brands are listed in these tables. Both publications employ inclusion rules, based on a brand achieving a certain proportion of total market share, the exact proportion varying from year to year; in all years, brands achieving at least 1 per cent of the total market are included.

LGC surveys: classification of manufactured cigarettes by tar yield

Since 1972 the Laboratory of the Government Chemist (LGC) has conducted surveys of the tar, nicotine, and, from 1978 onwards, carbon monoxide yields of many of the brands of manufactured cigarettes sold in the UK.

In this section the tar, nicotine, and carbon monoxide yields of the main brands of cigarettes sold in the UK have been tabulated across the LGC surveys. Carbon monoxide yields for surveys 10-15, 20, 21, 24, 26, and 27 were not published, but have been included in Table 8.10. The brands chosen are those whose market share is listed at least once in *Tobacco* or *World Tobacco* during the period of the surveys. In Appendix 2, LGC surveys 1-19, 22, 23, 25, and 27-29 have been reproduced as they were originally published, with surveys 20, 21, 24, and 26 which were not published.

In LGC surveys 2-21 (1973-1984) the cigarettes were classified by tar band as follows (data rounded):

Low tar	0-10 mg tar/cigarette
Low to middle tar	11-16 mg tar/cigarette
Middle tar	17-22 mg tar/cigarette
Middle to high tar	23-28 mg tar/cigarette
High tar	29+ mg tar/cigarette.

The number of brands and the percentage of sales in the low and low to middle tar bands rose during this period. By survey 12, no brands tested fell into the high tar category, and few brands were in the middle to high tar category.

The definition of the bands was altered in survey 22 (1985) as follows:

Low tar	0-9.99 mg tar/cigarette
Low to middle tar	10.0-14.99 mg tar/cigarette
Middle tar	15.0-17.99 mg tar/cigarette
High tar	18+ mg tar/cigarette

(data truncated, i.e. less than 10 mg, 10 mg but less than 15 mg, 15 mg but less than 18 mg, and 18 mg and above).

Because of this change in classification, data from surveys 22 through 29 have been tabulated separately from data from surveys 1-21.

Despite the growing popularity of low tar cigarettes, in 1988 the percentage of sales was greatest in the low/middle tar band (10.0-14.99 mg).

Tar, nicotine, and carbon monoxide yields of manufactured cigarettes

In a study by Wald, Doll, and Copeland[f], the tar, nicotine, and carbon monoxide yields of cigarettes manufactured in the UK between 1934 and 1979 were analysed by the LGC, and sales-weighted yields calculated. These calculations have since been extended to 1988, and are included in this section. Data for the years 1934-1971 were obtained from old cigarettes analysed in 1977. TAC sales-weighted tar and nicotine yields for 1965-1987 are included for comparison, and are similar to the yields based on analysis by the LGC (differences partly arising from different sources of sales data used).

Tar yield

Between 1934-40 and 1988, the sales-weighted tar yield of all brands of manufactured cigarettes declined, slowly at first, and more rapidly after 1970, from 33 mg/cigarette to 13 mg/cigarette.

In 1934-40, the sales-weighted tar yield of plain cigarettes was about 33 mg/cigarette. It declined to 30 mg/cigarette by about 1960, and then declined further to about 17 mg/

cigarette in 1988. The sales-weighted tar yield of unventilated filter cigarettes fell from 24 mg/cigarette during the 1960s to 14 mg/cigarette in 1988. The sales-weighted tar yield of ventilated filter cigarettes fell from 12 mg/cigarette in 1972 to 9 mg/cigarette in 1974, and remained at about this level until 1982. By 1988 the sales-weighted yield of ventilated filter cigarettes had risen to 12 mg/cigarette, as more unventilated brands with somewhat higher tar yields became ventilated.

Nicotine yield

The sales-weighted nicotine yield of all brands of cigarettes was just over 2 mg/cigarette between 1934-40 and about 1960, and fell to 1.2 mg/cigarette in 1988.

Between 1934 and 1960 the sales-weighted nicotine yield of plain cigarettes was about 2 mg/cigarette. During the 1960s and early 1970s the sales-weighted nicotine yield of plain cigarettes declined to 1.7 mg/cigarette, rose again to nearly 2 mg/cigarette in 1976, and then declined to 1.3 mg/cigarette in 1988. The sales-weighted nicotine yield of unventilated cigarettes declined between 1962 and 1973 from 1.7 to 1.2 mg/cigarette; thereafter the yield rose to nearly 1.5 mg/cigarette in 1979, declined to 1.4 mg/cigarette in 1980, and stayed close to this level until 1987 to decline again in 1988 to 1.25 mg/cigarette. The sales-weighted nicotine yield of ventilated cigarettes rose from 0.8 mg/cigarette in 1972 to 1.1 mg/cigarette in 1988.

Carbon monoxide yield

The sales-weighted carbon monoxide yield of all brands of cigarettes was about 19 mg/cigarette between 1934-40 and 1960, and thereafter declined, slowly until about 1970 and then more rapidly, to about 14 mg/cigarette in 1988.

Between 1934-40 and 1960, the sales-weighted carbon monoxide yield of plain cigarettes was about 19 mg/cigarette. During the 1960s, the sales-weighted carbon monoxide yields of both plain and unventilated filter cigarettes were about 18 mg/cigarette. Between 1970 and 1988 the sales-weighted carbon monoxide yield of plain cigarettes fell from 17 mg/cigarette to 11 mg/cigarette. During this period there was little decline in the carbon monoxide yield of unventilated filter cigarettes, which had a sales-weighted yield of 16 mg/cigarette in 1988. The sales-weighted carbon monoxide yield of ventilated cigarettes was 13 mg/cigarette when introduced in 1972, varied between 10 and 12 mg/cigarette between 1976 and 1984, and by 1988 had risen to 13.1 mg/cigarette, as unventilated brands with slightly higher carbon monoxide yields became ventilated.

In 1979 the LGC determined the tar, nicotine, and carbon monoxide yields from 24 brands of cigarettes, and repeated these measurements in 1989 from the same stock of cigarettes in order to compare the variation of yields with age of cigarettes. The yields of tar, nicotine, and carbon monoxide were similar in 1979 and 1989 (see Table 8.22). These results provide support for the validity of the analyses of old cigarettes to determine tar, nicotine, and carbon monoxide yields over time (used in the study reported by Wald, Doll, and Copeland[f], and cited in Tables 8.4-8.6).

Yields of other analytes from manufactured cigarettes

The LGC has estimated the yields of a variety of other analytes (thought potentially injurious to health). From 75 brands of cigarettes examined during the period of survey 18 (October 1982-March 1983), five additional analytes were examined. In 1986 the LGC repeated the testing of these analytes on 14 of the 75 brands together with one reformulated and four new brands. Details of these results have been included in Tables 8.14 and 8.17 respectively.

In two further small surveys directed to particular components of the 'tar' phase LGC determined six low molecular weight phenols from 25 brands sampled in 1986 (see Table 8.20) and three polycyclic aromatic hydrocarbons in 23 brands from survey 29 (March-August 1989) (see Table 8.21). There was a close association between the tar and polycyclic aromatic hydrocarbons yields of these different brands.

Table 8.1 Percentage market share of plain and filter manufactured cigarettes, 1934-40 to 1988 United Kingdom

Year	Plain	Filter (unventilated + ventilated)	Unventilated filter	Ventilated filter
1934-40	>99	< 1	< 1	0
1941-47	>99	< 1	< 1	0
1948-54	99	1	1	0
1955-61	90	10	10	0
1962-68	50	50	50	0
1969	25	75	75	0
1970	22	78	78	0
1971	20	80	80	< 1
1972	18	82	81	1
1973	17	83	79	4
1974	16	84	78	6
1975	13	87	80	7
1976	12	88	77	11
1977	11	89	74	15
1978	10	90	76	14
1979	9	91	77	14
1980	7	93	77	16
1981	6	94	79	15
1982	6	94	77	17
1983	5	95	71	24
1984	4	96	69	27
1985	4	96	59	37
1986	3	97	59	38
1987	3	97	57	40
1988	2	98	52	46

Source: 1934-40 to 1979 from Wald, Doll, and Copeland, *British Medical Journal,* 1981, **282**: 763-5; 1980-1988 derived from market shares quoted in *Tobacco*

Fig. 8.1 Percentage market share of (i) plain and filter cigarettes, 1934-1988 and (ii) unventilated and ventilated filter cigarettes, 1970-1988 United Kingdom. *Source*: 1934-40 to 1979 from Wald, Doll, and Copeland, *British Medical Journal,*1981, **282**: 763-5; 1980-1988 derived from market shares quoted in *Tobacco*

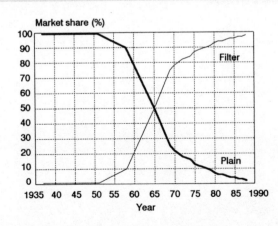
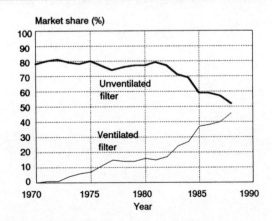

Table 8.2 Number of cigarette brands in each tar band of the LGC surveys, 1972-1989
United Kingdom

Survey	Date	Low 0-10 mg tar/cig	Low/middle 11-16 mg tar/cig	Middle 17-22 mg tar/cig	Middle/high 23-28 mg tar/cig	High 29+ mg tar/cig	Total number of brands
1[1]	Jul 1972 - Dec 1972	5	19	53	13	11	101
2	Jun 1973 - Nov 1973	10	22	53	14	6	105
3	Jan 1974 - Jun 1974	9	24	56	15	7	111
4	Aug 1974 - Jan 1975	11	18	56	17	7	109
5	Mar 1975 - Aug 1975	12	19	56	17	6	110
6	Oct 1975 - Mar 1976	13	31	59	13	5	121
7	May 1976 - Oct 1976	14	37	50	15	5	121
8	Dec 1976 - May 1977	19	32	48	12	3	114
9	Jul 1977 - Dec 1977	26	33	47	11	3	120
10	Feb 1978 - Jul 1978	24	30	53	11	3	121
11	Sep 1978 - Feb 1979	25	29	62	5	2	123
12	Apr 1979 Sep 1979	25	40	57	6	0	128
13	Nov 1979 - Apr 1980	28	44	62	6	0	140
14	Jun 1980 - Nov 1980	30	46	62	5	0	143
15	Jan 1981 - Jun 1981	33	41	61	4	0	139
16	Aug 1981 - Jan 1982	33	51	52	3	0	139
17	Mar 1982 - Aug 1982	37	62	37	3	0	139
18	Oct 1982 - Mar 1983	35	66	37	3	0	141
19	May 1983 - Oct 1983	31	73	31	4	0	139
20[2]	Dec 1983 - May 1984	31	70	34	4	0	139
21[2]	Jul 1984 - Dec 1984	33	72	30	2	0	137

Survey	Date	Low 0-9.99 mg tar/cig	Low/middle 10.0-14.99 mg tar/cig	Middle 15.0-17.99 mg tar/cig	High 18.0+ mg tar/cig	Total number of brands
22	Feb 1985 - Jul 1985	32	51	52	5	140
23	Sep 1985 - Feb 1986	33	53	42	10	138
24[2]	Apr 1986 - Sep 1986	36	63	39	7	145
25	Nov 1986 - Apr 1987	39	66	36	6	147
26[2]	Jun 1987 - Nov 1987	42	73	34	2	151
27	Jan 1988 - Jun 1988	36	77	33	3	149
28	Aug 1988 - Jan 1989	38	78	25	4	145
29	Mar 1989 - Aug 1989	38	90	16	2	146

1 In survey 1, brands were listed in order of tar level, but no bands were stated
2 Surveys 20, 21, 24, and 26 were not published by the Health Departments of the UK

Source: LGC

Fig. 8.2 Distribution of cigarette brands: by tar yield, LGC surveys 1 and 29
United Kingdom. *Source*: LGC

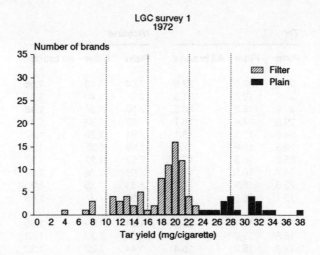

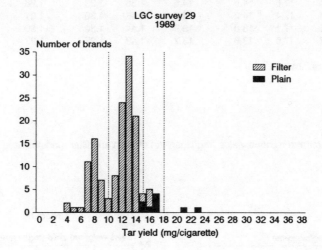

Table 8.3 Annual sales-weighted tar and nicotine yields (mg/cigarette) of plain and filter
manufactured cigarettes, 1965-1987
United Kingdom

	Tar			Nicotine		
Year	Plain	Filter	All brands	Plain	Filter	All brands
1965	35.0	29.3	31.5	2.21	2.00	2.08
1966	33.9	28.6	30.3	2.13	1.93	2.00
1967	32.6	23.2	26.0	2.14	1.67	1.82
1968	30.1	21.6	23.9	2.07	1.59	1.72
1969	30.3	21.8	23.9	2.07	1.53	1.67

Table 8.3 (*continued*) Annual sales-weighted tar and nicotine yields (mg/cigarette) of plain and filter manufactured cigarettes, 1965-1987
United Kingdom

Year	Tar			Nicotine		
	Plain	Filter	All brands	Plain	Filter	All brands
1970	29.6	20.6	22.5	2.04	1.43	1.56
1971	27.7	19.8	21.3	1.96	1.40	1.51
1972	27.8	18.9	20.5	2.00	1.36	1.48
1973	24.6	17.4	18.7	1.92	1.33	1.44
1974	24.6	17.1	18.1	1.94	1.28	1.37
1975	24.8	16.9	17.9	1.98	1.25	1.34
1976	25.0	16.8	17.8	2.07	1.27	1.37
1977	24.7	16.5	17.4	2.07	1.28	1.33
1978	22.6	16.9	17.4	1.83	1.35	1.39
1979	19.1	16.6	16.8	1.53	1.37	1.38
1980	18.6	16.1	16.3	1.44	1.29	1.30
1981	18.5	15.6	15.8	1.50	1.32	1.33
1982	17.9	15.2	15.4	1.44	1.32	1.32
1983	17.8	14.9	15.0	1.41	1.31	1.31
1984	17.6	14.5	14.6	1.38	1.28	1.28
1985	17.4	14.2	14.4	1.46	1.30	1.31
1986	17.1	13.8	13.9	1.44	1.30	1.30
1987	17.0	13.6	13.7	1.43	1.27	1.27

Source: TAC

Fig. 8.3 Annual sales-weighted tar and nicotine yields (mg/cigarette) of plain and filter manufactured cigarettes, 1965-1987
United Kingdom. *Source*: TAC

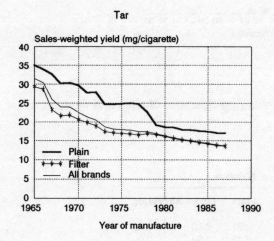

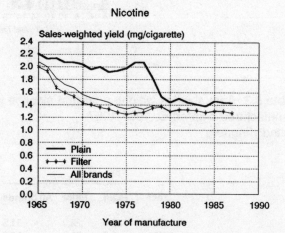

Fig. 8.4 Annual sales-weighted tar, nicotine, and carbon monoxide yields (mg/cigarette) of manufactured cigarettes: all brands, 1934-40 to 1988
United Kingdom. *Source*: Wald, Doll, and Copeland, 1981, and unpublished data

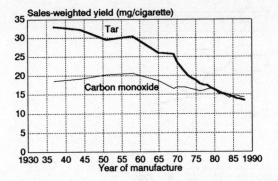 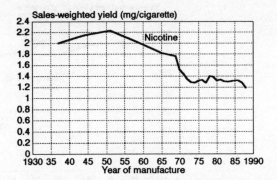

Table 8.4 Annual sales-weighted tar yield (mg/cigarette): by type of manufactured cigarette, 1934-40 to 1988
United Kingdom

Year	Plain	Unventilated filter	Ventilated filter	All brands
1934-40	32.9			32.9
1941-47	32.2			32.2
1948-54	29.5			29.5
1955-61	30.4			30.4
1962-68	29.0	24.0		26.0
1969	29.0	22.0		25.7
1970	29.4	21.2		23.6
1971	28.5	20.6		22.3
1972	28.0	19.5	12.0	21.0
1973	26.5	18.9	11.0	19.9
1974	25.4	18.8	9.4	19.3
1975	25.3	18.5	9.3	18.8
1976	24.7	18.0	9.3	17.9
1977	24.6	18.2	9.8	17.6
1978	22.3	18.3	9.8	17.5
1979	18.7	17.9	9.7	16.8
1980	18.2	17.7	9.5	16.4
1981	18.3	16.9	9.3	15.9
1982	17.8	16.5	9.6	15.4
1983	17.5	16.2	10.7	15.1
1984	17.6	15.8	11.9	14.8
1985	17.1	15.6	12.1	14.4
1986	16.8	15.4	11.4	13.9
1987	16.8	15.0	12.0	13.8
1988	16.6	14.5	12.0	13.4

Source: 1934-40 to 1979, from Wald, Doll, and Copeland, *British Medical Journal*, 1981, **282**: 763-5, based on analysis by LGC; 1980-1988, calculated from LGC surveys, with market-share data from *Tobacco*

Fig. 8.5 Annual sales-weighted tar yield (mg/cigarette): by type of manufactured cigarette, 1934-40 to 1988 United Kingdom. *Source*: Wald, Doll, and Copeland, 1981, and unpublished data

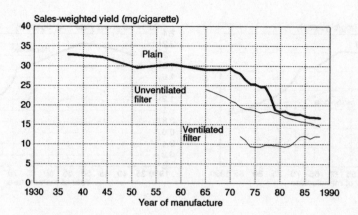

Table 8.5 Annual sales-weighted nicotine yield (mg/cigarette): by type of manufactured cigarette, 1934-40 to 1988
United Kingdom

Year	Plain	Unventilated filter	Ventilated filter	All brands
1934-40	2.00			2.00
1941-47	2.14			2.14
1948-54	2.23			2.23
1955-61	2.03			2.03
1962-68	2.03	1.68		1.82
1969	1.99	1.51		1.76
1970	1.96	1.34		1.52
1971	1.91	1.32		1.44
1972	1.82	1.25	0.80	1.35
1973	1.72	1.22	0.75	1.29
1974	1.76	1.24	0.65	1.28
1975	1.91	1.27	0.76	1.32
1976	1.96	1.31	0.81	1.33
1977	1.95	1.28	0.86	1.28
1978	1.81	1.44	0.89	1.40
1979	1.54	1.46	0.85	1.39
1980	1.44	1.40	0.88	1.32
1981	1.47	1.41	0.93	1.34
1982	1.42	1.39	0.91	1.31
1983	1.37	1.37	1.05	1.30
1984	1.36	1.37	1.14	1.31
1985	1.42	1.40	1.17	1.32
1986	1.41	1.41	1.18	1.32
1987	1.39	1.35	1.18	1.28
1988	1.32	1.25	1.12	1.19

Source: 1934-40 to 1979, from Wald, Doll, and Copeland, *British Medical Journal,* 1981, **282**: 763-5, based on analysis by LGC; 1980-1988, calculated from LGC surveys, with market-share data from *Tobacco*

Fig. 8.6 Annual sales-weighted nicotine yield (mg/cigarette): by type of manufactured cigarette, 1934-40 to 1988 United Kingdom. *Source*: Wald, Doll, and Copeland, 1981, and unpublished data

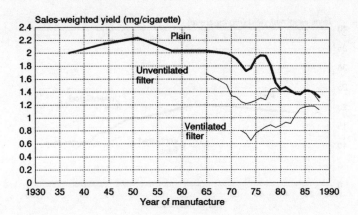

Table 8.6 Annual sales-weighted carbon monoxide yield (mg/cigarette): by type of manufactured cigarette, 1934-40 to 1988
United Kingdom

Year	Plain	Unventilated filter	Ventilated filter	All brands
1934-40	18.6			18.6
1941-47	19.2			19.2
1948-54	20.3			20.3
1955-61	20.6			20.6
1962-68	18.4	18.9		18.7
1969	17.2	16.0		16.6
1970	17.4	17.0		17.1
1971	17.1	17.0		17.0
1972	16.6	17.2	13.0	17.0
1976	13.7	17.1	10.7	16.0
1977	13.6	17.6	11.1	16.1
1978	12.8	18.0	11.5	16.5
1979	10.9	18.1	12.0	16.6
1980	11.2	17.9	12.1	16.6
1981	11.0	16.6	10.1	15.3
1982	11.5	16.6	10.2	15.2
1983	11.3	16.1	10.9	14.7
1984	11.0	15.2	11.7	14.1
1985	11.1	16.1	12.5	14.7
1986	11.1	16.4	12.5	14.7
1987	10.9	15.8	12.7	14.4
1988	11.0	15.8	13.1	14.4

Source: 1934-40 to 1979, from Wald, Doll, and Copeland, *British Medical Journal,* 1981, **282**: 763-5, based on analysis by LGC; 1980-1988, calculated from LGC surveys, with market-share from *Tobacco*

Fig. 8.7 Annual sales-weighted carbon monoxide yield (mg/cigarette): by type of manufactured cigarette, 1934-40 to 1988
United Kingdom. *Source*: Wald, Doll, and Copeland, 1981, and unpublished data

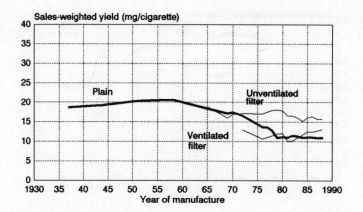

Table 8.7 Percentage market share and proportion of market share tested: by type of cigarette, for Tables 8.4, 8.5, and 8.6
United Kingdom

| Year | Plain | | Unventilated filter | | Ventilated filter | | All brands |
	Market share %	Prop. tested %	Market share %	Prop. tested %	Market share %	Prop. tested %	Prop. tested %
1934-40	>99	79	< 1		0		79
1941-47	>99	68	< 1		0		68
1948-54	99	62	1		0		62
1955-61	90	76	10		0		69
1962-68	50	42	50	62	0		52
1969	25	90	75	26	0		42
1970	22	97	78	66	0		73
1971	20	96	80	90	< 1		91
1972	18	98	80	95	1	>90	94
1973	17	94	79	96	4	>90	96
1974	16	94	78	98	6	98	98
1975	13	99	80	96	7	96	96
1976	12	97	77	>99	11	95	99
1977	11	97	74	98	15	96	97
1978	10	98	76	98	14	97	98
1979	9	98	77	99	14	96	98

Table 8.7 (*continued*) Percentage market share and proportion of market share tested: by type of cigarette, for Tables 8.4, 8.5, and 8.6
United Kingdom

| Year | Plain | | Unventilated filter | | Ventilated filter | | All brands |
	Market share %	Prop. tested %	Market share %	Prop. tested %	Market share %	Prop. tested %	Prop. tested %
1980	7	85	77	95	16	95	94
1981	6	90	79	96	15	96	96
1982	6	90	77	94	17	94	94
1983	5	92	71	96	24	96	96
1984	4	85	69	88	27	88	88
1985	4	81	59	93	37	93	92
1986	3	81	59	88	38	88	88
1987	3	81	57	88	40	88	88
1988	2	88	52	90	46	90	90

Source: 1934-40 to 1979, from Wald, Doll, and Copeland, *British Medical Journal*, 1981, **282**:763-5; 1980-1988, derived from *Tobacco*

Table 8.8.1 Tar yield (mg/cigarette) of selected cigarette brands from LGC surveys 1-14, 1972-1980
United Kingdom

	LGC survey													
	1	2	3	4	5	6	7	8	9	10	11	12	13	14
	Year of survey													
Brand	1972	73	74	74/75	75	75/76	76	76/77	77	78	78/79	79	79/80	80
Plain														
Capstan Full Strength	38	38	36	35	34	34	35	34	33	31	31	28	26	24
Capstan Medium	32	25	26	26	27	27	27	26	26	25	19	19	19	19
Park Drive Plain	28	23	24	25	25	25	24	23	24	23	19	19	19	18
Piccadilly No. 1	28	28	24	23	24	22	23	22	21	18	20	18	18	17
Player's Medium Navy Cut	27	26	26	27	26	26	27	27	26	25	25	18	18	18
Player's No. 6 Plain	25	24	24	24	24	22	21	21	22	22	19	18	19	18
Senior Service Plain	31	23	26	26	26	26	25	25	25	26	19	19	19	19
Weights Plain	26	24	23	25	25	25	24	24	25	24	20	18	18	18
Woodbine Plain	27	26	27	24	24	24	24	26	24	24	19	18	18	18
Ventilated filter														
Belair Menthol Kings	*	u	u	u	u	u	u	u	10	9	9	10	10	9
B and H Longer Length	*	*	*	*	*	*	*	*	*	*	*	*	*	*
Berkeley Extra Mild KS	*	*	*	*	*	*	*	*	*	*	*	*	*	*
Berkeley Luxury Length	*	*	*	*	*	*	*	*	*	*	*	*	*	*
Consulate Menthol	u	u	u	u	u	u	u	u	u	u	u	u	u	u
Consulate No. 2	*	*	*	*	u	u	u	u	u	u	u	u	u	u
Du Maurier KS	*	*	*	*	*	*	*	*	*	*	*	*	u	u
Dunhill KS Superior Mild	*	*	*	*	*	*	*	*	*	8+	8	9	9	9
Embassy Extra Mild	11	11	11	11	12	11	11	9	9	10	9	9	10	9
Embassy No. 1 Extra Mild	*	*	*	*	*	*	*	10+	9	9	9	9	10	10

	LGC survey													
	1	2	3	4	5	6	7	8	9	10	11	12	13	14
Year of survey														
Brand	1972	73	74	74/ 75	75	75/ 76	76	76/ 77	77	78	78/ 79	79	79/ 80	80
Ventilated filter														
Embassy No. 3 Standard Size	*	*	*	*	*	*	*	u	u	u	u	u	u	u
Embassy No. 5 Extra Mild	*	*	*	*	*	*	12	10	10	9	10	10	9	10
J P Carlton Long Size	u	u	u	u	u	u	u	u	12	13	13	13	13	13
J P Carlton Premium	u	u	u	u	u	u	u	u	12	12	12	12	13	13
J P KS Extra Mild	*	*	*	*	*	*	..	8	9	9	9	9	9	9
J P Special Filter	u	u	u	u	u	u	u	u	20	19	18	18	18	18
J P Superkings	*	*	*	*	*	*	*	*	*	*	*	*	*	*
J P Vanguard KS	*	*	*	*	*	*	*	*	*	*	*	*		9
Lambert and Butler Sp Mild KS	*	*	*	*	*	*	*	*	*	*	*	*	9	9
Marlboro KS	u	u	u	u	u	u	u	u	u	u	u	u	u	u
Marlboro 100s	*	*	*	*	*	*	*	*	*	*	*	*	*	*
Peter Stuy Lux Length Ex Mild	*	*	*	*	*	*	*	*	*	*	*	*	*	10
Player's No. 6 Extra Mild	12	8	8	10	9	10	9	9	9	9	9	9	10	10
Player's No. 10 Extra Mild	*	*	*	*	..	13	13	13	12	13	13	12	13	13
Raffles	*	*	*	*	*	*	*	*	*	*	*	*	*	*
State Express 555 Sp Mild KS	*	*	*	*	*	*	*	*	*	*	*	*	*	*
Silk Cut	12	11	11	9	8	9	8	9	9	9	9	9	9	9
Silk Cut KS	11	9	9	8	9	9	8	9	9	9	9	9	10	9
Silk Cut No. 3	12	11	11	9	8	9	8	9	9	9	10	10	10	10
Silk Cut No. 5	*	*	*	*	*	*	8	9	8	9	9	9	9	9
Unventilated filter														
Albany	19	*	*	*	*	*	*	*	*	*	*	*	*	*
Ardath KS	*	*	*	*	*	*	*	*	*	*	*	*	*	*
Belair Menthol Kings	*	14	13	12	13	12	12	11	v	v	v	v	v	v
B and H Gold Bond Filter	19	19	18	18	17	17	17	17	16	18	19	18	18	18
B and H Sovereign Filter	18	18	19	18	18	18	18	18	19	19	19	19	19	18
B and H Sovereign KS	*	*	*	*	*	*	*	*	*	*	*	*	*	15+
B and H (Special F) KS	20	20	19	19	19	18	19	19	18	19	19	18	18	18
B and H Sterling Filter	21	20	19	19	19	19	19	18	19	20	19	19	19	19
Black Cat No. 9	*	*	*	*	*	*	12	12	12	14	14	15	14	14
Cadets	18	18	18	18	18	18	15	15	16	17	16	15	16	15
Cambridge	16	15	16	17	17	16	15	16	*	*	*	*	*	*
Consulate Menthol	14	13	13	13	13	12	11	10	9	10	9	8	9	9
Consulate No. 2	*	*	*	*	..	12	11	11	9	10	10	9	10	9
Craven A KS	*	*	*	*	*	*	*	*	*	*	*	17+	17	17
Du Maurier KS	*	*	*	*	*	*	*	*	*	*	*	*	14+	13
Dunhill International	19	19	19	19	18	20	19	19	19	18	17	17	16	16
Dunhill KS	*	*	..	..	18	17	16	17	18	17	17	15	16	16
Dunhill Luxury Length	*	*	*	*	*	*	*	*	*	*	*	*	*	*
Embassy Envoy	*	*	*	*	*	*	..	17	18	17	18	18	18	17
Embassy Filter	20	19	19	19	19	19	18	18	18	18	19	18	18	18
Embassy Gold	18	18	18	18	18	18	19	19	19	19	18	19	19	19

	LGC survey													
	1	2	3	4	5	6	7	8	9	10	11	12	13	14
	Year of survey													
Brand	1972	73	74	74/75	75	75/76	76	76/77	77	78	78/79	79	79/80	80
Unventilated filter														
Embassy KS	*	*	*	*	*	*	..	19	18	18	19	19	18	18
Embassy No. 1 KS	*	*	*	*	*	*	*	18+	18	19	19	18	19	18
Embassy No. 3 Standard Size	*	*	*	*	*	*	*	17+	18	18	18	18	18	18
Embassy Regal	18	17	17	18	17	17	17	17	18	18	18	18	18	17
Gold Leaf F Va	21	19	20	20	20	20	20	19	21	20	19	18	19	18
Guards	20	19	18	18	17	16	16	16	16	16	16	16	16	16
J P Carlton Long Size	15+	16	16	16	16	16	16	15	v	v	v	v	v	v
J P Carlton Premium	16+	18	16	16	15	16	16	15	v	v	v	v	v	v
John Player KS	*	*	*	*	*	*	18	18	18	18	18	18	19	18
J P Special Filter	22	20	21	20	19	19	18	19	v	v	v	v	v	v
J P Special KS	*	*	*	*	*	*	*	*	*	*	*	*	19+	18
Kensitas Club F Va	19	20	19	18	19	18	18	19	17	18	19	19	19	19
Kensitas Club KS	*	*	*	*	*	*	*	*	*	18	18	18	18	17
Kensitas Corsair F Va	19	18	18	19	19	19	18	18	19	20	20	19	18	17
Kensitas Mild	*	13	14	14	14	13	16	14	13	16	..	*	*	*
Kensitas Tipped	21	19	19	19	19	19	19	19	19	*	*	*	*	*
Kensitas F Va KS	*	*	*	*	*	*	*	*	*	19	18	18	18	18
Lambert and Butler KS	*	*	*	*	*	*	*	*	*	*	19+	18	19	18
London KS	*	*	*	*	*	*	*	*	*	*	*	*	*	..
Marlboro KS	20	19	18	16	16	15	15	15	15	16	16	16	16	16
Park Drive Tipped	21	19	19	19	18	18	18	18	18	20	19	19	19	19
Peter Stuyvesant KS	17	16	16	17	15	15	14	14	14	14	15	14	14	14
Peter Stuy Luxury Length	20	17	16	18	17	16	*	*	*	*	*	*	*	14
Piccadilly Filter De Luxe	19	17	18	18	17	17	18	18	16	16	17	16	16	16
Piccadilly KS	18	19	19	20	20	19	19	19	19	19	17	17	16	16
Piccadilly No. 7	15	14	15	14	13	13	12	12	13	14	14	14	14	14
Player's No. 6 F Va	20	18	19	20	20	19	19	18	19	19	19	18	19	18
Player's No. 6 KS	22	19	19	20	20	20	18	18	18	19	19	18	19	19
Player's No. 10 F Va	20	19	19	19	20	20	19	20	20	19	19	19	19	18
Regal KS (Embassy)	*	*	*	*	*	*	*	*	18+	18	19	18	19	18
Rothmans KS	19	19	20	20	21	21	20	19	19	19	19	18	18	17
Senior Service Filter	20	20	20	19	19	19	19	19	..	*	*	*	*	*
Silk Cut No. 1	*	*	..	9	9	8	9	9	..	*	*	*	*	*
State Express 555 Filter Kings	*	*	*	*	*	*	*	*	18+	18	17	17	18	17
State Express 555 Med Mild KS	*	*	*	*	*	*	*	*	*	*	14+	14	15	14
St Moritz Lux Length Menthol	14	13	13	13	12	12	12	11	11	13	12	11	12	11
Winston KS	*	*	*	*	*	*	*	18	18	18	18	19	18	18

+ Manufacturer's estimate. Brand recently introduced; not then analysed by LGC for a period of 6 months
* Brand not on market during the survey
u Cigarette filter unventilated during the survey
v Cigarette filter ventilated during the survey
.. Brand not tested by LGC

Source: LGC

Table 8.8.2 Tar yield (mg/cigarette) of selected cigarette brands from LGC surveys 15-29, 1981-1989 United Kingdom

Brand	LGC survey														
	15	16	17	18	19	20	21	22	23	24	25	26	27	28	29
Year of survey	1981	81/82	82	82/83	83	83/84	84	85	85/86	86	86/87	87	88	88/89	89
Plain															
Capstan Full Strength	26	26	25	25	25	25	25	25	25	24	23	24	23	23	23
Capstan Medium	19	19	18	17	17	18	17	17	18	16	18	16	17	17	*
Park Drive Plain	18	18	18	18	18	18	18	16	17	16	16	16	16	16	15
Piccadilly No. 1	18	18	16	16	16	17	16	16	16	16	16	16	16	16	16
Player's Medium Navy Cut	19	18	18	17	17	17	17	16	17	16	16	15	16	17	17
Player's No. 6 Plain	18	18	17	17	17	19	17	16	16	16	16	15	16	*	*
Senior Service Plain	19	19	18	18	18	19	18	17	18	18	18	17	17	18	17
Weights Plain	18	17	17	17	17	19	17	16	16	15	15	15	16	15	*
Woodbine Plain	18	19	18	18	17	17	17	16	16	16	16	16	16	15	15
Ventilated filter															
Belair Menthol Kings	9	10	9	10	10	9	9	8	8	7	7	8	8	8	*
B and H Longer Length/ B and H 100s[1]	*	*	..	16	16	16	16	14	14	14	13	14	14	13	13
B and H XL	*	*	*	*	*	*	*	*	*	*	13+	13	13	14	14
Berkeley Extra Mild KS	9	9	9	9	9	9	9	8	8	8	8	9	..	*	*
Berkeley Luxury Length/ Berkeley Superkings[2]	*	*	15+	16	15	15	*	14	14	14	13	13	13	12	12
Berkeley Superkings Mild	*	*	*	*	*	*	*	*	*	*	9+	9	9	8	8
Consulate Menthol	u	10	9	9	8	8	8	7	8	7	8	8	8	9	9
Consulate No. 2	u	9	9	9	8	9	7	7	8	7	7	7	8	8	7
Dorchester Extra Mild KS	*	*	*	*	*	*	*	9+	8	8	8	8	8	8	8
Du Maurier KS	u	u	10	9	9	9	9	7	9	*	*	*	*	*	*
Dunhill KS Superior Mild	8	9	8	9	9	8	8	7	8	9	9	9	9	9	9
Embassy Extra Mild	10	9	9	9	9	9	9	8	7	7	7	8	8	7	7
Embassy Filter	u	u	u	u	u	u	u	14	14	13	13	13	13	13	12
Embassy No. 1 Extra Mild	9	9	9	9	9	10	9	8	9	8	8	8	8	8	7
Embassy No. 3 Standard Size	u	u	u	u	14	15	14	14	13	13	13	13	12	*	*
Embassy No. 5 Extra Mild	10	9	9	10	9	9	9	8	8	9	8	9	*	*	*
Embassy Regal/ Regal Filter[3]	u	u	u	u	u	u	u	u	14	13	13	13	13	13	12
J P Carlton Long Size	13	13	13	13	12	12	12	12	13	12	12	12	12	*	*
J P Carlton Premium	14	13	13	13	13	13	12	12	12	12	12	12	11	*	*
J P King Size	u	u	u	u	u	u	u	u	13	12	12	12	12	12	13
J P KS Extra Mild	9	9	9	10	9	9	9	8	8	8	8	8	8	8	7
J P Special Filter	17	16	16	17	16	15	15	15	16	14	16	15	15	*	*
J P Superkings	*	*	*	16+	15	15	15	15	13	13	13	13	13	13	13
J P Superkings Low Tar	*	*	*	*	*	*	8	8	9	8	8	9	9	9	8
J P Vanguard KS	9	9	9	9	9	9	9	8	8	7	8	8	8	*	*
Lambert and Butler Sp Mild KS	9	9	9	10	6	4	4	4	4	4	4	4	4	4	4
Marlboro KS	u	u	u	u	u	15	14	13	13	13	13	13	13	13	13
Marlboro 100s	14+	15	15	14	14	..	13	13	13	14	13	13	14	14	14
Peter Stuy Lux Length Ex Md	10	10	10	9	9	9	9	8	9	9	8	8	8	8	8

	LGC survey														
	15	16	17	18	19	20	21	22	23	24	25	26	27	28	29
Year of survey															
Brand	1981	81/82	82	82/83	83	83/84	84	85	85/86	86	86/87	87	88	88/89	89
Ventilated filter															
Player's No. 6 Extra Mild	10	10	10	9	10	10	9	9	9	8	8	7	7	*	*
Player's No. 10 Extra Mild	13	12	13	13	12	10	9	8	8	8	8	8	*	*	*
Raffles 100s	*	*	*	*	*	15	14	14	14	14	13	14	13	13	13
Rothmans Special	*	*	*	*	*	*	*	*	9+	10	9	9	8	8	8
State Express 555 Sp Mild KS	9	9	10	10	9	..	*	*	*	*	*	*	*	*	*
Silk Cut	10	9	9	9	9	8	8	8	8	8	8	7	8	7	7
Silk Cut Extra	*	*	*	*	*	*	*	9+	9	8	9	9	9	9	8
Silk Cut KS	9	9	9	9	8	10	9	9	9	8	9	9	9	9	8
Silk Cut No. 3	10	10	10	10	9	10	9	8	9	8	8	8	8	8	8
Silk Cut No. 5	9	10	10	10	10	10	10	8	8	7	8	8	8	8	7
Unventilated filter															
Ardath KS	*	*	16+	17	16	17	15	14	15	*	*	*	*	*	*
B and H Gold Bond Filter	18	18	18	18	19	18	18	16	16	16	14	14	14	13	14
B and H Sovereign Filter	18	18	17	16	16	17	18	16	17	16	14	15	15	14	12
B and H Sovereign KS	15	15	16	15	16	15	15	14	15	14	13	13	13	14	13
B and H (Special F) KS	17	17	18	18	18	17	17	16	16	16	16	14	14	14	14
B and H Sterling Filter	*	*	*	*	*	*	*	*	*	*	*	*	*	*	*
Black Cat No. 9	*	*	*	*	*	*	*	*	*	*	*	*	*	*	*
Cadets	*	*	*	*	*	*	*	*	*	*	*	*	*	*	*
Consulate Menthol	9	v	v	v	v	v	v	v	v	v	v	v	v	v	v
Consulate No. 2	9	v	v	v	v	v	v	v	v	v	v	v	v	v	v
Craven A KS	16	*	*	*	*	18	17	16	17	16	16	16	16	17	16
Dorchester KS	*	*	*	*	*	17	16	15	15	15	15	15	15	14	15
Du Maurier KS	14	12	v	v	v	v	v	v	v	v	v	v	v	v	v
Dunhill International	17	16	16	15	16	16	16	16	16	16	15	15	15	16	16
Dunhill KS	15	15	14	14	14	16	15	15	14	14	14	14	14	15	14
Dunhill Luxury Length	*	*	13+	14	15	15	14	14	15	14	14	13	14	15	15
Embassy Filter	17	17	16	16	15	15	15	v	v	v	v	v	v	v	v
Embassy Gold	19	18	17	17	16	17	16	15	15	15	15	15	15	*	*
Embassy KS	18	16	..	*	*	*	*	*	*	*	*	*	*	*	*
Embassy No. 1 KS	18	17	16	16	15	15	14	13	13	13	13	14	14	14	13
Embassy No. 3 Standard Size	17	16	16	16	v	v	v	v	v	v	v	v	v	*	*
Embassy Regal	17	16	16	16	14	14	15	14	v	v	v	v	v	v	v
Gold Leaf F Va	17	17	17	17	17	17	16	16	16	16	16	16	16	13	13
Goldmark KS	*	*	*	*	*	*	*	*	..	14+	13	13	13	13	13
Guards	16	17	15	15	15	14	14	13	13	13	13	13	13	13	13
John Player KS	17	17	16	16	14	14	13	12	v	v	v	v	v	v	v
J P Special Filter	v	v	v	v	v	v	v	v	v	v	v	v	v	v	v
J P Special KS	18	18	17	17	17	16	16	16	16	15	15	15	15	15	14
Kensitas Club F Va	18	19	18	17	18	18	17	15	15	16	15	14	14	13	14
Kensitas Club KS	17	17	17	18	18	18	17	16	16	16	15	15	15	14	14

Brand	LGC survey														
	15	16	17	18	19	20	21	22	23	24	25	26	27	28	29
Year of survey															
	1981	81/ 82	82	82/ 83	83	83/ 84	84	85	85/ 86	86	86/ 87	87	88	88/ 89	89
Unventilated filter															
Kensitas Corsair F Va	18	17	17	17	17	17	17	16	17	16	13	14	14	14	12
Kensitas F Va KS	17	17	17	17	17	18	17	16	16	16	16	15	14	14	14
Kingsmen	*	*	*	*	*	*	..	16	15	13	14	14	13	13	13
Lambert and Butler KS	18	17	16	15	15	15	14	13	13	13	13	13	13	13	12
London KS	19	20	19	18	15	14	13	14	16	15	16	17	16	15	13
Marlboro KS	16	16	15	16	16	v	v	v	v	v	v	v	v	v	v
Park Drive Tipped	*	*	*	*	*	*	*	*	*	*	*	*	*	*	*
Peter Stuyvesant KS	14	14	15	13	13	12	12	11	11	10	11	11	11	11	11
Peter Stuy Lux Length	15	14	13	13	13	15	15	15	14	13	12	12	13	13	13
Piccadilly Filter De Luxe	17	17	16	15	14	15	14	13	13	12	12	13	13	13	13
Piccadilly KS	15	15	13	16	15	16	15	14	14	14	13	14	14	14	14
Piccadilly No. 7	14	15	*	*	*	*	*	*	*	*	*	*	*	*	*
Player's No. 6 F Va	18	18	17	16	16	16	15	15	15	14	15	15	14	15	14
Player's No. 6 KS	17	17	16	16	15	14	14	14	14	14	14	14	13	13	13
Player's No. 10 F Va	17	17	16	17	17	16	16	16	16	15	15	15	15	15	14
Red Band KS	*	*	*	*	*	*	*	..	14	13	13	13	13	13	12
Regal KS (Embassy)	18	17	17	16	15	15	14	13	13	13	14	14	14	13	13
Rothmans KS	17	17	16	17	17	17	17	15	16	16	16	15	16	16	16
Spar KS	*	*	*	*	*	*	..	16	14	13	13	13	13	13	13
State Express 555 Filter Kings	17	17	16	17	16	16	15	15	15	*	*	*	*	*	*
State Express 555 Med Mild KS	14	14	14	14	13	..	*	*	*	*	*	*	*	*	*
St Moritz Lux Length Menthol	12	13	12	11	11	11	10	10	11	10	10	10	10	10	13
Victoria Wine KS/ Victoria Wine Spec F[4]	*	*	*	*	14+	13	15	13	15	15	16	15	17	16	14
Winston KS	17	15	15	15	15	16	15	13	13	13	13	13	13	13	11

+ Manufacturer's estimate. Brand recently introduced; not then analysed by LGC for a period of 6 months
* Brand not on market during the survey
u Cigarette filter unventilated during the survey
v Cigarette filter ventilated during the survey
.. Brand not tested by LGC

1 Renamed B and H 100s during survey 24
2 Renamed Berkeley Superkings during survey 22
3 Renamed Regal Filter during survey 28
4 Renamed Victoria Wine Spec F during survey 28

Source: LGC

Brand	LGC survey													
	1	2	3	4	5	6	7	8	9	10	11	12	13	14
	Year of survey													
	1972	73	74	74/ 75	75	75/ 76	76	76/ 77	77	78	78/ 79	79	79/ 80	80
Plain														
Capstan Full Strength	3.2	3.4	3.2	3.2	3.4	3.5	3.6	3.7	3.5	3.5	3.6	3.1	2.7	2.4
Capstan Medium	2.0	1.6	1.8	1.7	1.9	1.9	2.0	2.0	1.9	1.9	1.4	1.4	1.3	1.2
Park Drive Plain	1.9	1.6	1.7	1.8	2.0	1.9	1.9	1.9	2.0	2.0	1.6	1.6	1.5	1.4
Piccadilly No. 1	1.6	1.7	1.4	1.3	1.5	1.3	1.4	1.4	1.3	1.4	1.5	1.4	1.4	1.3
Player's Medium Navy Cut	1.7	1.6	1.8	1.7	1.9	1.8	2.0	2.1	1.9	1.9	1.9	1.4	1.4	1.4
Player's No. 6 Plain	1.6	1.5	1.6	1.6	1.7	1.6	1.6	1.6	1.5	1.6	1.2	1.2	1.2	1.1
Senior Service Plain	1.9	1.4	1.6	1.7	1.9	1.8	1.9	2.0	1.9	2.1	1.6	1.5	1.6	1.5
Weights Plain	1.6	1.5	1.5	1.6	1.7	1.7	1.7	1.8	1.7	1.7	1.2	1.2	1.2	1.2
Woodbine Plain	1.7	1.6	1.7	1.7	1.8	1.8	2.0	2.2	1.9	2.0	1.6	1.6	1.5	1.4
Ventilated filter														
Belair Menthol Kings	*	u	u	u	u	u	u	u	0.6	0.6	0.6	0.7	0.6	0.6
B and H Longer Length	*	*	*	*	*	*	*	*	*	*	*	*	*	*
Berkeley Extra Mild KS	*	*	*	*	*	*	*	*	*	*	*	*	*	*
Berkeley Luxury Length	*	*	*	*	*	*	*	*	*	*	*	*	*	*
Consulate Menthol	u	u	u	u	u	u	u	u	u	u	u	u	u	u
Consulate No. 2	*	*	*	*	u	u	u	u	u	u	u	u	u	u
Du Maurier KS	*	*	*	*	*	*	*	*	*	*	*	*	u	u
Dunhill KS Superior Mild	*	*	*	*	*	*	*	*	*	0.7+	0.7	0.7	0.7	0.7
Embassy Extra Mild	0.8	0.8	0.8	0.8	0.9	0.8	0.9	0.8	0.8	0.8	0.8	0.8	0.8	0.7
Embassy No. 1 Extra Mild	*	*	*	*	*	*	*	0.8+	0.7	0.7	0.7	0.7	0.8	0.8
Embassy No. 3 Standard Size	*	*	*	*	*	*	*	u	u	u	u	u	u	u
Embassy No. 5 Extra Mild	*	*	*	*	*	*	1.0	0.9	0.8	0.8	0.8	0.8	0.7	0.7
J P Carlton Long Size	u	u	u	u	u	u	u	u	1.3	1.3	1.3	1.4	1.4	1.4
J P Carlton Premium	u	u	u	u	u	u	u	u	1.1	1.1	1.1	1.2	1.2	1.2
J P KS Extra Mild	*	*	*	*	*	*	..	0.7	0.7	0.7	0.7	0.7	0.7	0.8
J P Special Filter	u	u	u	u	u	u	u	u	1.6	1.6	1.5	1.6	1.5	1.5
J P Superkings	*	*	*	*	*	*	*	*	*	*	*	*	*	*
J P Vanguard KS	*	*	*	*	*	*	*	*	*	*	*	*	*	1.0
Lambert and Butler Sp Mild KS	*	*	*	*	*	*	*	*	*	*	*	*	0.7	0.8
Marlboro KS	u	u	u	u	u	u	u	u	u	u	u	u	u	u
Marlboro 100s	*	*	*	*	*	*	*	*	*	*	*	*	*	*
Peter Stuy Lux Length Ex Md	*	*	*	*	*	*	*	*	*	*	*	*	*	0.9
Players's No. 6 Extra Mild	0.8	0.5	0.5	0.7	0.6	0.7	0.7	0.7	0.7	0.7	0.7	0.7	0.7	0.7
Players's No. 10 Extra Mild	*	*	*	*	..	0.7	0.9	0.9	0.7	0.8	0.8	0.8	0.8	0.8
Raffles	*	*	*	*	*	*	*	*	*	*	*	*	*	*
State Express 555 Sp Md KS	*	*	*	*	*	*	*	*	*	*	*	*	*	*
Silk Cut	0.8	0.7	0.8	0.6	0.7	0.8	0.8	0.8	0.8	0.9	0.8	0.8	0.8	0.7
Silk Cut KS	0.8	0.7	0.7	0.6	0.8	0.8	0.8	0.9	0.9	1.0	1.0	0.9	0.9	0.9
Silk Cut No. 3	0.8	0.8	0.8	0.6	0.7	0.7	0.7	0.8	0.8	0.8	0.9	0.8	0.8	0.8
Silk Cut No. 5	*	*	*	*	*	*	0.7	0.8	0.7	0.8	0.7	0.8	0.7	0.6

Brand	LGC survey													
	1	2	3	4	5	6	7	8	9	10	11	12	13	14
	Year of survey													
	1972	73	74	74/ 75	75	75/ 76	76	76/ 77	77	78	78/ 79	79	79/ 80	80
Unventilated filter														
Albany	1.2	*	*	*	*	*	*	*	*	*	*	*	*	*
Ardath KS	*	*	*	*	*	*	*	*	*	*	*	*	*	*
Belair Menthol Kings	*	0.8	0.8	0.7	0.8	0.8	0.8	0.8	v	v	v	v	v	v
B and H Gold Bond Filter	1.2	1.2	1.1	1.2	1.2	1.1	1.2	1.2	1.2	1.5	1.5	1.5	1.5	1.4
B and H Sovereign Filter	1.2	1.1	1.2	1.1	1.2	1.2	1.3	1.3	1.3	1.5	1.4	1.5	1.4	1.3
B and H Sovereign KS	*	*	*	*	*	*	*	*	*	*	*	*	*	1.2+
B and H (Special F) KS	1.4	1.3	1.2	1.2	1.3	1.2	1.4	1.5	1.5	1.7	1.7	1.7	1.6	1.6
B and H Sterling Filter	1.3	1.2	1.2	1.2	1.4	1.2	1.3	1.4	1.4	1.5	1.6	1.6	1.6	1.5
Black Cat No. 9	*	*	*	*	*	*	0.7	0.7	0.7	1.0	1.0	1.1	1.0	1.0
Cadets	1.1	1.1	1.1	1.1	1.2	1.1	1.0	1.1	1.1	1.2	1.3	1.2	1.2	1.1
Cambridge	1.0	0.9	0.9	1.0	1.0	0.9	0.9	1.0	*	*	*	*	*	*
Consulate Menthol	0.8	0.8	0.8	0.9	0.8	0.8	0.7	0.8	0.5	0.6	0.6	0.6	0.6	0.6
Consulate No. 2	*	*	*	*	..	0.7	0.7	0.7	0.5	0.6	0.6	0.5	0.6	0.6
Craven A KS Filter	*	*	*	*	*	*	*	*	..	..	..	1.4+	1.3	1.3
Du Maurier KS	*	*	*	*	*	*	*	*	*	*	*	*	1.2+	1.1
Dunhill International	1.4	1.4	1.3	1.3	1.3	1.4	1.4	1.3	1.4	1.4	1.4	1.5	1.4	1.3
Dunhill KS	*	*	..	..	1.3	1.1	1.2	1.3	1.3	1.3	1.4	1.3	1.3	1.3
Dunhill Luxury Length	*	*	*	*	*	*	*	*	*	*	*	*	*	*
Embassy Envoy	*	*	*	*	*	*	..	1.3	1.3	1.2	1.3	1.4	1.2	1.2
Embassy Filter	1.3	1.2	1.3	1.3	1.3	1.3	1.4	1.4	1.3	1.4	1.4	1.5	1.4	1.3
Embassy Gold	1.2	1.1	1.2	1.2	1.2	1.2	1.3	1.4	1.3	1.4	1.3	1.4	1.3	1.3
Embassy KS	*	*	*	*	*	*	..	1.6	1.4	1.4	1.4	1.4	1.4	1.3
Embassy No. 1 KS	*	*	*	*	*	*	*	1.5+	1.4	1.4	1.4	1.4	1.4	1.3
Embassy No. 3 Standard Size	*	*	*	*	*	*	*	1.4+	1.3	1.3	1.4	1.5	1.4	1.4
Embassy Regal	1.2	1.1	1.1	1.1	1.2	1.2	1.3	1.3	1.3	1.3	1.4	1.5	1.4	1.3
Gold Leaf F Va	1.5	1.3	1.4	1.3	1.4	1.4	1.5	1.5	1.6	1.6	1.6	1.5	1.5	1.4
Guards	1.3	1.2	1.2	1.2	1.2	1.0	1.1	1.0	1.1	1.1	1.1	1.1	1.1	1.1
J P Carlton Long Size	1.2+	1.3	1.3	1.2	1.4	1.4	1.4	1.4	v	v	v	v	v	v
J P Carlton Premium	1.3+	1.3	1.3	1.3	1.3	1.2	1.3	1.3	v	v	v	v	v	v
John Player KS	*	*	*	*	*	*	1.4	1.5	1.3	1.3	1.4	1.5	1.5	1.4
JP Special Filter	1.4	1.2	1.3	1.3	1.3	1.3	1.4	1.5	v	v	v	v	v	v
JP Special KS	*	*	*	*	*	*	*	*	*	*	*	*	1.4+	1.4
Kensitas Club F Va	1.2	1.2	1.2	1.2	1.3	1.2	1.2	1.3	1.3	1.5	1.5	1.5	1.5	1.4
Kensitas Club KS	*	*	*	*	*	*	*	*	*	1.6	1.6	1.6	1.5	1.4
Kensitas Corsair F Va	1.2	1.2	1.2	1.2	1.3	1.2	1.3	1.3	1.3	1.6	1.5	1.4	1.3	1.2
Kensitas Mild	*	0.8	0.8	0.9	0.9	0.8	1.2	1.2	1.2	1.5	..	*	*	*
Kensitas Tipped	1.4	1.2	1.1	1.2	1.3	1.2	1.3	1.4	1.5	*	*	*	*	*
Kensitas F Va KS	*	*	*	*	*	*	*	*	*	1.7	1.6	1.6	1.5	1.5
Lambert and Butler KS	*	*	*	*	*	*	*	*	*	*	1.4+	1.5	1.5	1.4
London KS	*	*	*	*	*	*	*	*	*	*	*	*	*	..

Brand	LGC survey													
	1	2	3	4	5	6	7	8	9	10	11	12	13	14
	Year of survey													
	1972	73	74	74/75	75	75/76	76	76/77	77	78	78/79	79	79/80	80
Unventilated filter														
Marlboro KS	1.7	1.4	1.3	1.1	1.2	1.2	1.2	1.2	1.1	1.2	1.2	1.3	1.3	1.2
Park Drive Tipped	1.4	1.3	1.3	1.3	1.3	1.2	1.3	1.4	1.4	1.7	1.5	1.5	1.5	1.4
Peter Stuyvesant KS	1.0	1.1	1.2	1.4	1.2	1.2	1.3	1.2	1.0	1.1	1.1	1.1	1.2	1.2
Peter Stuy Luxury Length	1.2	1.2	1.2	1.5	1.3	1.2	*	*	*	*	*	*	*	1.2
Piccadilly Filter De Luxe	1.1	1.0	1.1	1.1	1.1	1.0	1.1	1.1	1.0	1.2	1.3	1.3	1.4	1.3
Piccadilly KS	1.1	1.2	1.2	1.2	1.4	1.2	1.3	1.3	1.4	1.5	1.4	1.5	1.3	1.4
Piccadilly No. 7	0.8	0.8	0.9	0.8	0.7	0.7	0.7	0.7	0.7	1.0	1.0	1.0	1.1	1.0
Player's No. 6 F Va	1.2	1.2	1.3	1.3	1.3	1.2	1.3	1.3	1.2	1.3	1.3	1.3	1.3	1.3
Player's No. 6 KS	1.4	1.2	1.1	1.3	1.3	1.3	1.4	1.5	1.3	1.5	1.6	1.6	1.6	1.5
Player's No. 10 F Va	1.3	1.2	1.3	1.3	1.4	1.2	1.3	1.4	1.3	1.3	1.3	1.3	1.3	1.2
Regal KS (Embassy)	*	*	*	*	*	*	*	*	1.4+	1.5	1.4	1.4	1.4	1.4
Rothmans KS	1.4	1.3	1.3	1.3	1.5	1.4	1.4	1.3	1.4	1.4	1.5	1.4	1.4	1.4
Senior Service Filter	1.3	1.2	1.2	1.2	1.3	1.2	1.4	1.4	..	*	*	*	*	*
Silk Cut No. 1	*	*	..	0.6	0.7	0.7	0.8	0.8	..	*	*	*	*	*
State Exp 555 Filter Kings	*	*	*	*	*	*	*	*	1.3+	1.4	1.4	1.4	1.5	1.3
State Exp 555 Med Mild KS	*	*	*	*	*	*	*	*	*	*	1.2+	1.2	1.3	1.2
St Moritz Lux Length Menthol	1.0	0.9	0.9	1.0	0.9	0.9	0.9	0.9	0.8	0.9	0.9	0.8	0.9	0.8
Winston KS	*	*	*	*	*	*	*	1.3	1.4	1.5	1.4	1.5	1.4	1.3

+ Manufacturer's estimate. Brand recently introduced; not then analysed by LGC for a period of 6 months
* Brand not on market during the survey
u Cigarette filter unventilated during the survey
v Cigarette filter ventilated during the survey
.. Brand not tested by LGC

Source: LGC

Table 8.9.2 Nicotine yield (mg/cigarette) of selected cigarette brands from LGC surveys 15-29, 1981-1989
United Kingdom

	LGC survey														
	15	16	17	18	19	20	21	22	23	24	25	26	27	28	29
	Year of survey														
Brand	81	81/82	82	82/83	83	83/84	84	85	85/86	86	86/87	87	88	88/89	89
Plain															
Capstan Full Strength	2.7	2.6	2.6	2.4	2.5	2.5	2.6	2.6	2.7	2.5	2.5	2.4	2.3	2.3	2.3
Capstan Medium	1.4	1.3	1.3	1.3	1.3	1.3	1.3	1.3	1.5	1.2	1.4	1.2	1.4	1.3	*
Park Drive Plain	1.5	1.5	1.5	1.5	1.5	1.4	1.4	1.4	1.5	1.4	1.5	1.4	1.3	1.3	1.2
Piccadilly No. 1	1.6	1.5	1.4	1.4	1.4	1.4	1.4	1.3	1.4	1.4	1.5	1.4	1.3	1.4	1.4
Player's Medium Navy Cut	1.4	1.4	1.3	1.3	1.2	1.3	1.3	1.3	1.4	1.2	1.3	1.4	1.4	1.2	1.3
Player's No. 6 Plain	1.2	1.1	1.1	1.1	1.1	1.2	1.3	1.3	1.3	1.3	1.3	1.3	1.2	*	*
Senior Service Plain	1.6	1.5	1.5	1.4	1.4	1.4	1.5	1.4	1.5	1.5	1.5	1.4	1.4	1.3	1.3
Weights Plain	1.2	1.1	1.1	1.1	1.1	1.2	1.3	1.3	1.3	1.2	1.3	1.2	1.2	1.2	*
Woodbine Plain	1.5	1.5	1.4	1.5	1.3	1.3	1.3	1.3	1.3	1.3	1.3	1.2	1.2	1.2	1.1
Ventilated filter															
Belair Menthol Kings	0.6	0.7	0.6	0.6	0.6	0.6	0.6	0.6	0.6	0.5	0.5	0.5	0.6	0.6	*
B and H Longer Length/ B and H 100s[1]	*	*	..	1.5	1.5	1.5	1.5	1.3	1.4	1.4	1.4	1.4	1.3	1.2	1.2
B and H XL	*	*	*	*	*	*	*	*	*	*	1.5+	1.4	1.4	1.3	1.4
Berkeley Extra Mild KS	1.0	0.9	0.9	0.9	0.9	0.9	0.9	0.8	0.9	0.8	0.8	0.9	..	*	*
Berkeley Luxury Length/ Berkeley Superkings[2]	*	*	1.4+	1.4	1.3	1.4	*	1.3	1.4	1.4	1.3	1.2	1.2	1.1	1.1
Berkeley Superkings Mild	*	*	*	*	*	*	*	*	*	*	1.0+	1.0	0.9	0.8	0.8
Consulate Menthol	u	0.9	0.8	0.8	0.8	0.8	0.8	0.7	0.8	0.8	0.8	0.8	0.8	0.8	0.9
Consulate No. 2	u	0.7	0.8	0.8	0.8	0.8	0.7	0.6	0.8	0.7	0.7	0.7	0.7	0.7	0.7
Dorchester Extra Mild KS	*	*	*	*	*	*	*	1.0+	0.8	0.8	0.9	0.8	0.9	0.8	0.8
Du Maurier KS	u	u	0.9	0.9	0.9	1.0	0.8	0.7	0.9	*	*	*	*	*	*
Dunhill KS Superior Mild	0.8	0.8	0.8	0.8	0.9	0.8	0.7	0.7	0.8	0.9	0.8	0.8	0.8	0.8	0.8
Embassy Extra Mild	0.8	0.7	0.7	0.8	0.8	0.9	0.8	0.8	0.8	0.7	0.8	0.8	0.8	0.7	0.7
Embassy Filter	u	u	u	u	u	u	u	1.3	1.3	1.2	1.2	1.2	1.2	1.1	1.1
Embassy No. 1 Extra Mild	0.9	0.8	0.8	0.8	0.9	0.9	0.9	0.9	0.9	0.9	0.9	0.8	0.8	0.8	0.8
Embassy No. 3 Standard Size	u	u	u	u	1.3	1.3	1.3	1.3	1.3	1.3	1.2	1.2	1.1	*	*
Embassy No. 5 Extra Mild	0.8	0.7	0.7	0.8	0.7	0.7	0.8	0.7	0.7	0.9	0.7	0.8	*	*	*
Embassy Regal/ Regal Filter[3]	u	u	u	u	u	u	u	u	1.3	1.2	1.3	1.2	1.2	1.1	1.1
J P Carlton Long Size	1.4	1.3	1.3	1.2	1.2	1.2	1.2	1.1	1.3	1.1	1.2	1.1	1.1	*	*
J P Carlton Premium	1.2	1.2	1.1	1.1	1.1	1.1	1.1	1.1	1.1	1.0	1.0	1.0	0.9	*	*
J P King Size	u	u	u	u	u	u	u	u	1.2	1.1	1.1	1.1	1.1	1.0	1.1
J P KS Extra Mild	0.8	1.0	1.0	1.0	1.0	0.9	0.9	0.8	0.9	0.9	0.8	0.8	0.8	0.8	0.8
J P Special Filter	1.5	1.4	1.4	1.4	1.4	1.3	1.3	1.4	1.5	1.4	1.5	1.3	1.3	*	*
J P Superkings	*	*	*	1.6+	1.5	1.6	1.5	1.5	1.4	1.4	1.4	1.4	1.3	1.3	1.4
J P Superkings Low Tar	*	*	*	*	*	*	0.9	0.9	1.0	0.9	0.9	0.9	0.9	0.9	0.8
J P Vanguard KS	1.0	1.0	1.0	0.9	0.9	0.9	0.9	0.9	0.8	0.9	0.8	0.8	0.7	*	*
Lambert and Butler Sp Mild KS	0.9	0.8	0.8	0.9	0.6	0.6	0.5	0.5	0.5	0.5	0.5	0.4	0.4	0.4	0.4
Marlboro KS	u	u	u	u	u	1.1	0.9	0.8	0.9	0.9	0.9	0.9	1.0	1.0	1.0
Marlboro 100s	1.5+	1.4	1.3	1.3	1.2	..	1.0	0.9	1.0	1.1	1.0	1.1	1.1	1.2	1.1

	LGC survey														
	15	16	17	18	19	20	21	22	23	24	25	26	27	28	29
Brand	Year of survey														
	81	81/ 82	82	82/ 83	83	83/ 84	84	85	85/ 86	86	86/ 87	87	88	88/ 89	89
Ventilated filter															
Peter Stuy Lux Length Ex Md	0.9	1.0	0.9	0.8	0.8	0.8	0.8	0.7	0.8	0.8	0.8	0.6	0.7	0.7	0.7
Players's No. 6 Extra Mild	0.7	0.7	0.8	0.7	0.8	0.8	0.8	0.8	0.9	0.7	0.7	0.6	0.7	*	*
Players's No. 10 Extra Mild	0.8	0.8	0.9	0.9	0.8	0.7	0.7	0.6	0.7	0.7	0.7	0.7	*	*	*
Raffles 100s	*	*	*	*	*	1.4	1.3	1.3	1.4	1.3	1.2	1.3	1.1	1.1	1.1
Rothmans Special	*	*	*	*	*	*	*	*	1.3+	1.1	1.1	1.1	0.8	0.9	0.9
State Express 555 Sp Md KS	0.9	0.9	0.9	0.9	0.9	..	*	*	*	*	*	*	*	*	*
Silk Cut	0.9	0.9	0.8	0.8	0.8	0.8	0.8	0.7	0.8	0.8	0.8	0.7	0.7	0.7	0.7
Silk Cut Extra	*	*	*	*	*	*	*	1.0+	1.0	0.9	1.0	0.9	0.8	0.9	0.8
Silk Cut KS	1.0	0.9	0.9	0.9	0.9	1.0	0.9	0.9	0.9	0.9	1.0	0.9	0.8	0.8	0.8
Silk Cut No. 3	0.8	0.8	0.8	0.8	0.8	0.8	0.7	0.7	0.7	0.8	0.8	0.8	0.8	0.7	0.8
Silk Cut No. 5	0.7	0.7	0.7	0.8	0.8	0.8	0.7	0.7	0.8	0.7	0.8	0.7	0.7	0.7	0.7
Unventilated filter															
Ardath KS	*	*	1.3+	1.3	1.3	1.3	1.2	1.2	1.3	*	*	*	*	*	*
B and H Gold Bond Filter	1.4	1.4	1.4	1.4	1.5	1.5	1.5	1.3	1.4	1.4	1.3	1.1	1.2	1.1	1.1
B and H Sovereign Filter	1.3	1.3	1.3	1.1	1.1	1.3	1.4	1.3	1.3	1.4	1.2	1.2	1.2	1.1	0.9
B and H Sovereign KS	1.3	1.2	1.4	1.3	1.4	1.3	1.3	1.2	1.3	1.3	1.2	1.2	1.2	1.2	1.2
B and H (Special F) KS	1.5	1.5	1.5	1.5	1.5	1.5	1.5	1.4	1.5	1.5	1.5	1.2	1.2	1.2	1.2
B and H Sterling Filter	*	*	*	*	*	*	*	*	*	*	*	*	*	*	*
Black Cat No. 9	*	*	*	*	*	*	*	*	*	*	*	*	*	*	*
Cadets	*	*	*	*	*	*	*	*	*	*	*	*	*	*	*
Consulate Menthol	0.7	v	v	v	v	v	v	v	v	v	v	v	v	v	v
Consulate No. 2	0.6	v	v	v	v	v	v	v	v	v	v	v	v	v	v
Craven A KS	1.3	*	*	*	*	1.4	1.3	1.3	1.5	1.4	1.3	1.2	1.3	1.4	1.4
Dorchester KS	*	*	*	*	*	1.2	1.1	1.0	1.1	1.1	1.1	1.2	1.1	1.0	1.1
Du Maurier KS	1.2	1.1	v	v	v	v	v	v	v	v	v	v	v	v	v
Dunhill International	1.5	1.5	1.4	1.4	1.4	1.4	1.4	1.5	1.7	1.5	1.5	1.4	1.5	1.5	1.5
Dunhill KS	1.3	1.2	1.2	1.2	1.2	1.3	1.3	1.3	1.3	1.3	1.3	1.2	1.2	1.3	1.3
Dunhill Luxury Length	*	*	1.3+	1.3	1.3	1.3	1.2	1.2	1.4	1.3	1.3	1.2	1.2	1.3	1.3
Embassy Filter	1.4	1.4	1.4	1.3	1.3	1.3	1.3	v	v	v	v	v	v	v	v
Embassy Gold	1.4	1.3	1.3	1.4	1.3	1.4	1.3	1.3	1.3	1.3	1.3	1.3	1.2	*	*
Embassy KS	1.4	1.3	..	*	*	*	*	*	*	*	*	*	*	*	*
Embassy No. 1 KS	1.5	1.4	1.3	1.3	1.3	1.3	1.3	1.2	1.2	1.2	1.2	1.3	1.3	1.2	1.1
Embassy No. 3 Standard Size	1.4	1.3	1.4	1.3	v	v	v	v	v	v	v	v	v	*	*
Embassy Regal	1.3	1.3	1.4	1.3	1.3	1.3	1.3	1.2	v	v	v	v	v	v	v
Gold Leaf F Va	1.4	1.4	1.4	1.3	1.4	1.3	1.3	1.3	1.4	1.4	1.3	1.4	1.3	1.1	1.1
Goldmark KS	*	*	*	*	*	*	*	*	..	1.1+	1.0	1.0	1.0	0.9	1.0
Guards	1.2	1.3	1.1	1.1	1.2	1.1	1.1	1.1	1.2	1.1	1.1	1.1	1.0	1.1	1.1
John Player KS	1.4	1.4	1.4	1.3	1.3	1.3	1.3	1.2	v	v	v	v	v	v	v
J P Special Filter	v	v	v	v	v	v	v	v	v	v	v	v	v	v	v
J P Special KS	1.4	1.4	1.4	1.5	1.4	1.4	1.4	1.4	1.4	1.4	1.4	1.4	1.3	1.3	1.2

	LGC survey														
	15	16	17	18	19	20	21	22	23	24	25	26	27	28	29
	Year of survey														
Brand	81	81/ 82	82	82/ 83	83	83/ 84	84	85	85/ 86	86	86/ 87	87	88	88/ 89	89
Unventilated filter															
Kensitas Club F Va	1.4	1.4	1.4	1.4	1.5	1.5	1.4	1.3	1.3	1.4	1.3	1.2	1.2	1.1	1.2
Kensitas Club KS	1.4	1.3	1.4	1.4	1.5	1.4	1.4	1.4	1.4	1.5	1.4	1.4	1.3	1.2	1.2
Kensitas Corsair F Va	1.3	1.2	1.3	1.3	1.3	1.3	1.3	1.2	1.3	1.4	1.1	1.1	1.2	1.2	0.9
Kensitas F Va KS	1.5	1.4	1.4	1.4	1.4	1.5	1.5	1.4	1.5	1.4	1.5	1.3	1.2	1.2	1.2
Kingsmen	*	*	*	*	*	*	..	1.2	1.3	1.0	1.1	1.1	1.0	0.9	1.0
Lambert and Butler KS	1.5	1.4	1.4	1.3	1.3	1.3	1.3	1.2	1.3	1.2	1.2	1.2	1.2	1.1	1.1
London KS	1.7	1.9	1.6	1.2	0.9	0.9	0.8	0.9	1.1	1.0	1.2	1.2	1.3	1.2	0.9
Marlboro KS	1.3	1.3	1.3	1.3	1.3	v	v	v	v	v	v	v	v	v	v
Park Drive Tipped	*	*	*	*	*	*	*	*	*	*	*	*	*	*	*
Peter Stuyvesant KS	1.2	1.3	1.3	1.2	1.1	1.0	1.1	1.0	1.0	0.8	0.9	0.9	0.9	1.0	0.9
Peter Stuy Luxury Length	1.4	1.4	1.3	1.2	1.3	1.3	1.4	1.4	1.4	1.4	1.3	1.3	1.3	1.4	1.3
Piccadilly Filter De Luxe	1.5	1.4	1.3	1.3	1.3	1.3	1.2	1.3	1.4	1.2	1.2	1.2	1.2	1.2	1.2
Piccadilly KS	1.3	1.2	1.1	1.2	1.3	1.3	1.2	1.1	1.4	1.3	1.2	1.2	1.2	1.2	1.2
Piccadilly No. 7	1.1	1.1	*	*	*	*	*	*	*	*	*	*	*	*	*
Player's No. 6 F Va	1.4	1.4	1.4	1.4	1.3	1.4	1.3	1.3	1.4	1.4	1.4	1.3	1.3	1.3	1.2
Player's No. 6 KS	1.5	1.4	1.5	1.4	1.3	1.3	1.3	1.3	1.3	1.3	1.3	1.3	1.2	1.2	1.2
Player's No. 10 F Va	1.2	1.2	1.2	1.2	1.2	1.2	1.2	1.2	1.3	1.2	1.2	1.2	1.1	1.1	1.0
Red Band KS	*	*	*	*	*	*	*	..	1.2	1.0	1.0	1.0	1.0	1.0	0.9
Regal KS (Embassy)	1.5	1.4	1.4	1.4	1.3	1.3	1.3	1.2	1.3	1.2	1.3	1.3	1.2	1.2	1.2
Rothmans KS	1.4	1.5	1.4	1.4	1.4	1.4	1.5	1.2	1.6	1.5	1.5	1.4	1.5	1.5	1.6
Spar KS	*	*	*	*	*	*	..	1.2	1.2	1.0	1.0	1.0	1.0	0.9	1.0
State Exp 555 Filter Kings	1.4	1.3	1.3	1.2	1.2	1.3	1.2	1.3	1.3	*	*	*	*	*	*
State Exp 555 Med Mild KS	1.2	1.2	1.2	1.1	1.2	..	*	*	*	*	*	*	*	*	*
St Moritz Lux Length Menthol	0.9	1.1	0.9	1.0	0.9	0.9	0.9	0.9	1.0	0.9	0.9	1.0	0.9	1.0	1.2
Victoria Wine KS/ Victoria Wine Spec F[4]	*	*	*	*	0.9+	0.9	1.0	0.9	1.2	1.2	1.3	1.2	1.6	1.4	1.3
Winston KS	1.4	1.2	1.2	1.2	1.3	1.3	1.3	1.2	1.1	1.1	1.1	1.1	1.1	1.0	0.8

+ Manufacturer's estimate. Brand recently introduced; not then analysed by LGC for a period of 6 months
* Brand not on market during the survey
u Cigarette filter unventilated during the survey
v Cigarette filter ventilated during the survey
.. Brand not tested by LGC

1 Renamed B and H 100s during survey 24
2 Renamed Berkeley Superkings during survey 22
3 Renamed Regal Filter during survey 28
4 Renamed Victoria Wine Spec F during survey 28

Source: LGC

Table 8.10.1 Carbon monoxide yield (mg/cigarette) of selected cigarette brands from LGC surveys 10-21, 1978-1984
United Kingdom

Brand	LGC survey											
	10	11	12	13	14	15	16	17	18	19	20	21
	Year of survey											
	1978	78/ 79	79	79/ 80	80	81	81/ 82	82	82/ 83	83	83/ 84	84
Plain												
Capstan Full Strength	16	16	16	15	14	13	14	14	14	14	14	14
Capstan Medium	15	11	11	11	12	11	11	11	11	11	12	10
Park Drive Plain	13	12	11	12	12	12	12	12	12	12	12	11
Piccadilly No. 1	12	12	10	11	11	10	11	10	10	10	11	11
Player's Medium Navy Cut	13	12	11	11	11	11	11	12	11	11	11	11
Player's No. 6	12	11	11	12	11	11	11	11	11	11	11	10
Senior Service Plain	15	11	11	12	12	12	11	11	11	11	12	11
Weights Plain	14	11	11	11	11	11	11	12	11	11	12	10
Woodbine Plain	13	9	9	10	10	9	10	11	11	11	11	10
Ventilated filter												
Belair Menthol Kings	14	14	14	15	15	14	14	13	13	13	13	13
B and H Longer Length	*	*	*	*	*	*	*	..	14	14	14	14
B and H XL	*	*	*	*	*	*	*	*	*	*	*	*
Berkeley Extra Mild KS	*	*	*	*	*	9	9	9	9	9	9	9
Berkeley Luxury Length	*	*	*	*	*	*	*	14+	15	13	13	..
Berkeley Superkings Mild	*	*	*	*	*	*	*	*	*	*	*	*
Consulate Menthol	u	u	u	u	u	u	10	9	8	8	8	7
Consulate No. 2	u	u	u	u	u	u	8	8	8	7	8	6
Dorchester Extra Mild KS	*	*	*	*	*	*	*	*	*	*	*	*
Du Maurier KS	*	*	*	u	u	u	u	10	10	9	10	9
Dunhill KS Superior Mild	..	9	9	10	10	8	8	8	8	9	8	8
Embassy Extra Mild	11	10	10	11	10	10	10	10	10	10	9	9
Embassy Filter	u	u	u	u	u	u	u	u	u	u	u	u
Embassy No. 1 Extra Mild	13	13	13	14	11	10	10	10	10	11	11	9
Embassy No. 3 Standard Size	u	u	u	u	u	u	u	u	u	13	13	13
Embassy No. 5 Extra Mild	10	9	10	10	10	10	10	9	9	9	8	8
Embassy Regal	u	u	u	u	u	u	u	u	u	u	u	u
J P Carlton Long Size	12	12	12	12	12	11	11	12	10	11	10	10
J P Carlton Premium	11	10	11	12	12	11	11	12	11	11	11	10
J P King Size	u	u	u	u	u	u	u	u	u	u	u	u
J P KS Extra Mild	11	11	11	12	11	10	9	10	10	8	9	9
J P Special Filter	16	16	16	16	16	15	15	16	14	13	12	12
J P Superkings	*	*	*	*	*	*	*	*	15+	15	15	14
J P Superkings Low Tar	*	*	*	*	*	*	*	*	*	*	*	8
J P Vanguard KS	*	*	*	*	13	12	13	13	13	13	12	13
Lambert and Butler Sp Mild KS	*	*	*	14	12	10	10	10	11	7	6	5
Marlboro KS	u	u	u	u	u	u	u	u	u	u	14	13
Marlboro 100s	*	*	*	*	*	12+	13	14	13	12	..	13
Peter Stuy Lux Length Ex Mild	*	*	*	*	10	10	10	10	9	10	10	10
Player's No. 6 Extra Mild	10	11	11	12	12	12	11	11	9	10	9	9

	LGC survey											
	10	11	12	13	14	15	16	17	18	19	20	21
	Year of survey											
Brand	1978	78/79	79	79/80	80	81	81/82	82	82/83	83	83/84	84
Ventilated filter												
Player's No. 10 Extra Mild	12	12	12	13	13	12	12	13	13	12	9	9
Raffles 100s	*	*	*	*	*	*	*	*	*	*	16	15
Rothmans Special	*	*	*	*	*	*	*	*	*	*	*	*
State Express 555 Sp Mild KS	*	*	*	*	*	8	10	10	10	9	..	*
Silk Cut	11	12	10	11	11	10	10	10	10	9	9	9
Silk Cut Extra	*	*	*	*	*	*	*	*	*	*	*	*
Silk Cut KS	12	12	12	13	13	10	10	10	10	9	10	9
Silk Cut No. 3	10	9	10	10	10	9	9	10	9	9	10	9
Silk Cut No. 5	8	8	8	10	10	9	10	10	10	10	10	9
Unventilated filter												
Ardath KS	*	*	*	*	*	*	*	17+	17	16	17	15
B and H Gold Bond Filter	17	17	17	16	17	16	16	16	16	17	16	16
B and H Sovereign Filter	14	14	14	14	15	13	14	14	14	14	14	14
B and H Sovereign KS	*	*	*	*	16+	16	15	18	16	16	15	16
B and H (Special Filter) KS	18	18	18	18	18	17	17	19	19	19	18	16
B and H Sterling Filter	19	18	18	18	17	*	*	*	*	*	*	*
Black Cat No. 9	13	13	14	14	14	*	*	*	*	*	*	*
Cadets	13	11	11	12	13	*	*	*	*	*	*	*
Consulate Menthol	15	15	14	15	12	14	v	v	v	v	v	v
Consulate No. 2	14	13	12	13	13	12	v	v	v	v	v	v
Craven A KS	*	*	16+	16	16	15	*	*	*	*	17	15
Dorchester KS	*	*	*	*	*	*	*	*	*	*	19	17
Du Maurier KS	*	*	*	14+	13	13	12	v	v	v	v	v
Dunhill International	19	15	15	16	15	15	15	15	15	16	16	16
Dunhill KS	17	15	14	15	15	15	14	14	14	14	15	15
Dunhill Luxury Length	*	*	*	*	*	*	*	16+	16	16	17	16
Embassy Envoy	16	17	17	17	17	*	*	*	*	*	*	*
Embassy Filter	18	18	18	18	18	17	17	15	15	14	13	14
Embassy Gold	15	14	15	15	15	15	14	15	14	13	14	13
Embassy KS	19	19	19	20	18	17	16	..	*	*	*	*
Embassy No. 1 KS	19	19	19	20	18	17	16	16	15	15	14	14
Embassy No. 3 Standard Size	18	18	18	18	18	16	17	15	15	v	v	v
Embassy Regal	17	17	17	18	18	17	16	14	14	13	13	13
Gold Leaf F Va	18	18	18	19	18	16	17	17	16	15	16	15
Goldmark KS	*	*	*	*	*	*	*	*	*	*	*	*
Guards	16	16	15	17	15	16	16	15	15	15	15	14
John Player KS	19	19	19	20	20	17	18	16	15	15	13	13
J P Special KS	*	*	*	20+	19	18	19	18	16	15	15	15
Kensitas Club F Va	17	16	15	16	17	15	16	16	15	16	16	15
Kensitas Club KS	19	18	17	18	18	16	17	18	18	18	18	17

	LGC survey											
	10	11	12	13	14	15	16	17	18	19	20	21
	Year of survey											
Brand	1978	78/ 79	79	79/ 80	80	81	81/ 82	82	82/ 83	83	83/ 84	84
Unventilated filter												
Kensitas Corsair F Va	16	15	15	15	14	14	14	14	15	13	14	14
Kensitas Mild	13	..	*	*	*	*	*	*	*	*	*	*
Kensitas F Va KS	18	18	16	17	18	16	17	18	18	18	19	18
Kingsmen	*	*	*	*	*	*	*	*	*	*	*	..
Lambert and Butler KS	*	19+	20	20	19	17	17	16	15	15	14	15
London KS	*	*	*	*	..	16	17	16	16	17	16	16
Marlboro KS	16	15	15	16	16	15	15	16	16	15	v	v
Park Drive Tipped	16	15	15	15	15	*	*	*	*	*	*	*
Peter Stuyvesant KS	15	14	14	15	14	14	14	15	13	14	13	13
Peter Stuyvesant Lux Length	*	*	*	*	16	15	15	16	15	15	16	17
Piccadilly Filter De Luxe	18	16	13	14	14	14	14	15	14	14	13	13
Piccadilly KS	19	15	15	15	15	14	14	14	15	15	15	15
Piccadilly No. 7	13	13	13	14	14	13	13	*	*	*	*	*
Player's No. 6 F Va	18	18	18	18	18	16	18	17	15	14	14	13
Player's No. 6 KS	19	19	20	20	19	17	17	16	16	14	14	14
Player's No. 10 F Va	15	15	15	16	16	15	15	15	15	15	15	15
Red Band KS	*	*	*	*	*	*	*	*	*	*	*	*
Regal KS (Embassy)	19	19	19	20	19	17	17	16	16	15	14	14
Rothmans KS	20	19	18	20	18	15	15	15	16	17	15	15
Spar KS	*	*	*	*	*	*	*	*	*	*	*	..
State Express 555 Filter Kings	17	17	17	17	17	16	16	17	17	15	16	15
State Express 555 Med Mild KS	*	13+	13	14	14	13	13	14	14	14	..	*
St Moritz Lux Length Menthol	16	16	14	15	15	14	15	15	14	14	14	13
Victoria Wine KS	*	*	*	*	*	*	*	*	*	19+	17	16
Winston KS	18	17	17	17	18	16	14	14	15	14	15	15

+ Manufacturer's estimate. Brand recently introduced; not then analysed by LGC for a period of 6 months
* Brand not on market during the survey
u Cigarette filter unventilated during the survey
v Cigarette filter ventilated during the survey
.. Brand not tested by LGC

Source: LGC

Table 8.10.2 Carbon monoxide yield (mg/cigarette) of selected cigarette brands from LGC surveys 22-29, 1985-1989
United Kingdom

	LGC survey							
	22	23	24	25	26	27	28	29
	Year of survey							
Brand	1985	85/ 86	86	86/ 87	87	88	88/ 89	89
Plain								
Capstan Full Strength	14	14	14	13	14	14	14	14
Capstan Medium	11	11	11	11	11	11	11	*
Park Drive Plain	11	11	11	11	11	11	10	10
Piccadilly No. 1	11	11	11	11	10	11	10	11
Player's Medium Navy Cut	11	11	11	11	16	17	11	11
Player's No. 6 Plain	10	10	10	10	10	10	*	*
Senior Service Plain	10	11	11	11	10	10	11	10
Weights Plain	10	10	10	10	10	10	10	*
Woodbine Plain	10	10	10	10	10	10	10	9
Ventilated filter								
Belair Menthol Kings	14	14	13	12	13	13	13	*
B and H Longer Length/ B and H 100s[1]	14	14	15	15	16	17	15	16
B and H XL	*	*	*	13+	13	13	14	14
Berkeley Extra Mild KS	9	9	9	9	10	..	*	*
Berkeley Luxury Length/ Berkeley Superkings[2]	13	14	14	14	14	14	13	13
Berkeley Superkings Mild	*	*	*	9+	9	10	8	8
Consulate Menthol	8	7	8	8	8	7	8	8
Consulate No. 2	7	7	8	7	7	7	7	7
Dorchester Extra Mild KS	10+	9	9	10	10	9	9	9
Du Maurier KS	8	10	*	*	*	*	*	*
Dunhill KS Superior Mild	7	8	8	8	8	8	8	8
Embassy Extra Mild	9	9	9	9	10	9	9	9
Embassy Filter	13	14	13	13	14	13	13	13
Embassy No. 1 Extra Mild	9	9	9	8	9	9	9	8
Embassy No. 3 Standard Size	13	13	13	13	14	14	*	*
Embassy No. 5 Extra Mild	8	8	9	8	9	*	*	*
Embassy Regal/ Regal Filter[3]	u	14	13	13	14	13	13	13
J P Carlton Long Size	11	12	12	11	12	11	*	*
J P Carlton Premium	11	11	11	10	10	10	*	*
J P King Size	u	14	13	13	13	13	13	15
J P KS Extra Mild	9	9	9	9	9	9	9	8
J P Special Filter	13	13	12	13	15	15	*	*
J P Superkings	15	14	14	14	14	13	14	14
J P Superkings Low Tar	8	8	8	8	9	9	9	8
J P Vanguard KS	11	11	11	11	11	11	*	*
Lambert and Butler Sp Mild KS	6	6	5	5	4	5	5	5
Marlboro KS	13	13	14	13	13	12	13	12
Marlboro 100s	14	13	13	12	13	14	14	15

Table 8.10.2 (*continued*) Carbon monoxide yield (mg/cigarette) of selected cigarette brands from LGC surveys 22-29, 1985-1989
United Kingdom

	LGC survey							
	22	23	24	25	26	27	28	29
	Year of survey							
Brand	1985	85/86	86	86/87	87	88	88/89	89
Ventilated filter								
Peter Stuy Lux Length Ex Mild	9	10	10	9	9	9	9	8
Player's No. 6 Extra Mild	9	9	8	8	7	8	*	*
Player's No. 10 Extra Mild	9	8	8	8	7	*	*	*
Raffles 100s	15	16	16	16	16	15	14	14
Rothmans Special	*	9+	9	8	8	7	8	7
State Express 555 Sp Mild KS	*	*	*	*	*	*	*	*
Silk Cut	9	9	10	9	9	9	9	9
Silk Cut Extra	9+	9	9	9	9	9	10	9
Silk Cut KS	10	9	9	9	10	10	10	10
Silk Cut No. 3	9	9	7	9	9	9	9	9
Silk Cut No. 5	9	8	7	8	8	9	8	8
Unventilated filter								
Ardath KS	15	15	*	*	*	*	*	*
B and H Gold Bond Filter	15	16	17	16	15	15	15	15
B and H Sovereign Filter	13	14	14	13	14	14	13	12
B and H Sovereign KS	15	16	16	16	16	17	17	17
B and H (Special Filter) KS	17	17	17	16	15	15	15	16
B and H Sterling Filter	*	*	*	*	*	*	*	*
Black Cat No. 9	*	*	*	*	*	*	*	*
Cadets	*	*	*	*	*	*	*	*
Consulate Menthol	v	v	v	v	v	v	v	v
Consulate No. 2	v	v	v	v	v	v	v	v
Craven A KS	15	17	17	16	15	15	16	16
Dorchester KS	17	17	17	16	17	17	16	16
Du Maurier KS	v	v	v	v	v	v	v	v
Dunhill International	16	16	16	15	15	15	15	15
Dunhill KS	14	15	15	14	13	14	15	14
Dunhill Luxury Length	16	16	16	15	15	16	16	16
Embassy Filter	v	v	v	v	v	v	v	v
Embassy Gold	13	14	13	14	13	12	*	*
Embassy KS	*	*	*	*	*	*	*	*
Embassy No. 1 KS	14	15	15	15	16	16	16	14
Embassy No. 3 Standard Size	v	v	v	v	v	v	*	*
Embassy Regal	13	v	v	v	v	v	v	v
Gold Leaf F Va	15	15	16	15	16	16	14	13
Goldmark KS	*	..	16+	16	15	16	15	16
Guards	15	16	16	15	15	15	14	15
John Player KS	13	v	v	v	v	v	v	v
J P Special F	v	v	v	v	v	v	v	v
J P Special KS	15	16	16	15	16	16	16	15
Kensitas Club F Va	15	15	14	16	15	15	15	14

Table 8.10.2 (*continued*) Carbon monoxide yield (mg/cigarette) of selected cigarette brands from LGC surveys 22-29, 1985-1989
United Kingdom

	LGC survey							
	22	23	24	25	26	27	28	29
	Year of survey							
Brand	1985	85/ 86	86	86/ 87	87	88	88/ 89	89
Unventilated filter								
Kensitas Club KS	17	17	17	16	17	17	17	17
Kensitas Corsair F Va	14	15	14	12	13	14	13	12
Kensitas F Va KS	17	17	17	16	16	15	17	17
Kingsmen	16	16	16	16	15	16	15	15
Lambert and Butler KS	15	16	15	15	15	15	15	15
London KS	16	16	15	15	15	15	14	14
Marlboro KS	v	v	v	v	v	v	v	v
Park Drive Tipped	*	*	*	*	*	*	*	*
Peter Stuyvesant KS	13	13	12	12	13	13	13	13
Peter Stuyvesant Lux Length	16	15	15	14	14	14	13	13
Piccadilly Filter De Luxe	13	13	13	12	12	12	12	12
Piccadilly KS	15	15	15	14	14	14	14	14
Piccadilly No. 7	*	*	*	*	*	*	*	*
Player's No. 6 F VA	14	15	14	14	15	15	15	14
Player's No. 6 KS	14	15	14	15	15	15	15	15
Player's No. 10 F Va	16	16	15	14	13	13	13	13
Red Band KS	..	16	16	16	15	15	15	15
Regal KS (Embassy)	15	15	15	15	16	16	15	15
Rothmans KS	17	15	16	14	14	15	14	14
Spar KS	17	16	17	16	16	15	15	15
State Express 555 Filter Kings	15	*	*	*	*	*	*	*
State Express 555 Med Mild KS	*	*	*	*	*	*	*	*
St Moritz Lux Length Menthol	13	15	15	14	15	15	14	15
Victoria Wine KS/ Victoria Wine Spec F[4]	12	14	16	15	14	14	13	13
Winston KS	15	15	15	16	16	17	16	16

+ Manufacturer's estimate. Brand recently introduced; not then analysed by LGC for a period of 6 months
* Brand not on market during the survey
u Cigarette filter unventilated during the survey
v Cigarette filter ventilated during the survey
.. Brand not tested by LGC

1 Renamed B and H 100s during survey 24
2 Renamed Berkeley Superkings during survey 22
3 Renamed Regal Filter during survey 28
4 Renamed Victoria Wine Spec F during survey 28

Source: LGC

Table 8.11 Percentage market share of cigarette brands, 1, 1972-1987
United Kingdom

Brand	1972	73	74	75	76	77	78	79	80	81	82	83	84	85	86	87
Plain																
Capstan Full Strength	0.5	0.4	0.4	0.3	0.3	0.3	0.3	0.2	..	..	0.3	0.3	..	..	..	..
Capstan Medium	0.5	0.4	0.4	0.3	0.2	0.2	0.1	0.2	..	..						
Park Drive Plain	4.9	4.5	4.4	4.0	3.7	3.4	3.0	2.8	2.5	2.2	1.9	1.5	1.4	1.2	1.0	1.0
Piccadilly No. 1	..	..	..	..	..	..	0.3	0.2	..	..	0.3	0.3	..	..	..	..
Player's Medium Navy Cut	3.5	3.0	2.6	2.2	1.9	1.5	1.5	1.2	1.0	..	0.8	0.5	0.5	..	..	..
Player's No. 6 Plain	1.2	1.2	1.0	0.9	0.8	0.6	0.5	0.4	0.3	..	0.3	0.3	0.3	..	..	..
Senior Service Plain	2.2	2.0	1.8	1.4	1.2	1.0	0.9	0.7	1.0	0.6	0.5	0.5	0.4	..	..	..
Weights Plain	0.8	0.8	0.8	0.6	0.6	0.4	0.4	0.4	0.3	..	0.3	0.3	..	..	..	..
Woodbine Plain	4.0	3.5	3.6	3.1	2.9	2.6	2.5	2.2	2.0	1.6	1.5	1.3	1.0	0.9	0.8	0.8
Ventilated filter																
Belair Menthol Kings	*	u	u	u	u		..	..	0.3	0.3	0.3	0.3	..	..	..	..
B and H Longer Length/ B and H 100s[1]	*	*	*	*	*	*	*	*	*	*	..	..	..	..	..	..
Berkeley Extra Mild KS/ Berkeley Special KS[2]	*	*	*	*	*	*	*	*	*	0.8	1.0	0.8	0.6	..	..	..
Berkeley Luxury Length/ Berkeley Superkings[3]	*	*	*	*	*	*	*	*	*	*	0.5	1.3	0.9	2.7	4.8	6.5
Consulate Menthol	u	u	u	u	u	u	u	u	u	..	0.5	0.8	0.6	0.8	0.8	
Consulate No. 2	*	*	*	u	u	u	u	u	u	..	..	..	0.1	1.3	1.3	
Du Maurier KS	*	*	*	*	*	*	*	*	u	u	1.5	0.8	..	..	*	*
Dunhill KS Superior Mild	*	*	*	*	*	*	..	..	..	..	0.5	0.5	0.5	..	..	..
Embassy Extra Mild	..	..	1.3	1.8	2.2	1.6	1.0	0.8	0.5	..	0.3	0.3	0.2	..	..	..
Embassy Filter	u	u	u	u	u	u	u	u	u	u	u	u	u	2.9	2.5	2.5
Embassy No. 1 Extra Mild	*	*	*	*	*	0.4	2.0	..	1.8	..	1.5	1.8	1.5	1.3	1.0	1.0
Embassy No. 3 Standard Size	*	*	*	*	*	u	u	u	u	u	u	0.3	..	..	..	..
Embassy No. 5 Extra Mild	*	*	*	*	0.5	0.3	0.1	0.1	..	..	..	..	..	..	..	..
Embassy Regal[4]	u	u	u	u	u	u	u	u	u	u	u	u	u	u	2.3	2.0
J P Carlton Long Size	u	u	u	u	u	1.4	1.0	0.8	0.5	..	0.3	0.3	0.3	..	..	..
J P Carlton Premium	u	u	u	u	u	1.0	0.4	0.2	..	..	..	..	..	..	..	..
J P King Size[4]	*	*	*	*	u	u	u	u	u	u	u	u	u	u	0.5	0.5
J P KS Extra Mild	*	*	*	0.5	1.3	1.5	..	..	..	..	..	..	..	..	..	..
J P Special Filter	u	u	u	u	u	0.1	0.1	0.1	..	..	..	..	..	..	..	..
J P Superkings	*	*	*	*	*	*	*	*	*	*	0.5	3.3	5.5	6.3	6.3	5.5
J P Superkings Low Tar	*	*	*	*	*	*	*	*	*	*	*	*	*	1.1	1.0	1.0
J P Vanguard KS	*	*	*	*	*	*	*	*	..	1.3	0.8	0.5	0.4	..	..	..
Lambert and Butler Sp Mild KS	*	*	*	*	*	*	*	..	0.8	1.0	0.5	0.8	0.8	1.0	1.3	1.3
Marlboro KS	u	u	u	u	u	u	u	u	u	u	u	2.0	2.5	2.3	2.0	1.8
Marlboro 100s	*	*	*	*	*	*	*	*	*	..	0.5	0.5	0.3	..	..	..
Peter Stuy Lux Length Ex Md	*	*	*	*	*	*	*	*	..	1.0	1.0	1.2	1.0	0.9	0.8	0.5
Player's No. 6 Extra Mild	..	..	0.3	0.3	0.5	0.5	0.1	0.2	..	..	..	..	..	..	..	..
Player's No. 10 Extra Mild	*	*	*	0.2	1.0	1.0	0.5	0.4	..	..	..	0.3	..	..	..	..
Raffles 100s	*	*	*	*	*	*	*	*	*	*	..	..	0.7	2.6	2.0	2.3
State Express 555 Sp Mild KS	*	*	*	*	*	*	*	*	*	..	0.3	0.3	..	*	*	*
Silk Cut	1.1	2.2	2.6	2.3	2.4	2.3	2.0	1.5	1.0	0.9	0.6	0.5	0.3	..	..	..
Silk Cut KS	..	0.5	0.6	0.6	0.8	1.2	3.5	4.1	4.9	5.0	5.3	5.3	5.6	5.6	5.8	6.3
Silk Cut No. 3	..	0.7	1.1	1.6	2.4	1.9	1.1	1.0	1.0	0.8	0.5	0.5	0.3	..	..	..
Silk Cut No. 5	*	*	*	*	0.3	0.7	0.4	0.3	..	..	..	..	..	..	..	..

Brand	1972	73	74	75	76	77	78	79	80	81	82	83	84	85	86	87
Unventilated filter																
Albany	0.5	*	*	*	*	*	*	*	*	*	*	*	*	*	*	*
Ardath KS	*	*	*	*	*	*	*	*	*	*	1.3	2.5	0.5	..	*	*
Belair Menthol Kings	*	..	..	v	v	v	v	v	v	v	v	v	v	v	v	v
B and H Gold Bond Filter	1.2	1.2	1.2	1.0	0.7	0.5	0.2	0.2	..	..	..	..	..	..	..	..
B and H Sovereign Filter	3.8	3.4	3.2	3.6	3.1	3.6	1.3	0.9	1.0	..	..	..	..	..	..	..
B and H Sovereign KS	*	*	*	*	*	*	*	*	..	..	..	..	..	..	..	..
B and H (Special F) KS	4.6	5.5	5.8	4.9	5.2	8.4	11.9	12.8	12.3	14.2	16.2	17.8	18.3	18.2	18.5	19.0
B and H Sterling Filter	0.6	0.5	0.4	0.3	0.2	0.1	0.1	0.1	*	*	*	*	*	*	*	*
Black Cat No. 9	*	*	*	*	0.3	0.4	..	*	*	*	*	*	*	*	*	*
Cadets	2.0	1.8	1.6	1.8	1.1	1.1	0.4	0.2	..	*	*	*	*	*	*	*
Cambridge	1.0	0.7	0.6	0.4	0.4	0.2	*	*	*	*	*	*	*	*	*	*
Consulate Menthol	1.0	1.0	1.0	0.9	0.7	0.6	0.6	0.7	..	v	v	v	v	v	v	v
Consulate No. 2	*	*	0.2	0.3	0.3	0.2	0.2		1.0	v	v	v	v	v	v	v
Craven A KS	*	*	*	*	*	*	*	*	..	..	..	..	..	..	*	*
Du Maurier KS	*	*	*	*	*	*	*	*	..	1.7	v	v	v	v	*	*
Dunhill International	..	..	0.6	0.5	0.4	0.4	0.5	0.6	..	..	0.5	0.3	0.5	..	..	..
Dunhill KS	*	*	..	..	..	..	3.4	3.4	2.0	2.7	3.0	3.5	3.3	2.6	1.8	1.5
Dunhill Luxury Length	*	*	*	*	*	*	*	*	..	..	1.5	1.0	0.8	..	..	..
Embassy Envoy	*	*	*	*	0.5	0.3	..	..	..	*	*	*	*	*	*	*
Embassy Filter	19.0	18.2	17.3	15.4	12.3	8.2	6.1	5.7	5.2	4.6	4.0	3.5	3.0	v	v	v
Embassy Gold	1.5	1.6	1.6	1.7	1.4	1.0	0.4	0.2	..	..	..	..	..	..	..	..
Embassy KS	*	*	*	*	0.5	0.7	..	..	..	*	*	*	*	*	*	*
Embassy No. 1 KS	*	*	*	*	*	3.0	5.5	4.7	4.2	3.3	3.3	3.3	3.2	3.1	3.0	2.8
Embassy No. 3 Standard Size	*	*	*	*	*	2.6	1.0	0.6	1.8	..	0.3	v	v	v	v	v
Embassy Regal[4]	6.2	7.2	8.4	10.5	10.3	8.7	6.2	5.8	4.7	4.7	4.0	3.5	3.0	2.7	v	v
Gold Leaf F Va	1.4	1.3	1.3	1.1	0.9	0.8	0.7	0.7	0.5	..	0.5	0.3	0.3	..	..	..
Guards	1.3	1.1	1.0	0.9	0.8	0.7	0.4	0.2	..	..	..	..	..	..	..	..
J P Carlton Long Size	..	0.8	1.2	1.3	1.4	v	v	v	v	v	v	v	v	v	v	v
J P Carlton Premium	..	0.5	0.5	0.8	0.9	v	v	v	v	v	v	v	v	v	v	v
John Player KS[4]	*	*	*	*	2.6	3.3	4.0	4.6	4.0	2.2	1.5	1.3	1.0	0.8	v	v
J P Special Filter	0.3	0.5	0.5	0.4	0.3	v	v	v	v	v	v	v	v	v	v	v
J P Special KS	*	*	*	*	*	*	*	*	..	9.5	11.3	8.5	7.0	6.0	5.0	4.5
Kensitas Club F Va	0.5	0.6	0.9	1.4	1.1	0.7	..	..	..	..	..	..	..	..	..	..
Kensitas Club KS	*	*	*	*	*	*	1.0	1.2	1.5	1.2	1.3	1.5	1.8	1.8	1.8	1.8
Kensitas Corsair F Va	0.5	0.5	0.5	0.4	0.7	0.3	0.2	0.1	..	..	..	..	..	..	..	..
Kensitas Mild	*	..	..	0.1	0.3	0.3	*	*	*	*	*	*	*	*	*	*
Kensitas Tipped	2.5	2.2	2.2	1.9	1.0	0.7	*	*	*	*	*	*	*	*	*	*
Kensitas F Va KS	*	*	*	*	*	*	*	..	..	..	0.3	0.3	..	..	..	..
Lambert and Butler KS	*	*	*	*	*	*	*	*	..	2.4	1.3	2.0	2.0	2.4	3.5	3.5
London KS	*	*	*	*	*	*	*	*	..	0.9	1.0	0.3	0.5	..	..	..
Marlboro KS	..	..	..	..	..	..	1.1	1.6	..	2.3	2.0	v	v	v	v	v
Park Drive Tipped	0.8	0.6	0.6	0.6	0.6	0.6	0.3	0.3	..	..	..	..	..	*	*	*
Peter Stuyvesant KS	..	..	0.3	0.3	0.4	0.6	0.4	0.3	1.0	..	..	..	..	..	..	..
Peter Stuyvesant Lux Length	*	*	*	*	*	*	*	..	..	2.0	2.5	2.0	1.7	1.3	1.0	0.8
Piccadilly Filter De Luxe	1.3	1.3	1.4	1.3	1.0	0.8	1.1	0.9	..	..	0.3	0.3	0.3	..	..	..
Piccadilly KS	..	..	..	..	0.4	0.9	0.3	..	..	..	..	..	..	..	..	..
Piccadilly No. 7	..	..	0.3	0.3	0.5	0.1	0.1	0.1	..	..	*	*	*	*	*	*

Brand	1972	73	74	75	76	77	78	79	80	81	82	83	84	85	86	87
Unventilated filter																
Player's No. 6 F Va	19.2	18.5	17.9	18.5	17.6	14.6	8.0	6.8	5.8	3.8	3.0	2.5	2.0	1.8	1.5	1.5
Player's No. 6 KS	..	..	..	..	..	..	5.0	5.2	4.0	3.9	3.3	2.5	2.0	1.5	1.0	1.0
Player's No. 10 F Va	4.6	4.0	4.5	5.0	4.3	4.7	1.8	1.1	0.8	..	0.5	0.2	..	..	..	..
Regal KS (Embassy)	*	*	*	*	*	..	3.8	3.0	2.7	4.1	5.2	5.8	6.0	6.1	5.8	6.0
Rothmans KS	1.4	1.4	1.6	1.5	2.0	3.7	4.0	4.5	4.2	3.3	3.3	3.5	3.0	2.7	2.8	2.5
Senior Service Filter	0.2	0.2	0.2	0.1	0.1	0.1	*	*	*	*	*	*	*	*	*	*
Silk Cut No. 1	*	*	..	..	0.4	0.1	*	*	*	*	*	*	*	*	*	*
State Express 555 Filter Kings	*	*	*	*	*	..	3.0	2.8	..	2.8	2.3	1.8	0.3	..	*	*
State Express 555 Med Mild KS	*	*	*	*	*	*	*	..	..	0.9	0.5	0.3	..	*	*	*
St Moritz Lux Length Menthol	..	..	..	..	..	..	..	..	..	..	0.3	0.3	0.3	*	*	*
Winston KS	*	*	*	*	*	..	0.3	0.3	..	..	..	..	..	..	..	..

* Brand not on market for entire year
u Cigarette filter unventilated for all or part of the year
v Cigarette filter ventilated for all or part of the year
.. Market share not published

1 Renamed B and H 100s in 1986
2 Renamed Berkeley Special KS in 1987
3 Renamed Berkeley Superkings in 1985
4 Embassy Regal and John Player KS had unventilated filters during survey 22, and ventilated filters during survey 23

Note: The market share quoted for a given brand in a given year sometimes varies according to the issue of *World Tobacco*. Some market shares may include the market share for a brand or brands of similar name to the one stated, and same manufacturer

Source: *World Tobacco* (Maxwell international estimates)

Brand	1972	73	74	75	76	77	78	79	80	81	82	83	84	85	86	87	88
Plain																	
Capstan Full Strength	..	..	..	..	..	..	..	..	..	..	..	..	..	..	..	..	..
Capstan Medium	..	..	..	..	..	..	..	..	..	..	..	..	..	..	..	..	..
Park Drive	4.7	4.5	4.5	4.2	3.7	3.0	3.0	2.8	2.5	2.0	2.0	1.6	1.4	1.2	1.1	0.9	0.8
Piccadilly No. 1	..	..	..	..	..	0.3	0.3	0.3	0.2	0.2	0.2	..	..	..	..	..	..
Player's Med Navy Cut	3.3	2.8	2.5	2.2	1.9	1.5	1.4	1.2	1.0	0.8	0.8	0.7	0.6	0.5	0.5	0.4	0.4
Player's No. 6 Plain	1.3	1.0	0.9	0.8	..	..	..	..	..	0.2	0.2	0.2	..	..	..	..	..
Senior Service Plain	2.3	2.0	2.0	1.5	1.2	1.0	0.8	0.7	0.5	0.5	0.5	0.5	0.4	0.4	0.3	0.3	0.3
Weights Plain	0.7	0.7	0.6	0.5	..	..	..	..	..	0.2	0.2	0.2	..	..	..	..	..
Woodbine Plain	4.3	3.7	3.5	3.4	2.9	2.5	2.5	2.2	1.8	1.5	1.5	1.2	1.0	0.9	0.7	0.6	0.6
Ventilated filter																	
Belair Menthol Kings	*	u	u	u	u	..	..	..	..	..	..	..	..	..	..	..	..
B and H Longer Length/ B and H 100s[1]	*	*	*	*	*	*	*	*	*	*	..	1.2	1.0	0.9	0.9	0.8	0.7
B and H XL	*	*	*	*	*	*	*	*	*	*	*	*	*	*	..	0.9	0.8
Berkeley Extra Mild KS/ Berkeley Spec KS[2]	*	*	*	*	*	*	*	*	*	0.7	0.8	0.8	0.6	..	..	..	..
Berkeley Luxury Length/ Berkeley Superkings[3]	*	*	*	*	*	*	*	*	*	*	0.5	1.2	1.3	2.7	4.8	6.4	7.4
Berkeley Superkings Mild	*	*	*	*	*	*	*	*	*	*	*	*	*	*	..	0.4	0.8
Consulate Menthol	u	u	u	u	u	u	u	u	u	0.5	0.3	0.5	0.7	0.5	0.5	0.5	0.5
Consulate No. 2	*	*	*	u	u	u	u	u	u	..	..	..	..	..	..	..	..
Dorchester Extra Mild KS	*	*	*	*	*	*	*	*	*	*	*	*	..	0.3	0.7	0.5	0.6
Du Maurier KS	*	*	*	*	*	*	*	*	u	1.5	0.8	..	..	..	..	..	..
Dunhill KS Superior Mild	*	*	*	*	*	*	..	..	0.3	0.3	0.5	0.3	..	..	..	..	..
Embassy Extra Mild	..	..	1.1	2.2	2.2	1.5	0.9	0.8	0.7	0.5	0.5	0.2	..	..	..	..	..
Embassy Filter	u	u	u	u	u	u	u	u	u	u	u	u	u	2.9	2.6	2.4	2.3
Embassy No. 1 Extra Mild	*	*	*	*	*	1.0	2.0	2.0	1.8	1.5	1.5	1.7	1.5	1.2	1.0	0.9	0.8
Embassy No. 3 Standard Size	*	*	*	*	*	u	u	u	u	u	u	..	..	..	..	..	..
Embassy No. 5 Extra Mild	*	*	*	*	*	..	..	..	..	..	..	..	..	..	..	..	*
Embassy Regal/ Regal Filter[4,5]	u	u	u	u	u	u	u	u	u	u	u	u	u	u	2.3	2.1	2.0
J P Carlton Long Size	u	u	u	u	u	1.3	0.9	0.8	0.7	0.5	0.5	0.2	..	..	..	..	*
J P Carlton Premium	u	u	u	u	u	1.1	..	..	..	..	..	..	..	..	..	..	..
J P King Size[5]	u	u	u	u	u	u	u	u	u	u	u	u	u	u	0.6	0.5	0.4
J P KS Extra Mild	*	*	*	*	..	1.4	1.5	1.8	1.3	0.7	0.8	0.8	1.0	..	..	..	..
J P Special Filter	u	u	u	u	u	..	..	..	..	..	..	..	..	..	..	..	*
J P Superkings	*	*	*	*	*	*	*	*	*	*	0.2	3.4	5.6	6.3	6.2	5.5	4.4
J P Superkings Low Tar	*	*	*	*	*	*	*	*	*	*	*	*	..	1.1	0.9	0.9	0.7
J P Vanguard KS	*	*	*	*	*	*	*	*	2.0	1.3	0.8	0.3	..	..	..	..	*
Lambert and Butler Sp Mild KS	*	*	*	*	*	*	*	0.3	0.9	1.0	0.3	0.8	0.7	1.0	1.2	1.1	1.1
Lambert and Butler 100s	*	*	*	*	*	*	*	*	*	*	*	*	*	*	0.6	1.5	2.6
Marlboro KS	u	u	u	u	u	u	u	u	u	u	u	2.0	2.0	2.4	2.1	1.8	1.7
Marlboro 100s	*	*	*	*	*	*	*	*	*	..	..	0.5	..	..	..	..	..
Peter Stuy Lux Length Ex Md	*	*	*	*	*	*	*	*	0.5	1.0	1.3	1.2	1.0	1.0	0.7	0.6	0.4
Player's No. 6 Extra Mild	..	..	..	..	..	..	..	..	..	..	..	..	..	..	..	..	*
Player's No. 10 Extra Mild	*	*	*	1.0	1.0	1.0	..	..	..	..	..	..	..	..	..	..	..
Raffles 100s	*	*	*	*	*	*	*	*	*	*	*	..	2.0	2.6	1.9	2.2	2.2
State Express 555 Sp Mild KS	*	*	*	*	*	*	*	*	*	0.3	..	..	..	*	*	*	*

Table 8.12 (*continued*) Percentage market share of cigarette brands, 2, 1972-1988
United Kingdom

Brand	1972	73	74	75	76	77	78	79	80	81	82	83	84	85	86	87	88
Ventilated filter																	
Silk Cut	1.3	2.0	2.5	2.3	2.3	2.1	1.8	1.5	1.2	1.0	0.8	0.5	0.3	0.3	0.2	0.2	0.2
Silk Cut Extra	*	*	*	*	*	*	*	*	*	*	*	*	*	0.4	0.8	0.9	0.9
Silk Cut KS	..	..	..	..	..	1.0	3.5	4.1	4.8	4.3	5.5	5.8	5.6	5.6	5.8	6.1	7.1
Silk Cut No. 3	..	..	1.0	2.0	2.4	1.9	1.3	1.0	0.9	0.7	0.7	0.4	0.3	..	..	..	..
Silk Cut No. 5	*	*	*	..	..	..	..	..	..	..	..	..	..	..	..	..	..
Unventilated filter																	
Albany	..	*	*	*	*	*	*	*	*	*	*	*	*	*	*	*	*
Ardath KS	*	*	*	*	*	*	*	*	*	*	1.2	2.5	0.4	..	*	*	*
Belair Menthol Kings	*	..	..	..	..	v	v	v	v	v	v	v	v	v	v	v	v
B and H Gold Bond Filter	1.0	1.0	1.0	1.0	0.7	..	..	..	..	..	..	..	..	..	..	..	..
B and H Sovereign Filter	3.7	3.5	3.5	3.6	3.5	3.9	1.3	0.9	0.7	..	..	..	..	..	..	..	..
B and H Sovereign KS	*	*	*	*	*	*	*	*	1.0	0.8	..	..	..	..	..	..	..
B and H (Special F) KS	4.0	6.0	6.0	4.8	5.2	9.0	11.8	12.8	14.3	14.5	16.0	17.5	18.3	18.2	18.4	18.9	19.8
B and H Sterling Filter	0.8	0.8	..	..	..	..	..	..	..	*	*	*	*	*	*	*	*
Black Cat No. 9	*	*	*	*	*	*	..	..	..	*	*	*	*	*	*	*	*
Cadets	1.8	2.0	1.5	1.6	1.1	1.0	..	..	..	..	..	..	..	..	..	..	..
Cambridge	0.9	1.0	..	..	..	..	*	..	..	..	..	..	..	..	..	..	..
Consulate Menthol	1.1	1.1	1.1	0.9	..	..	..	0.7	0.6	v	v	v	v	v	v	v	v
Consulate No. 2	*	*	*	*	..	..	..	..	..	v	v	v	v	v	v	v	v
Craven A KS	*	*	*	*	*	*	*	0.8	1.6	..	..	..	..	1.1	1.2	1.3	0.9
Dorchester KS	*	*	*	*	*	*	*	*	*	..	..	..	2.0	2.3	2.6	1.9	2.4
Du Maurier KS	*	*	*	*	*	*	*	*	*	0.6	1.8	v	v	*	*	*	*
Dunhill International	..	..	..	..	..	..	..	0.5	0.5	0.5	0.3	0.4	0.4	..	..	..	..
Dunhill KS	*	*	..	..	..	..	3.5	3.4	2.2	2.8	3.0	3.4	3.6	2.6	1.9	1.6	1.7
Dunhill Luxury Length	*	*	*	*	*	*	*	*	*	*	1.7	1.2	0.7	..	..	..	..
Embassy Envoy	*	*	*	*	*	*	..	..	..	..	..	..	..	..	..	..	..
Embassy Filter	19.5	18.5	16.8	15.3	12.3	7.5	6.2	5.8	5.3	4.5	4.0	3.5	3.2	v	v	v	v
Embassy Gold	1.7	1.7	1.6	1.9	1.4	1.1	..	..	..	..	..	..	..	..	..	..	*
Embassy KS	*	*	*	*	..	..	..	..	..	..	..	*	*	..	..	..	..
Embassy No. 1 KS	*	*	*	*	*	3.8	5.5	5.1	4.5	3.5	3.2	3.4	3.2	3.1	2.9	2.8	2.8
Embassy No. 3 Standard Size	*	*	*	*	*	2.0	1.0	..	..	..	..	..	v	v	v	v	v
Embassy Regal/ Regal Filter[4,5]	6.8	7.1	8.6	11.0	10.3	8.6	6.3	5.8	5.7	4.8	4.0	3.5	3.1	2.7	v	v	v
Gold Leaf F Va	1.3	1.1	1.1	0.9	..	..	0.7	0.8	0.7	0.5	0.5	0.4	0.3	0.2	0.2	0.2	0.2
Goldmark	*	*	*	*	*	*	*	*	*	*	*	*	*	0.3	0.5	0.4	0.3
Guards	1.2	1.1	1.0	1.0	0.7	..	..	..	..	..	..	..	..	..	..	..	..
J P Carlton Long Size	..	..	1.1	1.4	1.4	v	v	v	v	v	v	v	v	v	v	v	*
J P Carlton Premium	..	..	..	..	..	v	v	v	v	v	v	v	v	v	v	v	*
John Player KS[5]	*	*	*	*	2.6	3.4	4.0	4.6	3.9	2.2	1.5	1.2	1.0	0.8	0.6	0.5	0.4
J P Special Filter	..	..	..	..	..	v	v	v	v	v	v	v	v	v	v	v	*
J P Special KS	*	*	*	*	*	*	*	*	3.7	9.5	11.0	8.5	7.0	6.0	4.9	4.6	4.4
Kensitas Club F Va	..	..	1.0	1.4	1.5	..	..	..	..	..	..	..	..	..	..	..	..
Kensitas Club KS	*	*	*	*	*	*	1.0	1.2	1.4	1.3	1.2	1.7	1.8	1.8	1.8	1.8	1.8
Kensitas Corsair F Va	..	..	..	..	..	..	..	..	..	..	..	..	..	..	..	..	..
Kensitas Mild	*	..	..	..	..	..	*	*	*	*	*	*	*	*	*	*	*
Kensitas Tipped	1.2	2.5	2.5	1.8	1.0	..	..	..	..	..	..	..	..	..	..	..	..
Kensitas F Va KS	*	*	*	*	*	..	0.5	0.5	0.5	0.3	0.3	0.2	*	..	..	..	..
Kingsmen	*	*	*	*	*	*	*	*	*	*	*	*	*	0.9	0.8	0.7	0.7

Brand	1972	73	74	75	76	77	78	79	80	81	82	83	84	85	86	87	88
Unventilated filter																	
Lambert and Butler KS	*	*	*	*	*	*	*	3.8	2.2	2.5	1.2	2.0	2.0	2.4	3.5	3.5	3.5
London KS	*	*	*	*	*	*	*	*	..	1.0	0.5	0.2	0.4	..	..	..	..
Marlboro KS	..	..	..	1.0	..	..	1.1	1.5	1.9	2.2	2.3	v	v	v	v	v	v
Park Drive Tipped	0.4	..	..	..	..	..	..	..	..	..	..	..	..	*	*	*	*
Peter Stuyvesant KS	..	..	..	..	..	..	..	..	..	..	..	..	..	..	..	..	..
Peter Stuy Lux Length	..	..	..	..	*	*	*	*	1.2	2.0	1.8	2.0	1.7	1.1	0.9	0.7	0.6
Piccadilly Filter De Luxe	1.4	1.4	1.2	1.1	1.5	1.0	1.1	0.9	0.7	0.5	0.5	0.2	..	..	..	..	..
Piccadilly KS	..	..	..	..	..	..	1.0	..	..	..	..	..	..	..	..	..	..
Piccadilly No. 7	..	..	..	..	..	..	..	..	..	..	*	*	*	*	*	*	..
Player's No. 6 F Va	19.8	18.5	18.3	19.0	17.6	14.0	8.1	6.9	5.5	3.8	3.0	2.5	2.1	1.7	1.4	1.2	1.1
Player's No. 6 KS	..	..	..	..	..	..	5.3	4.9	3.8	4.0	3.2	2.5	2.0	1.5	1.1	0.9	0.8
Player's No. 10 F Va	4.7	4.2	4.2	4.8	4.3	4.7	1.7	1.0	0.8	0.5	0.5	0.4	..	..	..	..	..
Red Band KS	*	*	*	*	*	*	*	*	*	*	*	*	..	0.9	1.0	0.9	0.9
Regal KS (Embassy)	*	*	*	*	*	..	3.6	3.0	3.0	5.0	5.5	5.8	6.0	6.1	5.8	6.0	6.0
Rothmans KS	1.5	1.8	1.6	1.2	3.1	4.0	4.0	4.6	3.9	3.5	3.2	3.4	3.2	2.7	2.7	2.5	2.3
Senior Service Filter	..	..	..	..	..	..	*	*	*	*	*	*	*	*	*	*	*
Silk Cut No. 1	*	*	..	..	..	..	*	*	*	*	*	*	*	*	*	*	*
State Express 555 Filter Kings	*	*	*	*	*	*	..	2.9	1.7	2.2	3.0	2.3	1.7	0.4	..	*	*
State Express 555 Med M KS	*	*	*	*	*	*	*	..	1.1	0.8	1.0	0.5	0.3	..	*	*	*
St Moritz Lux Length Menthol	..	..	..	..	..	..	..	..	..	..	..	..	..	..	..	..	..
Winston KS	*	*	*	*	*	..	..	..	..	..	..	..	..	..	..	..	..

* Brand not on market for entire year
u Cigarette filter unventilated for all or part of the year
v Cigarette filter ventilated for all or part of the year
.. Market share not published

1 Renamed B and H 100s in 1986
2 Renamed Berkeley Special KS in 1987
3 Renamed Berkeley Superkings in 1985
4 Renamed Regal Filter in 1988
5 Embassy Regal and John Player KS had unventilated filters during survey 22, and ventilated filters during survey 23

Note: the market share quoted for a given brand in a given year sometimes varies according to the issue of *Tobacco*. Some market shares may include the market share for a brand or brands of similar name to the one stated, and same manufacturer

Source: *Tobacco* (brand shares of the UK cigarette market)

Table 8.13 Percentage market share of sales in each tar band, 1972-1988
United Kingdom

Year	Tar band					
	Low	Low/middle	Middle	Middle/high	High	Unspecified
Data derived from market shares listed in *World Tobacco*						
1972	0.0	3.1	73.4	14.4	3.2	5.9
1973	0.5	5.4	72.1	15.4	0.4	6.2
1974	0.9	8.9	72.7	14.6	0.4	2.5
1975	4.8	5.9	73.2	12.5	0.3	3.3
1976	7.3	10.8	67.6	10.5	0.3	3.5
1977	11.2	8.1	67.6	9.1	0.3	3.7
1978	12.5	5.0	70.9	8.4	0.3	2.9
1979	8.9	8.1	70.7	0.2	0.0	12.1
1980	11.3	3.5	59.8	0.0	*	25.4
1981	11.1	7.9	67.0	0.0	*	14.0
1982	14.6	36.5	45.4	0.3	*	3.2
1983	13.9	45.2	36.3	0.3	*	4.3
1984	12.3	47.6	26.7	0.0	*	13.4
1985[1]	12.2	28.7	45.5	-	0.2	13.1
1986[1]	12.0	38.0	29.9	-	0.0	20.1
1987[1]	12.2	57.2	10.6	-	0.0	20.0
1988[1]	..	..	..	-	..	..
Data derived from market shares listed in *Tobacco*						
1972	0.0	3.3	70.8	14.3	2.3	9.3
1973	0.0	4.1	71.2	14.7	0.0	10.0
1974	0.0	6.8	69.9	14.0	0.0	9.3
1975	4.3	6.5	70.4	12.6	0.0	6.2
1976	4.7	6.4	65.0	9.7	0.0	14.2
1977	8.9	5.4	62.0	8.0	0.0	15.7
1978	11.0	3.1	68.4	8.0	0.0	9.5
1979	12.2	7.7	71.9	0.0	0.0	8.2
1980	14.7	9.0	70.4	0.0	*	5.9
1981	13.8	9.3	72.6	0.0	*	4.3
1982	15.1	34.4	44.6	0.0	*	5.9
1983	14.3	45.2	36.3	0.0	*	4.2
1984	12.0	49.4	26.7	0.0	*	11.9
1985[1]	13.3	31.1	48.0	-	0.0	7.6
1986[1]	11.8	40.5	35.4	-	0.3	12.0
1987[1]	12.1	61.6	14.5	-	0.0	11.8
1988[1]	13.1	62.7	14.1	-	0.0	10.1

* Cigarettes in this tar band no longer on the market
1 The definitions of the tar bands altered in 1985:

	1972-1984	1985-
Low	0-10 mg tar/cigarette	0- 9.99 mg tar/cigarette
Low/middle	11-16 mg tar/cigarette	10.0-14.99 mg tar/cigarette
Middle	17-22 mg tar/cigarette	15.0-17.99 mg tar/cigarette
Middle/high	23-28 mg tar/cigarette	no middle/high band
High	29+ mg tar/cigarette	18.0+ mg tar/cigarette
	(data rounded)	(data truncated)

Source: *World Tobacco* (Maxwell international estimates)
Tobacco (brand shares of the UK cigarette market)

Table 8.14 Yields (mg/cigarette) of tar, nicotine, carbon monoxide, total aldehydes, nitrogen monoxide, total cyanide, acrolein, and formaldehyde: by cigarette brand (75 brands, survey period October 1982-March 1983), United Kingdom

Cigarette brand	Tar	Nicotine	Carbon monoxide CO	Total aldehydes RCHO	Nitrogen monoxide NO	Total cyanide HCN	Acrolein	Formaldehyde HCHO	Market share 1982 %
J Player KS Ultra Mild	1	0.2	<0.5	0.2	<0.01	0.01	<0.01	<0.01	0.0
Silk Cut Extra Mild	4	0.5	4	0.5	0.03	0.04	0.03	0.01	0.0
Peer Special Extra Mild	7	0.8	7	0.8	0.03	0.07	0.05	0.03	0.0
Consulate KS	9	0.9	8	0.9	0.04	0.09	0.05	0.03	0.4
J Player Vanguard	9	0.9	13	1.3	0.05	0.14	0.09	0.03	0.7
Dunhill KS Mild	9	0.8	8	1.0	0.07	0.09	0.06	0.03	0.4
Silk Cut	9	0.8	10	1.2	0.06	0.13	0.07	0.04	0.7
Peter Stuy Lux L Mild	9	0.8	9	1.1	0.07	0.10	0.06	0.03	1.1
Berkeley Extra Mild KS	9	0.9	9	1.1	0.07	0.12	0.05	0.03	0.8
Embassy No. 1 Extra Mild	9	0.8	10	1.3	0.04	0.10	0.09	0.05	1.5
Silk Cut King Size	9	0.9	10	1.1	0.07	0.12	0.06	0.03	5.3
Embassy Extra Mild	9	0.8	10	1.3	0.05	0.13	0.08	0.04	0.4
Du Maurier KS	9	0.9	10	1.2	0.05	0.12	0.07	0.04	1.5
L and B Special Mild	10	0.9	11	1.4	0.04	0.12	0.07	0.05	0.4
Silk Cut No. 3	10	0.8	9	1.2	0.06	0.14	0.08	0.05	0.6
J Player KS Extra Mild	10	1.0	10	1.3	0.05	0.11	0.09	0.05	0.8
555 Special Mild	10	0.9	10	1.1	0.06	0.13	0.07	0.03	0.3
St Moritz	11	1.0	14	1.4	0.07	0.16	0.10	0.05	0.3
Gitanes International	12	1.0	17	1.3	0.45	0.14	0.04	0.03	0.0
Gitanes Filter	12	0.6	18	1.7	0.40	0.23	0.08	0.02	0.0
Peer Special KS Mild	13	1.1	12	1.3	0.06	0.15	0.08	0.04	0.0
Carlton Long Size	13	1.2	10	1.4	0.05	0.14	0.08	0.05	0.4
Peter Stuyvesant KS	13	1.2	13	1.5	0.08	0.18	0.08	0.04	0.0
Disque Bleu	13	0.7	20	1.7	0.43	0.26	0.09	0.02	0.0
Peter Stuy Lux Length	13	1.2	15	1.6	0.05	0.18	0.08	0.07	2.0
More	14	1.3	15	1.3	0.32	0.27	0.06	0.03	0.0
555 Medium Mild	14	1.1	14	1.6	0.06	0.18	0.10	0.06	0.5
Kim	14	1.2	13	1.4	0.05	0.13	0.08	0.05	0.0
Dunhill Luxury Length	14	1.3	16	1.5	0.06	0.16	0.09	0.06	1.7
Dunhill KS	14	1.2	14	1.8	0.07	0.19	0.11	0.06	3.0
Carrolls No. 1 KS	14	1.2	17	1.9	0.06	0.20	0.11	0.06	0.0
Kensitas Club Mild	14	1.3	13	1.6	0.08	0.19	0.10	0.05	0.0
Piccadilly Filter De Luxe	15	1.3	14	1.6	0.05	0.16	0.09	0.06	0.4
J Player Superkings	15	1.5	14	1.7	0.05	0.18	0.11	0.05	0.4
Camel Filter	15	1.2	15	1.7	0.19	0.24	0.10	0.05	0.0
Pall Mall Filter	15	1.3	13	1.7	0.24	0.21	0.10	0.05	0.0
Sovereign KS	15	1.3	16	1.8	0.11	0.22	0.10	0.05	0.8
Dunhill International	15	1.4	15	1.8	0.07	0.17	0.12	0.06	0.4
L and B King Size	15	1.3	15	2.0	0.07	0.19	0.13	0.08	1.1
Winston KS	15	1.2	15	1.7	0.16	0.23	0.10	0.04	0.0
Embassy No. 1 KS	16	1.4	15	1.9	0.07	0.17	0.14	0.08	3.3
Embassy Filter	16	1.3	15	1.8	0.06	0.17	0.12	0.07	4.0
J Player KS	16	1.3	15	1.9	0.06	0.19	0.12	0.06	1.5
Player's No. 6 KS	16	1.4	16	2.0	0.07	0.22	0.13	0.07	3.3
Kent De Luxe	16	1.2	14	1.7	0.26	0.22	0.09	0.05	0.0
Rothmans Royals	16	1.5	14	1.8	0.06	0.16	0.11	0.08	0.0
Embassy Regal	16	1.3	14	1.8	0.05	0.17	0.11	0.07	4.0
Regal KS	16	1.4	16	2.1	0.06	0.19	0.13	0.08	5.2
B and H Supreme	16	1.5	13	1.6	0.10	0.17	0.10	0.04	0.0
Marlboro KS	16	1.3	16	1.8	0.22	0.25	0.10	0.05	2.2
Silva Thins	16	1.4	17	1.9	0.10	0.23	0.10	0.07	0.0
Sovereign Filter	16	1.1	14	1.8	0.09	0.22	0.11	0.06	0.0
B and H Longer Length	16	1.5	14	1.8	0.09	0.18	0.10	0.04	0.0
Player's No. 6 Filter	16	1.4	15	1.9	0.07	0.20	0.12	0.07	3.0

Table 8.14 (*continued*) Yields (mg/cigarette) of tar, nicotine, carbon monoxide, total aldehydes, nitrogen monoxide, total cyanide, acrolein, and formaldehyde: by cigarette brand (75 brands, survey period October 1982-March 1983), United Kingdom

Cigarette brand	Tar	Nicotine	Carbon monoxide CO	Total aldehydes RCHO	Nitrogen monoxide NO	Total cyanide HCN	Acrolein	Formaldehyde HCHO	Market share 1982 %
Lark	17	1.5	14	1.3	0.21	0.15	0.06	0.04	0.0
555 Filter Kings	17	1.3	17	1.9	0.07	0.23	0.08	0.07	2.3
Player's No. 10 Filter	17	1.2	15	1.9	0.05	0.20	0.11	0.09	0.5
Player's Gold Leaf	17	1.3	16	2.0	0.06	0.19	0.11	0.08	0.5
Kensitas Va KS	17	1.4	18	2.0	0.11	0.25	0.13	0.05	0.3
Woodbine Filter	17	1.4	14	1.6	0.06	0.17	0.10	0.09	0.0
Rothmans KS	17	1.4	16	2.0	0.09	0.20	0.11	0.07	3.3
Embassy Gold	17	1.4	14	1.9	0.06	0.19	0.12	0.09	0.0
MS Filter	17	1.3	15	1.7	0.34	0.27	0.10	0.03	0.0
Player's Med Navy Cut (P)	17	1.3	11	1.9	0.04	0.14	0.09	0.07	0.8
J Player Special KS	17	1.5	16	2.0	0.07	0.20	0.13	0.08	11.2
Major Extra Size	18	1.3	17	2.3	0.08	0.22	0.12	0.07	0.0
Kensitas Club KS	18	1.5	18	1.9	0.11	0.24	0.12	0.06	1.3
London KS	18	1.2	16	2.0	0.09	0.24	0.11	0.07	0.2
Park Drive (P)	18	1.5	12	1.7	0.06	0.20	0.08	0.04	2.0
Woodbine (P)	18	1.5	11	1.8	0.04	0.18	0.07	0.07	1.5
Senior Service (P)	18	1.4	11	1.8	0.05	0.16	0.09	0.05	0.5
Gold Flake (P)	18	1.3	11	1.8	0.04	0.15	0.08	0.06	0.0
B and H Special KS	18	1.5	19	2.0	0.11	0.26	0.11	0.06	16.1
Gauloises (P)	24	1.3	20	2.0	0.41	0.30	0.08	0.04	0.0
Capstan Full (P)	25	2.4	14	1.9	0.05	0.21	0.09	0.04	0.2

P plain cigarette
(Crown Copyright reserved in respect of data included in this table)
Note: The data in this table relate to a special series of analyses done on major brands of cigarettes by the LGC at the request of the Independent Scientific Committee on Smoking and Health, to investigate further how far some selected compounds of possible interest in relation to health are likely to decline in parallel with reductions in the routinely-measured components of the particulate or gaseous phases of cigarette smoke. Thus interrelationships with tar or carbon monoxide are of interest, and the full table is provided to allow research workers to classify groups of products in different ways (American blends and continental dark tobacco cigarettes, for example, tend to have relatively high nitrogen monoxide yields). As the analyses were based on samples taken in a particular survey period (Oct 1982 to March 1983) comparisons between brands on a long-term basis may not be valid
Total market share of all 75 brands in the table = 93.1%
Market share estimates are those used by LGC, based on figures published in *Tobacco* for 1982

Source: LGC

Table 8.15 Summary of yields (mg/cigarette) of tar, nicotine, total cyanide, total aldehydes, formaldehyde, acrolein, carbon monoxide, and nitrogen monoxide: data from Table 8.14 (75 brands, survey period October 1982 - March 1983), United Kingdom

	Particulate		Whole smoke			Vapour		
	Tar	Nicotine	Total cyanide HCN	Total aldehydes RCHO	Formaldehyde HCHO	Acrolein	Carbon monoxide CO	Nitrogen monoxide NO
Lowest mean	1	<0.2	<0.02	0.17	<0.01	<0.01	0.4	<0.01
Highest mean	25	2.4	0.30	2.3	0.09	0.14	20	0.45
Sales-weighted mean	15	1.3	0.19	1.8	0.06	0.11	15	0.08

See notes to Table 8.14: Crown Copyright reserved in respect of data included in this table
Source: LGC

Table 8.16 Sales-weighted yields (mg/cigarette) of tar, nicotine, total cyanide, total aldehydes, formaldehyde, acrolein, carbon monoxide, and nitrogen monoxide: by cigarette type, data from Table 8.14 (75 brands, survey period October 1982 - March 1983), United Kingdom

| Type[1] | Number of brands | Particulate | | Whole smoke | | | Vapour | | | Market share 1982 % |
		Tar	Nicotine	Total cyanide HCN	Total aldehydes RCHO	Form-aldehyde HCHO	Acrolein	Carbon monoxide CO	Nitrogen monoxide NO	
Plain	6	18	1.5	0.18	1.8	0.06	0.08	11	0.05	5.0
Mini and regular	14	15	1.3	0.18	1.8	0.07	0.11	14	0.06	14.1
KS and International	51	15	1.3	0.20	1.8	0.06	0.11	15	0.08	74.0
Ventilated Filter	22	9	0.9	0.12	1.2	0.04	0.07	10	0.06	15.3
Aircured tobacco[2]	4	15	0.9	0.23	1.7	0.03	0.07	19	0.42	0.0
Imported brands	11	16	1.3	0.25	1.8	0.06	0.10	16	0.22	2.2

1 The cigarette types overlap
2 Arithmetic means, not sales-weighted
See notes to Table 8.14: Crown Copyright reserved in respect of data included in this table

Source: LGC

Table 8.17 Yields (mg/cigarette) of tar, nicotine, total cyanide, total aldehydes, formaldehyde, acrolein, carbon monoxide, and nitrogen monoxide: by cigarette brand (19 brands, survey period January-July 1986), United Kingdom

| Cigarette brand | Particulate | | Whole smoke | | | Vapour | | | Market share 1986 % |
	Tar	Nicotine	Total cyanide HCN	Total aldehydes RCHO	Form-aldehyde HCHO	Acrolein	Carbon monoxide CO	Nitrogen monoxide NO	
Berkeley Extra Mild KS	9	0.9	0.10	1.1	0.02	0.06	10	0.07	0.0
Embassy No. 1 Extra Mild	9	0.9	0.12	1.2	0.02	0.06	10	0.07	1.0
Silk Cut King Size	9	0.9	0.11	1.2	0.02	0.06	9	0.07	5.8
J Player Superkings	14	1.5	0.16	1.7	0.04	0.09	14	0.10	6.2
Regal KS	14	1.3	0.17	2.1	0.08	0.11	16	0.09	5.8
Embassy Filter	14	1.3	0.16	2.0	0.08	0.10	14	0.09	2.6
Peter Stuy Lux Length	14	1.4	0.16	1.9	0.06	0.09	15	0.10	0.9
Dunhill KS	15	1.4	0.19	2.0	0.06	0.10	16	0.14	1.9
Player's No. 6 Filter	15	1.4	0.20	2.1	0.08	0.12	15	0.11	1.4
J Player Special KS	16	1.5	0.20	2.4	0.09	0.12	16	0.12	4.9
B and H Special KS	17	1.6	0.23	2.2	0.06	0.12	17	0.13	18.4
Woodbine (P)	17	1.4	0.13	1.9	0.10	0.08	11	0.05	0.7
Kensitas Club KS	17	1.5	0.22	2.1	0.06	0.11	18	0.13	1.8
Gauloises Caporal (P)	25	1.6	0.26	2.2	0.04	0.09	23	0.51	0.0
L and B Special Mild*	4	0.6	0.05	0.7	0.02	0.05	6	0.05	1.2
Rothmans Special*	11	1.3	0.12	1.3	0.03	0.07	10	0.11	0.0
Red Band KS*	13	1.1	0.17	1.9	0.07	0.09	17	0.10	1.0
Raffles 100's*	14	1.4	0.16	2.0	0.08	0.10	17	0.06	1.9
Dorchester F*	15	1.2	0.21	2.2	0.10	0.11	17	0.26	2.6

* New brand not previously tested for additional analytes (L and B Special Mild was reformulated)
See notes to Table 8.14: Crown Copyright reserved in respect of data included in this table

Source: LGC

Table 8.18 Correlation coefficients for tar, nicotine, carbon monoxide, total aldehydes, nitrogen monoxide, total cyanide, acrolein, and formaldehyde: data from Table 8.14 (75 brands, survey period October 1982 - March 1983), United Kingdom

Correlation coefficient

Compound	Tar	Nicotine	Carbon monoxide CO	Total aldehydes RCHO	Nitrogen monoxide NO	Total cyanide HCN	Acrolein	Formaldehyde HCHO
Tar	+1.00							
Nicotine	+0.88	+1.00						
Carbon monoxide CO	+0.73	+0.55	+1.00					
Total aldehydes RCHO	+0.88	+0.74	+0.83	+1.00				
Nitrogen monoxide NO	+0.21	-0.06	+0.48	+0.14	+1.00			
Hydrogen cyanide HCN	+0.78	+0.57	+0.88	+0.80	+0.53	+1.00		
Acrolein	+0.63	+0.60	+0.68	+0.85	-0.09	+0.60	+1.00	
Formaldehyde HCHO	+0.59	+0.58	+0.48	+0.74	-0.33	+0.37	+0.77	+1.00

See notes to Table 8.14: Crown Copyright reserved in respect of data included in this table

Source: LGC

Table 8.19 Comparison of 1982/3 and 1986 yields (mg/cigarette) of tar, nicotine, total aldehydes, total cyanide, formaldehyde, acrolein, carbon monoxide, and nitrogen monoxide: by cigarette brand (14 brands, survey periods October 1982-March 1983, and January-July 1986), United Kingdom

	Particulate		Whole smoke			Vapour			
	Tar	Nicotine	Total aldehydes RCHO	Total cyanide HCN	Form-aldehyde HCHO	Acrolein	Carbon monoxide CO	Nitrogen monoxide NO	Market share 1986 %
	1982/3 1986	1982/3 1986	1982/3 1986	1982/3 1986	1982/3 1986	1982/3 1986	1982/3 1986	1982/3 1986	
B and H Special KS	18.3 16.5	1.5 1.6	2.0 2.2	0.26 0.23	0.06 0.07	0.11 0.12	19 17	0.11 0.13	18.4
J Player Superkings	15.1 13.5	1.5 1.5	1.7 1.7	0.18 0.16	0.05 0.04	0.11 0.09	14 14	0.05 0.10	6.2
Regal KS	16.0 13.5	1.4 1.3	2.1 2.1	0.19 0.17	0.08 0.08	0.13 0.11	16 16	0.06 0.09	5.8
Silk Cut King Size	9.2 8.6	0.9 0.9	1.1 1.2	0.12 0.11	0.03 0.02	0.06 0.06	10 9	0.07 0.07	5.8
J Player Special KS	17.4 15.9	1.5 1.5	2.0 2.4	0.20 0.20	0.08 0.09	0.13 0.12	16 16	0.07 0.12	4.9
Embassy Filter	15.5 13.6	1.3 1.3	1.8 2.0	0.17 0.16	0.07 0.07	0.12 0.10	15 14	0.06 0.09	2.6
Dunhill KS	14.0 14.8	1.2 1.4	1.8 2.0	0.19 0.19	0.06 0.06	0.11 0.10	14 16	0.07 0.14	1.9
Kensitas Club KS	17.6 16.7	1.5 1.5	1.9 2.1	0.24 0.22	0.06 0.07	0.12 0.11	18 18	0.11 0.13	1.8
Player's No. 6 Filter	16.4 15.0	1.4 1.4	1.9 2.1	0.20 0.20	0.07 0.08	0.12 0.12	15 15	0.07 0.11	1.4
Embassy No. 1 Extr Mld	9.2 8.6	0.8 0.9	1.3 1.2	0.10 0.12	0.05 0.03	0.09 0.06	10 10	0.04 0.07	1.0

Table 8.19 (*continued*) Comparison of 1982/3 and 1986 yields (mg/cigarette) of tar, nicotine, total aldehydes, total cyanide, formaldehyde, acrolein, carbon monoxide, and nitrogen monoxide: by cigarette brand (14 brands, survey periods October 1982-March 1983, and January-July 1986), United Kingdom

	Particulate		Whole smoke			Vapour			
	Tar	Nicotine	Total aldehydes RCHO	Total cyanide HCN	Form-aldehyde HCHO	Acrolein	Carbon monoxide CO	Nitrogen monoxide NO	Market share 1986 %
	1982/3 1986	1982/3 1986	1982/3 1986	1982/3 1986	1982/3 1986	1982/3 1986	1982/3 1986	1982/3 1986	
Peter Stuy Lux Length	13.4	1.2	1.6	0.18	0.06	0.08	15	0.05	0.9
	13.8	1.4	1.9	0.16	0.06	0.09	15	0.10	
Woodbine (P)	18.1	1.5	1.8	0.18	0.07	0.07	11	0.04	0.7
	16.6	1.4	1.9	0.13	0.10	0.08	11	0.05	
Berkeley Extra Mild KS	9.0	0.9	1.1	0.12	0.03	0.05	9	0.07	0.0
	8.6	0.9	1.1	0.10	0.03	0.06	10	0.07	
Gauloises Caporal (P)	24.0	1.3	2.0	0.3	0.04	0.08	20	0.41	0.0
	24.7	1.6	2.2	0.26	0.04	0.09	23	0.51	
Means (of 14)	15.2	1.3	1.7	0.19	0.06	0.10	14.4	0.09	(Total share 51.4%)
	14.3	1.3	1.9	0.17	0.06	0.09	14.6	0.13	
Ratio of means	0.94	1.04	1.08	0.92	1.04	0.95	1.01	1.40	

See notes to Table 8.14: Crown Copyright reserved in respect of data included in this table

Source: LGC

Table 8.20 Yields (mg/cigarette) of tar, nicotine, and phenols: guaicol, ortho-Cresol, unresolved meta and para-Cresol, phenol, catechol, and hydroquinone in mainstream smoke: by cigarette brand (25 brands), 1986, United Kingdom

Cigarette brand	Tar	Nicotine	Guaicol	Ortho-Cresol	Unresolved meta and para-Cresol	Phenol	Catechol	Hydro-quinone	Market share[2] 1986 %
Ventilated (KS and international)									
Silk Cut Extra Mild	4	0.5	0.01	0.02	0.01	0.01	0.06	0.04	<0.2[3]
L and B Special Mild	5	0.6	<0.01	<0.01	<0.01	0.01	0.07	0.03	1.2
Consulate Menthol	8	0.8	<0.01	0.02	0.02	0.04	0.12	0.10	0.6
Embassy No. 1 Extra Mild	8	0.9	<0.01	0.01	0.01	0.03	0.12	0.07	1.0
Rothmans Special	9	1.2	0.01	0.02	0.01	0.04	0.10	0.06	<0.2[3]
Silk Cut	10	1.0	0.01	0.01	0.01	0.03	0.10	0.05	5.8
Gitanes International*	12	1.0	0.01	0.01	0.03	0.04	0.05	0.05	<0.2[3]
Marlboro KS*	13	1.0	0.01	0.02	0.01	0.04	0.16	0.07	2.1
J Player Superkings	13	1.4	0.01	0.02	0.02	0.04	0.20	0.09	6.2
Other Filter (KS and international)									
Peter Stuy Lux Length	13	1.4	0.01	0.02	0.04	0.05	0.16	0.12	0.9
Red Band KS*	13	1.0	0.01	0.03	0.01	0.03	0.22	0.10	1.0
Embassy No. 1 KS	14	1.2	<0.01	0.01	0.02	0.05	0.20	0.09	2.9
Dunhill KS	14	1.3	0.01	0.03	0.02	0.04	0.22	0.18	1.9
Ronson KS*	14	1.2	0.02	0.02	0.02	0.05	0.18	0.12	0.5
Dorchester F*	15	1.2	0.01	0.03	0.03	0.05	0.22	0.14	2.6
Camel F Tip*	15	1.4	<0.01	0.03	0.02	0.05	0.20	0.10	<0.2[3]
J Player Special KS	16	1.4	0.01	0.03	0.01	0.04	0.24	0.16	4.9
B and H Spec F KS	16	1.5	0.01	0.02	0.02	0.04	0.22	0.12	18.4
Filter (regular size)									
Gauloises Caporal F*	12	0.7	0.01	0.02	0.03	0.04	0.05	0.03	<0.2[3]
Gitanes Caporal F*	12	0.8	0.02	0.01	0.04	0.05	0.05	0.04	<0.2[3]
Embassy F	13	1.3	<0.01	0.03	0.02	0.05	0.20	0.12	2.6
Plain									
Senior Service	18	1.5	0.05	0.03	0.04	0.12	0.34	0.18	0.3
Sweet Afton*	22	2.1	0.04	0.04	0.04	0.12	0.30	0.22	<0.2[3]
Gauloises P*	24	1.5	<0.01	0.04	0.08	0.09	0.10	0.10	<0.2[3]
Capstan Full Strength	25	2.6	0.05	0.05	0.04	0.12	0.30	0.20	<0.2[4]
Lowest mean	4	0.5	<0.01	<0.01	<0.01	0.01	0.05	0.03	
Sales-weighted mean (25)	14	1.3	0.01	0.02	0.02	0.04	0.19	0.11	53
Highest mean	25	2.6	0.05	0.05	0.08	0.12	0.34	0.22	
Tests per brand[1]	30	30	5	5	5	5	5	5	
Partitioned data[5]									
Ventilated F (9)	11	1.1	0.01	0.01	0.01	0.03	0.14	0.07	
KS and International F (18)	14	1.3	0.01	0.02	0.02	0.04	0.19	0.11	
Mini and Regular F (3)	13	1.3	0.01	0.03	0.02	0.05	0.20	0.12	
Plain (4)	19	1.7	0.05	0.03	0.04	0.12	0.32	0.18	
Air-cured (4)	15	1.0	0.05	0.05	0.05	0.06	0.06	0.06	
Imported brands (10)	14	1.1	0.01	0.02	0.02	0.04	0.19	0.11	

1 Each test comprised machine-smoking three cigarettes and mean values for each brand have been rounded
2 From *Tobacco*
3 For calculation of sales-weighted mean 0.02% had been assumed
4 For calculation of sales-weighted mean 0.05% had been assumed
5 The unrounded mean yield data were partitioned to indicate sales-weighted mean values for each cigarette type
* Imported cigarette brand

Note: four brands which were tested for polycyclic aromatic hydrocarbons (see Table 8.21), were not examined in the phenols study:
Vogue Super Slims 100s, Berkeley Superkings, Rothmans F and Gauloises Disque Bleu F
See notes to Table 8.14: Crown Copyright reserved in respect of data included in this table

Source: LGC

Table 8.21 Yields of tar, nicotine, and polycyclic aromatic hydrocarbons (PAHs): benzo[b]fluoranthene (BbF), benzo[k]fluoranthene (BkF), and benzo[a]pyrene (BaP) in mainstream smoke: by cigarette brand (23 brands, survey period March-August 1989), United Kingdom

Cigarette brand	Tar mg/cig	Nicotine mg/cig	BbF ng/cig	BkF ng/cig	BaP ng/cig	Market share[2] 1988 %
Ventilated (KS and international)						
Lambert and Butler LT	4	0.45	4	2	4	1.1
Silk Cut deLuxe Mild	5	0.6	4	2	6	<0.2[3]
Consulate Menthol	9	0.9	9	5	11	0.5
Vogue Super Slims	7	0.7	4	2	5	<0.2[3]
Rothmans Special	9	0.9	8	4	10	<0.2[3]
Silk Cut	9	0.9	7	3	9	7.1
Berkeley Superkings	12	1.2	10	4	13	7.4
J Player Superkings	14	1.4	11	5	14	4.4
Marlboro KS*	14	1.0	7	3	10	1.7
Other Filter (KS and international)						
Peter Stuy Lux Length	13	1.4	11	5	14	0.6
Red Band KS*	13	1.0	10	5	13	0.9
Embassy No. 1 KS	13	1.2	11	5	13	2.8
Camel F Tip*	14	1.2	10	5	11	<0.2[3]
J Player Special KS	14	1.3	12	5	15	4.4
Dorchester F*	15	1.1	15	8	18	2.4
B and H Spec F KS	15	1.2	11	6	14	19.8
Ronson KS*	16	1.4	11	5	14	<0.2[3]
Rothmans F	17	1.6	15	8	18	2.3
Filter (regular size)						
Gauloises Disque Bleu F*	12	0.7	9	3	11	<0.2[3]
Gitanes Caporal F*	12	0.8	10	3	9	<0.2[3]
Embassy F	13	1.1	10	5	12	2.3
Plain						
Senior Service	17	1.4	13	6	17	0.3
Capstan Full Strength	24	2.3	16	9	20	<0.2[4]
Lowest mean	4	0.45	4	2	4	
Sales-weighted mean (23)	13	1.2	10	5	13	58
Highest mean	24	2.3	16	9	20	
Tests per brand[1]	30	30	6-8	6-8	6-8	
Partitioned data[5]						
Ventilated F (9)	11	1.1	9	4	11	
KS and International F (18)	13	1.2	11	5	13	
Mini and Regular F (3)	13	1.1	10	5	12	
Plain (2)	18	1.5	13	6	17	
Air-cured (2)	12	0.8	10	3	10	
Imported brands (7)	14	1.0	12	6	15	

1 Each test comprised machine-smoking five cigarettes and mean values for each brand have been rounded
2 From *Tobacco*
3 For calculation of sales-weighted mean 0.02% had been assumed
4 For calculation of sales-weighted mean 0.05% had been assumed
5 The unrounded mean yield data were partitioned to indicate sales-weighted mean values for each cigarette type
* Imported cigarette brand

Note: six brands which were tested for phenols (see Table 8.20), were not examined in the PAHs study:
Embassy No. 1 EM, Dunhill KS, Gauloises deLuxe P, Caporal F, Gitanes International and Sweet Afton
See notes to Table 8.14: Crown Copyright reserved in respect of data included in this table

Source: LGC

Table 8.22 Comparison of yields (mg/cigarette) of 1979 cigarettes as determined in 1979[1] and 1989[2] for tar, nicotine, and carbon monoxide: by cigarette brand (24 brands), United Kingdom

Brand	Average puffs		Tar		Nicotine		Carbon monoxide	
	1979	1989	1979	1989	1979	1989	1979	1989
Embassy Premier (NSM* 25%)	9.5	10.2	7.8	7.8	0.6	0.5	12.0	13.8
Silk Cut	8.0	8.0	8.7	9.2	0.9	0.8	11.0	12.3
Embassy No. 1 Ex Mld	9.3	10.2	9.1	8.5	0.7	0.7	12.9	12.8
Silk Cut KS	9.2	9.8	9.4	9.9	1.0	1.0	12.3	13.0
Silk Cut No. 3	7.1	7.3	9.4	7.6	0.8	0.7	10.1	8.6
State Express 555 Ex Mld	8.4	9.1	14.4	13.1	1.2	1.0	13.4	13.2
Marlboro KS	7.9	7.8	15.6	16.0	1.2	1.2	15.6	15.4
President (NSM* 25%)	9.1	10.1	15.6	16.4	1.2	1.1	18.6	21.0
Dunhill KS	9.4	9.3	16.8	15.3	1.4	1.3	15.0	17.2
Piccadilly KS	9.1	9.4	17.1	14.6	1.4	1.1	15.3	15.9
Piccadilly No. 1 (P)	9.1	9.5	17.9	19.2	1.4	1.4	10.2	11.6
Players No. 6	8.2	8.5	18.0	17.2	1.3	1.1	17.7	19.6
John Player KS	9.1	9.9	18.1	19.1	1.4	1.3	19.2	21.2
State Express 555 KS	9.0	9.1	18.1	18.1	1.4	1.4	17.3	18.9
Embassy No. 3	8.2	8.2	18.4	17.0	1.3	1.2	17.7	18.5
Embassy Regal KS	9.4	9.5	18.4	18.2	1.5	1.3	19.1	21.2
Lambert and Butler KS	9.6	10.1	18.4	19.6	1.5	1.4	19.7	22.6
Embassy No. 1 KS	9.1	9.7	18.5	19.7	1.4	1.5	19.2	21.2
Players Gold Leaf	8.4	9.0	18.5	17.6	1.6	1.4	18.0	18.8
Embassy F	8.2	8.5	18.7	16.8	1.4	1.2	17.8	19.5
Benson and Hedges KS	9.4	9.9	18.8	17.7	1.7	1.6	17.9	20.5
Players No. 6 KS	9.5	10.3	18.8	19.7	1.6	1.5	19.5	21.9
Rothmans KS	9.1	9.3	19.0	19.0	1.4	1.3	19.5	21.8
Capstan Full Strength (P)	9.3	10.4	30.9	30.0	3.5	3.3	15.5	15.6
Monitor	8.7	9.1	23.6	23	1.6	1.4	17.6	18.4
Average	8.85	9.29	16.72	16.41	1.37	1.26	16.09	17.38

* New Smoking Material
1 Rounded average of 30 tests each comprising five cigarettes
2 Rounded average of four tests each comprising five cigarettes

See notes to Table 8.14: Crown Copyright reserved in respect of data included in this table

Source: LGC

Plain/filter cigarettes

TAC data show that, in 1961, 83 per cent of men and 64 per cent of women smokers of manufactured cigarettes usually smoked plain cigarettes. The switch to filter cigarettes began in the 1950s, quickened in the 1960s, and by 1971 plain cigarettes were smoked by only 23 per cent of men and 10 per cent of women who smoked manufactured cigarettes. This change to filters took place most quickly among young adults; by 1987 most plain cigarette smokers were aged 50 and over. Plain cigarettes are more popular with men than with women and more popular with social classes IV, V and VI than with other classes.

Hand-rolled cigarettes

GHS data in this section show that the proportion of male cigarette smokers smoking mainly hand-rolled cigarettes rose from 13 to 18 per cent between 1972 and 1988, while the proportion of those smoking mainly plain cigarettes fell from 20 to 3 per cent.

A higher proportion of male cigarette smokers who are manual workers smoke hand-rolled cigarettes than do non-manual workers (Table 9.11.1). Hand-rolled cigarettes have not been popular with women or with young men.

Data on hand-rolled cigarettes can also be found in Sections 3,4, and 5.

Tar yield of manufactured cigarettes

The classification of manufactured cigarettes by tar band started with the second LGC survey in 1973. The NOP surveys have collected data on tar yields of cigarettes smoked since 1974. The GHS included a question about tar yields for the first time in 1984.

Between 1974 and 1984 there were considerable changes in the tar yield distribution of the cigarette market. According to NOP data, the proportion of cigarette smokers smoking low tar cigarettes (0-10 mg tar/cigarette) increased from 1 to 8 per cent among men and from 2 to 24 per cent among women, and the proportion of smokers smoking cigarettes yielding 11-16 mg tar rose from 5 to 45 per cent among men, and from 15 to 47 per cent among women during this period. At the same time the proportion of smokers smoking cigarettes yielding 17-22 mg tar fell from 66 to 26 per cent among men, and from 72 to 23 per cent among women. Cigarettes of very high tar (29+ mg) disappeared from the market

151

altogether by 1979, and very few smokers continued to smoke cigarettes in the middle to high tar category (23-28 mg). In 1988, the percentage of male cigarette smokers smoking cigarettes with tar yields of less than 10 mg, 10 mg but less than 15 mg, and 15 mg but less than 18 mg, were 13, 56, and 16 per cent respectively; corresponding values for women were 23, 55, and 13 per cent.

Tar yield: by age

Men

The proportion of male cigarette smokers who smoke low tar cigarettes rises with age until 1986, while this is not as clear for 1987 and 1988. In 1988 NOP estimated that 8 per cent of male cigarette smokers aged 16-24 smoked cigarettes yielding less than 10 mg tar/cigarette and 11 per cent of male cigarette smokers aged 65 years and over. In the same survey, the proportion of cigarette smokers smoking cigarettes yielding 15 but less than 18 mg was 9 per cent among men aged 16-24 years, compared to about 27 per cent among men aged 65 years and over. A decrease took place in the proportion of cigarette smokers smoking middle tar cigarettes for all age groups in favour of the low/middle tar cigarettes.

Women

The proportion of female cigarette smokers smoking low tar cigarettes rises with age, while the proportion smoking higher tar cigarettes falls. NOP estimate that, in 1988, the proportions of female cigarette smokers aged 16-24 years smoking cigarettes yielding less than 10 mg tar, 10 mg but less than 15 mg tar, and 15 mg but less than 18 mg tar, were 21, 67, and 8 per cent respectively; the corresponding proportions for smokers aged 55-64 years were 35, 45, and 15 per cent.

Tar yield: by social class

Men

Male cigarette smokers who are manual workers less often smoke low tar cigarettes than do non-manual workers. In 1988, NOP estimated that 36 per cent of professional male cigarette smokers smoked cigarettes yielding less than 10 mg tar, while 5-11 per cent of manual workers did so. A decrease was shown in the proportion of cigarette smokers smoking middle tar cigarettes in all classes in favour of low/middle tar cigarettes, apart from social class AB where more smokers smoke low tar cigarettes.

Women

Professional women have a higher prevalence of low tar cigarette smoking, and a lower prevalence of higher tar smoking than all other women in NOP surveys. There is less variation as regards tar level smoked among women than among men.

Consumption of cigarettes: by tar yield

The average number of cigarettes smoked daily fluctuates slightly between tar bands, but there is no obvious pattern to the variation over the years. Women, however, consistently report smoking fewer cigarettes per day than men, although the difference has narrowed.

Table 9.1 Percentages[1] of manufactured cigarette smokers: by type of cigarette (plain or filter) usually smoked, 1961-1987
Manufactured cigarette smokers, men and women aged 16 and over, Great Britain

	Men		Women	
Year	Plain	Filter	Plain	Filter
1961	83	17	64	36
1965	51	49	29	71
1968	35	65	15	85
1971	23	77	10	90
1975	19	81	6	94
1976	15	85	6	94
1977	13	87	6	94
1978	13	87	5	95
1979	11	89	3	97
1980	9	91	3	97
1981	8	92	3	97
1982	7	93	3	97
1983	7	93	2	98
1984	4	96	2	98
1985	4	96	1	99
1986	4	96	1	99
1987	4	96	1	99

1 The percentages have been calculated from data on all manufactured cigarette smokers who stated a preference for plain or filter cigarettes

Source: TAC

Fig. 9.1 Percentages of cigarette smokers: by type of cigarette (plain, filter, or hand-rolled) usually smoked, 1988
Cigarette smokers, men and women aged 16 and over, Great Britain. *Source*: GHS

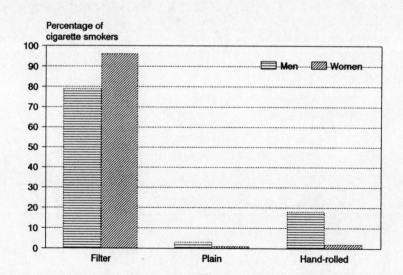

Table 9.2 Percentages[1] of men and women who smoke manufactured cigarettes: by type of cigarette (plain or filter) usually smoked, 1961-1987
Men and women aged 16 and over, Great Britain

| | | Percentage usually smoking | | | |
| | | Plain | | Filter | |
Year		Men	Women	Men	Women
1961		47.5	26.8	9.7	14.8
1965		27.0	11.8	25.6	29.4
1968		18.7	6.2	35.5	36.0
1971		11.7	4.0	38.2	37.3
1975		8.7	2.5	37.5	39.9
1976		6.8	2.3	37.6	39.2
1977		5.4	2.4	35.4	38.4
1978		5.5	2.0	35.5	37.4
1979		4.5	1.3	36.7	37.6
1980		3.9	1.1	37.7	37.6
1981		2.9	1.0	33.9	35.2
1982		2.4	0.9	33.3	34.4
1983		2.5	0.6	32.2	34.6
1984		1.3	0.7	33.8	31.4
1985		1.3	0.5	33.2	33.9
1986		1.3	0.3	31.8	32.7
1987		1.2	0.4	32.3	33.3

1 The percentages in this table exclude those who did not express a preference for a particular brand of cigarette. All respondents are included in Tables · 3.2.1/2 under the category 'All smokers of manufactured cigarettes'.

Source: TAC

Table 9.3 Percentages of cigarette smokers: by type of cigarette (plain, filter, or hand-rolled) usually smoked, 1972-1988
Cigarette smokers, men and women aged 16 and over, Great Britain

| | Men | | | Women | | |
Year	Mainly filter	Mainly plain	Mainly hand-rolled	Mainly filter	Mainly plain	Mainly hand-rolled
1972	67	20	13	90	9	1
1974	69	18	13	91	8	1
1976	71	15	14	93	6	1
1978	75	11	14	95	4	1
1980	77	8	15	95	3	1
1982	72	7	21	94	3	3
1984	77	6	17	95	2	3
1986	78	4	18	96	1	2
1988	79	3	18	96	1	2

Source: GHS

Table 9.4 Percentages[1] of men and women who smoke manufactured cigarettes: by age, and type of cigarette (plain or filter) usually smoked, 1961-1987
Men and women aged 16 and over, Great Britain

Percentage usually smoking plain cigarettes at ages

Year	Men 16-24	25-34	35-59	60+	16+	Women 16-24	25-34	35-59	60+	16+
1961	53	46	50	38	47.5	29	32	31	14	26.8
1965	18	24	30	25	27.0	5	13	16	8	11.8
1968	8	13	23	24	18.7	1	5	10	5	6.2
1971	4	9	14	16	11.7	1	2	6	3	4.0
1975	2	4	11	14	8.7	1	1	4	3	2.5

Year	Men 16-24	25-34	35-49	50-64	65+	16+	Women 16-24	25-34	35-49	50-64	65+	16+
1975	2.5	4.1	9.0	13.8	14.2	8.7	0.6	1.0	3.1	4.3	2.7	2.5
1978	1.7	4.0	5.6	8.9	6.8	5.5	0.3	0.6	2.5	3.6	2.4	2.0
1981	0.4	1.1	1.8	5.5	6.2	2.9	0.1	0.1	1.2	2.0	1.0	1.0
1982	0.1	0.9	1.7	4.9	4.7	2.4	0.1	0.6	0.7	1.7	1.4	0.9
1983	0.1	0.9	2.8	3.5	5.3	2.5	0.0	0.3	0.5	1.8	0.4	0.6
1984	0.2	0.7	0.9	2.9	2.0	1.3	0.0	0.3	0.3	1.6	1.0	0.7
1985	0.2	0.6	1.2	1.9	3.1	1.3	0.0	0.2	0.4	1.1	0.8	0.5
1986	0.2	0.2	1.3	1.6	3.3	1.3	0.0	0.1	0.2	0.7	0.3	0.3
1987	0.0	0.0	1.0	2.9	2.0	1.2	0.0	0.1	0.3	0.8	0.8	0.4

Percentage usually smoking filter cigarettes at ages

Year	Men 16-24	25-34	35-59	60+	16+	Women 16-24	25-34	35-59	60+	16+
1961	8	12	10	7	9.7	17	18	17	9	14.8
1965	37	31	25	18	25.6	39	37	33	14	29.4
1968	49	43	33	22	35.5	47	42	41	18	36.0
1971	50	45	36	27	38.2	49	45	42	19	37.3
1975	48	42	37	26	37.5	49	47	45	24	39.9

Year	Men 16-24	25-34	35-49	50-64	65+	16+	Women 16-24	25-34	35-49	50-64	65+	16+
1975	47.8	41.6	37.2	35.4	23.1	37.5	48.8	47.1	46.3	41.6	19.7	39.9
1978	44.4	40.2	36.7	31.3	23.3	35.5	44.6	46.6	44.6	36.7	18.3	37.4
1981	40.4	40.3	36.8	29.5	20.0	33.9	39.3	41.9	41.2	37.8	18.4	35.2
1982	42.2	36.9	35.5	27.3	22.6	33.3	38.1	36.9	40.0	39.3	19.5	34.4
1983	40.7	34.9	33.6	29.3	20.1	32.2	41.7	39.5	38.5	37.1	19.0	34.6
1984	38.0	41.2	34.2	32.3	21.5	33.8	35.6	37.3	33.7	35.4	17.6	31.4
1985	41.9	38.9	35.0	27.2	21.2	33.2	39.7	41.3	38.0	35.5	18.3	33.9
1986	41.2	35.9	33.7	29.0	16.3	31.8	40.8	36.6	39.1	33.5	16.2	32.7
1987	41.8	38.2	33.8	26.4	19.1	32.3	41.9	37.9	36.3	34.0	19.4	33.3

1 The percentages in this table exclude those who did not express a preference for a particular brand of cigarette. All respondents are included in Tables 4.1.1/2

Source: TAC

Table 9.5 Percentages[1] of men and women who smoke manufactured cigarettes: by tar yield of brand of cigarette usually smoked, 1978-1987
Men and women aged 16 and over, Great Britain

Percentage usually smoking

Year	Low tar		Low/middle tar		Middle tar		Middle/high or high tar	
	Men	Women	Men	Women	Men	Women	Men	Women
1978	3.0	6.6	1.8	2.6	34.0	28.7	0.9	0.3
1979	3.9	7.6	2.3	3.0	33.9	27.8	0.7	0.2
1980	5.2	9.3	4.5	5.6	31.1	23.2	0.1	0.0
1981	4.0	8.3	5.5	5.7	26.4	21.5	0.0	0.0
1982	3.7	7.4	3.9	5.0	27.4	21.4	0.0	0.0
1983	3.0	7.4	16.9	15.9	14.1	11.0	0.0	0.0
1984	3.9	6.5	15.7	15.2	14.4	10.4	0.0	0.0
1985[2]	4.1	7.7	12.8	11.8	16.4	13.5	0.0	0.0
1986[3]	3.7	6.8	13.6	12.6	14.5	12.0	0.0	0.0
1987[3]	3.8	7.7	13.5	13.7	14.6	10.7	0.0	0.0

1 The percentages in this table exclude those who did not express a preference for a particular brand of cigarette. All respondents are included in Tables 3.2.1/2 under the category 'All smokers of manufactured cigarettes'
2 1985 data are given according to the tar bands that applied for 1972-1984
3 The definitions of the tar bands altered in 1985:

	1972-1984	1985-
Low	0-10 mg tar/cigarette	0- 9.99 mg tar/cigarette
Low/middle	11-16 mg tar/cigarette	10.0-14.99 mg tar/cigarette
Middle	17-22 mg tar/cigarette	15.0-17.99 mg tar/cigarette
Middle/high	23-28 mg tar/cigarette	no middle/high band
High	29+ mg tar/cigarette	18.0+ mg tar/cigarette
	(data rounded)	(data truncated)

Source: TAC

Fig. 9.2 Percentages of men and women who smoke manufactured cigarettes: by tar yield of brand of cigarette usually smoked, 1987
Men and women aged 16 and over, Great Britain. *Source*: TAC

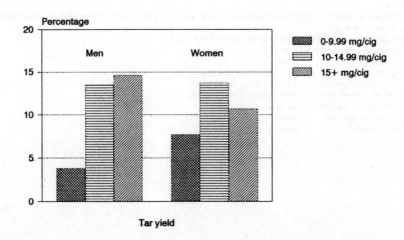

Table 9.6 Percentages[1] of men and women who smoke manufactured cigarettes: by age, and tar yield[2] of brand of cigarette usually smoked, 1978-1987
Men and women aged 16 and over, Great Britain

	Men						Women					
Year	16-24	25-34	35-49	50-64	65+	16+	16-24	25-34	35-49	50-64	65+	16+
Percentage usually smoking low tar cigarettes												
1978	0.9	2.2	4.0	3.9	3.7	3.0	3.1	6.4	9.1	9.3	4.3	6.6
1981	1.7	3.9	5.7	5.0	3.3	4.0	2.9	6.8	10.4	14.1	6.2	8.3
1982	1.9	2.2	4.8	5.4	3.9	3.7	2.3	5.6	10.3	10.0	7.6	7.4
1983	1.2	1.6	3.2	4.5	4.5	3.0	3.2	6.1	8.5	10.3	7.8	7.4
1984	1.5	3.6	3.7	5.1	5.8	3.9	3.0	5.3	8.9	8.5	5.9	6.5
1985[3]	2.4	3.1	5.2	4.8	4.6	4.1	3.8	7.6	7.9	10.4	8.0	7.7
1986[4]	3.0	2.8	4.0	5.3	3.4	3.7	5.6	5.5	8.6	9.4	4.8	6.8
1987[4]	4.2	3.1	3.7	3.7	4.6	3.8	7.2	5.2	10.6	8.6	6.3	7.7
Percentage usually smoking low/middle tar cigarettes												
1978	2.3	2.1	1.3	1.9	1.0	1.8	2.3	3.4	3.2	2.4	1.7	2.6
1981	5.9	8.0	4.8	4.0	4.9	5.5	5.6	6.6	7.7	6.2	3.0	5.7
1982	5.0	4.3	4.9	1.9	3.5	3.9	3.1	5.3	5.6	7.6	3.3	5.0
1983	19.0	18.5	19.4	14.4	11.6	16.9	17.5	20.0	19.6	16.3	7.6	15.9
1984	16.3	19.9	16.8	15.4	8.6	15.7	17.3	19.1	16.5	17.4	7.2	15.2
1985[3]	16.6	15.2	13.7	9.8	8.3	12.8	14.7	15.1	13.4	11.2	5.9	11.8
1986[4]	17.3	15.2	15.8	11.2	6.8	13.6	14.8	16.7	15.0	13.0	5.0	12.6
1987[4]	15.4	17.8	14.9	11.0	7.0	13.5	17.2	17.0	15.4	14.5	6.0	13.7
Percentage usually smoking middle tar cigarettes												
1978	41.5	39.0	34.5	31.3	22.0	34.0	38.8	36.3	32.8	26.0	13.7	28.7
1981	32.6	28.5	27.2	24.8	17.1	26.4	30.9	28.3	24.0	18.6	9.3	21.5
1982	35.3	30.5	27.1	23.9	19.2	27.4	32.6	25.1	23.1	20.5	9.3	21.4
1983	20.3	15.2	12.9	13.4	8.0	14.1	20.5	12.8	9.5	11.0	3.8	11.0
1984	19.5	17.3	13.4	13.0	8.1	14.4	16.5	12.8	9.0	11.0	4.9	10.4
1985[3]	22.5	20.0	15.9	13.2	9.6	16.4	20.5	17.5	14.9	12.9	4.3	13.5
1986[4]	20.3	17.0	14.4	12.4	7.6	14.5	19.5	12.8	14.1	9.4	5.7	12.0
1987[4]	21.4	16.4	14.0	12.4	8.3	14.6	16.8	14.2	9.2	9.4	5.9	10.7

1 The percentages in this table exclude those who did not express a preference for a particular brand of cigarette. All respondents are included in Tables 4.1.1/2
2 Data on population smoking cigarettes with middle/high or high tar are not included in this table as the percentages are too small for trends by age group to be meaningful
3 1985 data are given according to the tar bands that applied for 1972-1984
4 The definitions of the tar bands altered in 1985:

	1972-1984	1985-
Low	0-10 mg tar/cigarette	0- 9.99 mg tar/cigarette
Low/middle	11-16 mg tar/cigarette	10.0-14.99 mg tar/cigarette
Middle	17-22 mg tar/cigarette	15.0-17.99 mg tar/cigarette
Middle/high	23-28 mg tar/cigarette	no middle/high band
High	29+ mg tar/cigarette	18.0+ mg tar/cigarette
	(data rounded)	(data truncated)

Table 9.7 Percentages[1] of men and women who smoke manufactured cigarettes: by social class, and (i) type of cigarette (plain or filter), and (ii) tar yield[2] of brand of cigarette usually smoked, 1975-1987
Men and women aged 16 and over, Great Britain

	Social class									
	I+II	IIINM	IIIM	IV+V+VI	All classes	I+II	IIINM	IIIM	IV+V+VI	All classes
Year	Men					Women				
Percentage usually smoking plain cigarettes										
1975	5.2	8.4		12.2	8.7	1.5	2.2		3.7	2.5
1978	2.6	3.4	6.1	7.8	5.5	0.4	0.7	2.4	3.9	2.0
1981	0.7	0.4	3.0	4.9	2.9	0.3	0.4	1.6	1.4	1.0
1982	0.9	1.4	2.4	3.8	2.4	0.7	0.6	0.6	1.7	0.9
1983	1.4	2.9	2.2	3.4	2.5	0.5	0.3	0.9	0.8	0.6
1984	0.4	0.5	1.2	2.5	1.3	0.4	0.6	0.4	1.2	0.7
1985	1.0	0.8	1.1	2.1	1.3	0.2	0.2	1.0	0.6	0.5
1986	0.8	2.1	1.5	1.0	1.3	0.2	-	0.4	0.4	0.3
1987	0.8	0.6	1.1	1.7	1.2	0.3	0.2	0.5	0.7	0.4
Percentage usually smoking filter cigarettes										
1975	34.8	38.6		37.3	37.5	34.2	42.8		38.4	39.9
1978	28.3	30.1	38.9	38.2	35.5	32.7	40.3	40.5	35.5	37.4
1981	29.7	36.8	33.6	37.4	33.9	28.5	36.8	37.4	36.5	35.2
1982	26.6	33.2	34.3	37.2	33.3	26.6	34.5	39.9	35.4	34.4
1983	23.8	26.5	34.1	38.1	32.2	27.6	33.1	39.2	37.0	34.6
1984	26.8	28.2	36.1	38.1	33.8	24.3	32.4	33.9	33.6	31.4
1985	25.2	31.3	34.4	38.6	33.2	27.7	32.4	36.1	37.3	33.9
1986	25.1	25.4	30.6	40.5	31.8	25.1	30.8	35.3	36.9	32.7
1987	22.2	27.8	34.4	39.7	32.3	25.1	32.0	34.5	38.9	33.3
Percentage usually smoking low tar cigarettes										
1978	3.6	3.1	3.3	1.9	3.0	8.0	7.2	5.1	4.7	6.6
1981	5.5	5.1	3.6	3.0	4.0	9.0	8.3	8.1	8.3	8.3
1982	5.0	3.9	3.7	2.7	3.7	8.9	7.5	6.6	7.0	7.4
1983	3.4	3.1	3.1	2.5	3.0	8.4	7.9	8.0	5.9	7.4
1984	4.4	4.8	4.2	2.7	3.9	7.5	7.7	6.0	5.4	6.5
1985[3]	4.2	5.5	4.2	3.4	4.1	8.5	7.9	7.9	6.9	7.7
1986[4]	5.5	4.6	3.0	3.0	3.7	7.6	6.9	6.6	6.5	6.8
1987[4]	4.6	3.8	3.6	3.5	3.8	9.0	8.6	7.1	6.6	7.7

Table 9.7 (*continued*) Percentages[1] of men and women who smoke manufactured cigarettes: by social class, and (i) type of cigarette (plain or filter), and (ii) tar yield[2] of brand of cigarette usually smoked, 1975-1987
Men and women aged 16 and over, Great Britain

	Social class									
Year	I+II	IIINM	IIIM	IV+V+VI	All classes	I+II	IIINM	IIIM	IV+V+VI	All classes
	Men					Women				
Percentage usually smoking low/middle tar cigarettes										
1978	2.0	2.1	1.6	1.6	1.8	2.8	2.5	1.6	2.8	2.6
1981	5.3	7.8	5.3	5.1	5.5	5.8	6.4	6.2	4.8	5.7
1982	4.8	5.2	3.9	3.0	3.9	4.2	5.1	6.1	4.7	5.0
1983	11.7	13.2	18.6	19.9	16.9	10.8	15.0	18.7	18.1	15.9
1984	11.3	13.4	16.5	18.7	15.7	9.4	14.0	17.5	18.2	15.2
1985[3]	7.6	9.9	13.1	17.6	12.8	7.0	9.6	13.7	14.9	11.8
1986[4]	9.3	10.1	13.3	18.5	13.6	7.7	10.5	15.2	15.2	12.6
1987[4]	7.8	11.3	14.4	17.8	13.5	9.5	12.6	13.9	17.2	13.7
Percentage usually smoking middle tar cigarettes										
1978	22.5	26.6	37.8	40.3	34.0	20.4	29.5	23.5	30.6	28.7
1981	18.9	23.7	26.6	33.2	26.4	13.6	21.9	24.0	24.4	21.5
1982	17.3	25.1	28.4	34.7	27.4	12.7	20.7	26.3	24.1	21.4
1983	9.2	12.9	13.9	18.5	14.1	7.7	9.7	12.4	13.2	11.0
1984	10.5	8.8	15.5	17.8	14.4	7.1	11.0	11.6	11.4	10.4
1985[3]	13.3	16.2	17.0	18.1	16.4	11.1	14.1	13.1	14.9	13.5
1986[4]	9.7	10.6	14.8	19.3	14.5	8.3	12.2	12.4	13.9	12.0
1987[4]	8.8	12.1	15.7	19.1	14.6	5.8	9.8	12.4	13.3	10.7

1 The percentages in this table exclude those who did not express a preference for a particular brand of cigarette. All respondents are included in Table 5.2
2 Data on population smoking cigarettes with middle/high or high tar are not included in this table as the percentages are too small for trends by social class to be meaningful
3 1985 data are given according to the tar bands that applied for 1972-1984
4 The definitions of the tar bands altered in 1985:

	1972-1984	1985-
Low	0-10 mg tar/cigarette	0- 9.99 mg tar/cigarette
Low/middle	11-16 mg tar/cigarette	10.0-14.99 mg tar/cigarette
Middle	17-22 mg tar/cigarette	15.0-17.99 mg tar/cigarette
Middle/high	23-28 mg tar/cigarette	no middle/high band
High	29+ mg tar/cigarette	18.0+ mg tar/cigarette
	(data rounded)	(data truncated)

Source: TAC

Table 9.8 Percentages[1] of manufactured cigarette smokers: by age, and tar yield of brand of cigarette usually smoked, 1988
Manufactured cigarette smokers, men and women aged 16 and over, Great Britain

	Tar yield (mg/cigarette)				No regular brand	New brand/ don't know
Age	0-9.99	10.0-14.99	15.0-17.99	18.0+		
Men						
16-19	10	65	10	-	1	15
20-24	15	67	15	-	1	3
25-34	15	66	16	-	2	1
35-49	16	64	16	0	2	3
50-59	18	53	23	1	1	3
60+	17	49	29	0	1	4
16+	16	61	18	0	1	3
Women						
16-19	19	55	12	-	-	14
20-24	20	63	15	-	-	2
25-34	18	63	17	-	0	1
35-49	27	56	14	-	1	2
50-59	27	55	14	-	0	4
60+	34	44	16	-	1	5
16+	25	56	15	-	1	3

1 18% of male smokers and 2% of female smokers said they mainly smoked hand-rolled cigarettes and have been excluded from this analysis

Source: GHS

Table 9.9 Percentages of cigarette smokers: by tar yield of brand of cigarette usually smoked, 1974-1988
Cigarette smokers, men and women aged 16 and over, Great Britain

Survey date	Manufactured cigarettes, tar band					Hand-rolled	Other/don't know
	Low	Low/middle	Middle	Middle/high	High		
Men							
Nov 1974	1	5	66	17	1	10	2
Mar 1976	3	5	63	14	1	12	2
Nov 1976	7	5	63	11	1	14	0
Nov/Dec 1977	8	6	57	14	0	12	2
Nov/Dec 1978	9	4	64	8	1	12	3
Nov/Dec 1979	8	5	71	0	*	12	3
Nov/Dec 1980	10	7	65	0	*	13	4
Nov 1982	7	19	54	1	*	16	4
Nov 1983	9	42	28	0	*	15	5
Nov 1984	8	45	26	0	*	16	5
Nov 1985[1]	8	29	42	-	0	16	5
Nov 1986[1]	12	32	35	-	1	18	3
Nov 1987[1]	13	39	31	-	0	12	4
Nov 1988[1]	13	56	16	-	1	13	4
Women							
Nov 1974	2	15	72	7	0	1	3
Mar 1976	10	11	70	7	0	1	2
Nov 1976	13	14	67	5	0	1	1
Nov/Dec 1977	19	13	61	2	0	2	3
Nov/Dec 1978	19	7	65	4	0	1	4
Nov/Dec 1979	19	8	66	0	*	1	6
Nov/Dec 1980	20	15	60	0	*	1	5
Nov 1982	20	24	49	0	*	2	6
Nov 1983	20	45	28	0	*	1	5
Nov 1984	24	47	23	0	*	1	5
Nov 1985[1]	22	32	38	-	0	2	6
Nov 1986[1]	27	41	24	-	0	2	6
Nov 1987[1]	20	46	29	-	0	1	4
Nov 1988[1]	23	55	13	-	0	2	6

* Cigarettes with this tar yield no longer on the market
1 The definitions of the tar bands altered in 1985:

	1972-1984	1985-
Low	0-10 mg tar/cigarette	0- 9.99 mg tar/cigarette
Low/middle	11-16 mg tar/cigarette	10.0-14.99 mg tar/cigarette
Middle	17-22 mg tar/cigarette	15.0-17.99 mg tar/cigarette
Middle/high	23-28 mg tar/cigarette	no middle/high band
High	29+ mg tar/cigarette	18.0+ mg tar/cigarette
	(data rounded)	(data truncated)

Source: NOP

Fig. 9.3 Percentages of cigarette smokers: by tar yield of brand of cigarette usually smoked, 1974, 1985, and 1988
Cigarette smokers, men and women aged 16 and over, Great Britain. *Source*: NOP
Note: percentages may not total 100 due to 'Other/don't know' replies

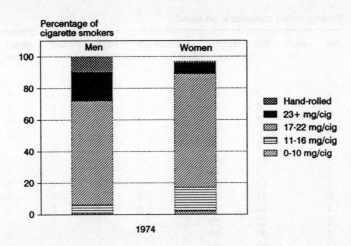

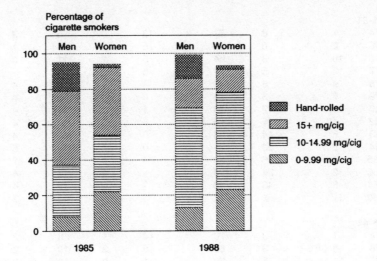

Table 9.10.1 Percentage of cigarette smokers: by age, and tar yield of brand of cigarette usually smoked, 1974-1988
Cigarette smokers, men aged 16 and over, Great Britain

Survey date	Manufactured cigarettes, tar band					Hand-rolled	Other/ don't know	All cigarettes
	Low	Low/middle	Middle	Middle/high	High			
Men aged 16-24								
Nov 1974	1	3	87	5	0	3	1	100
Mar 1976	3	6	80	4	0	6	1	100
Nov 1976	6	2	87	1	0	5	0	100
Nov/Dec 1977	3	6	81	3	0	5	2	100
Nov/Dec 1978	3	0	87	3	0	6	1	100
Nov/Dec 1979	1	10	83	0	*	4	2	100
Nov/Dec 1980	3	8	80	0	*	6	3	100
Nov 1982	5	19	65	0	*	8	5	100
Nov 1983	6	47	35	0	*	9	3	100
Nov 1984	2	50	38	0	*	8	2	100
Nov 1985[1]	3	32	56	-	0	8	1	100
Nov 1986[1]	4	35	51	-	0	7	3	100
Nov 1987[1]	17	39	39	-	0	4	0	100
Nov 1988[1]	8	81	9	-	0	3	0	100
Men aged 25-34								
Nov 1974	1	8	71	12	0	6	3	100
Mar 1976	2	6	79	5	0	8	1	100
Nov 1976	10	8	64	5	1	11	0	100
Nov/Dec 1977	10	5	73	5	0	5	1	100
Nov/Dec 1978	9	6	72	4	1	6	4	100
Nov/Dec 1979	7	3	76	0	*	10	4	100
Nov/Dec 1980	4	12	69	1	*	10	4	100
Nov 1982	4	26	52	0	*	14	4	100
Nov 1983	6	44	33	0	*	13	4	100
Nov 1984	5	50	21	0	*	18	5	100
Nov 1985[1]	4	36	38	-	0	15	7	100
Nov 1986[1]	12	34	34	-	0	17	4	100
Nov 1987[1]	8	46	36	-	0	12	4	100
Nov 1988[1]	11	52	17	-	0	13	7	100
Men aged 35-44								
Nov 1974	1	3	70	14	1	8	2	100
Mar 1976	5	3	62	15	3	10	2	100
Nov 1976	11	5	60	11	0	12	0	100
Nov/Dec 1977	7	5	55	13	0	18	1	100
Nov/Dec 1978	8	5	60	4	0	19	6	100
Nov/Dec 1979	7	2	70	1	*	16	4	100
Nov/Dec 1980	15	5	66	0	*	11	3	100
Nov 1982	6	19	49	0	*	23	4	100
Nov 1983	11	38	17	0	*	25	9	100
Nov 1984	9	49	23	0	*	14	6	100
Nov 1985[1]	13	26	37	-	0	19	4	100
Nov 1986[1]	10	29	36	-	0	22	2	100
Nov 1987[1]	11	42	29	-	2	13	3	100
Nov 1988[1]	14	55	16	-	0	12	3	100
Men aged 45-54								
Nov 1974	1	3	62	17	2	14	1	100
Mar 1976	3	6	50	20	3	16	3	100
Nov 1976	3	6	60	15	1	15	0	100
Nov/Dec 1977	10	10	47	19	1	13	1	100

Table 9.10.1 (*continued*) Percentage of cigarette smokers: by age, and tar yield of brand of cigarette usually smoked, 1974-1988
Cigarette smokers, men aged 16 and over, Great Britain

| Survey date | Manufactured cigarettes, tar band | | | | | Hand-rolled | Other/ don't know | All cigarettes |
	Low	Low/middle	Middle	Middle/high	High			
Men aged 45-54								
Nov/Dec 1978	11	4	57	10	1	14	3	100
Nov/Dec 1979	11	6	70	0	*	11	2	100
Nov/Dec 1980	12	7	61	1	*	14	5	100
Nov 1982	7	18	51	0	*	19	4	100
Nov 1983	9	48	28	0	*	13	2	100
Nov 1984	8	44	27	0	*	17	4	100
Nov 1985[1]	7	26	48	-	0	13	7	100
Nov 1986[1]	10	30	32	-	3	23	2	100
Nov 1987[1]	11	37	30	-	0	17	5	100
Nov 1988[1]	13	41	14	-	0	25	7	100
Men aged 55-64								
Nov 1974	1	4	49	33	0	13	0	100
Mar 1976	6	6	52	21	1	13	3	100
Nov 1976	7	2	52	19	2	18	0	100
Nov/Dec 1977	13	3	42	22	0	17	2	100
Nov/Dec 1978	11	7	56	14	0	10	2	100
Nov/Dec 1979	14	8	63	1	*	10	4	100
Nov/Dec 1980	13	7	58	0	*	16	5	100
Nov 1982	10	16	53	4	*	15	3	100
Nov 1983	13	46	19	3	*	17	2	100
Nov 1984	15	35	22	0	*	19	8	100
Nov 1985[1]	10	30	36	-	1	14	10	100
Nov 1986[1]	16	35	25	-	2	18	4	100
Nov 1987[1]	21	27	28	-	0	16	8	100
Nov 1988[1]	18	54	14	-	0	14	0	100
Men aged 65+								
Nov 1974	1	11	41	27	1	17	2	100
Mar 1976	3	4	51	22	1	20	0	100
Nov 1976	5	6	48	18	2	21	0	100
Nov/Dec 1977	7	7	43	21	2	15	4	100
Nov/Dec 1978	9	0	46	18	2	18	6	100
Nov/Dec 1979	8	6	62	0	*	22	2	100
Nov/Dec 1980	13	4	52	1	*	24	6	100
Nov 1982	9	12	56	3	*	18	2	100
Nov 1983	13	28	33	0	*	18	9	100
Nov 1984	13	37	26	0	*	19	5	100
Nov 1985[1]	16	17	37	-	0	29	2	100
Nov 1986[1]	22	26	22	-	2	24	5	100
Nov 1987[1]	17	35	28	-	0	14	5	100
Nov 1988[1]	11	44	27	-	3	11	3	100

* Cigarettes with this tar yield no longer on the market
1 The definitions of the tar bands altered in 1985:

	1972-1984	1985-
Low	0-10 mg tar/cigarette	0- 9.99 mg tar/cigarette
Low/middle	11-16 mg tar/cigarette	10.0-14.99 mg tar/cigarette
Middle	17-22 mg tar/cigarette	15.0-17.99 mg tar/cigarette
Middle/high	23-28 mg tar/cigarette	no middle/high band
High	29+ mg tar/cigarette	18.0+ mg tar/cigarette
	(data rounded)	(data truncated)

Source: NOP

Table 9.10.2 Percentage of cigarette smokers: by age, and tar yield of brand of cigarette usually smoked, 1974-1988
Cigarette smokers, women aged 16 and over, Great Britain

Survey date	Manufactured cigarettes, tar band					Hand-rolled	Other/ don't know	All cigarettes
	Low	Low/middle	Middle	Middle/high	High			
Women aged 16-24								
Nov 1974	1	13	81	1	0	1	2	100
Mar 1976	6	4	89	0	0	0	2	100
Nov 1976	4	11	84	0	0	1	0	100
Nov/Dec 1977	10	10	75	0	0	2	3	100
Nov/Dec 1978	10	7	80	0	0	0	3	100
Nov/Dec 1979	10	6	77	0	*	0	8	100
Nov/Dec 1980	15	9	70	0	*	1	7	100
Nov 1982	9	27	56	0	*	4	3	100
Nov 1983	11	39	41	0	*	3	6	100
Nov 1984	7	49	34	0	*	3	7	100
Nov 1985[1]	13	33	43	-	0	7	5	100
Nov 1986[1]	20	43	29	-	0	0	8	100
Nov 1987[1]	11	50	36	-	0	0	4	100
Nov 1988[1]	21	67	8	-	0	1	1	100
Women aged 25-34								
Nov 1974	1	11	81	3	0	0	3	100
Mar 1976	6	9	78	4	0	0	2	100
Nov 1976	12	8	76	2	0	1	0	100
Nov/Dec 1977	16	14	62	1	1	3	4	100
Nov/Dec 1978	13	7	74	1	0	2	3	100
Nov/Dec 1979	13	8	72	0	*	1	6	100
Nov/Dec 1980	14	20	62	0	*	1	4	100
Nov 1982	12	23	56	0	*	1	8	100
Nov 1983	13	48	32	1	*	0	6	100
Nov 1984	15	56	24	0	*	3	3	100
Nov 1985[1]	14	36	43	-	0	0	8	100
Nov 1986[1]	20	44	31	-	0	2	3	100
Nov 1987[1]	14	52	29	-	0	2	4	100
Nov 1988[1]	16	57	18	-	0	3	7	100
Women aged 35-44								
Nov 1974	3	17	70	5	1	0	4	100
Mar 1976	14	10	71	2	0	1	2	100
Nov 1976	14	13	63	5	0	3	1	100
Nov/Dec 1977	23	14	56	2	0	2	2	100
Nov/Dec 1978	28	5	60	3	0	4	3	100
Nov/Dec 1979	20	10	63	0	*	1	7	100
Nov/Dec 1980	22	13	62	0	*	0	2	100
Nov 1982	19	24	51	0	*	1	4	100
Nov 1983	20	54	19	0	*	2	5	100
Nov 1984	22	47	20	0	*	1	9	100
Nov 1985[1]	23	30	44	-	0	0	2	100
Nov 1986[1]	30	47	19	-	0	1	3	100
Nov 1987[1]	24	49	20	-	0	2	5	100
Nov 1988[1]	21	49	17	-	0	7	6	100
Women aged 45-54								
Nov 1974	1	21	65	11	0	1	1	100
Mar 1976	8	15	63	11	1	1	1	100
Nov 1976	17	16	57	8	0	0	1	100
Nov/Dec 1977	20	13	61	2	0	1	4	100

Table 9.10.2 (*continued*) Percentage of cigarette smokers: by age, and tar yield of brand of cigarette usually smoked, 1974-1988
Cigarette smokers, women aged 16 and over, Great Britain

Survey date	Manufactured cigarettes, tar band					Hand-rolled	Other/ don't know	All cigarettes
	Low	Low/middle	Middle	Middle/high	High			
Women aged 45-54								
Nov/Dec 1978	22	7	64	5	0	0	2	100
Nov/Dec 1979	29	8	55	0	*	0	8	100
Nov/Dec 1980	18	16	58	0	*	0	7	100
Nov 1982	31	19	47	0	*	1	3	100
Nov 1983	29	44	23	2	*	0	2	100
Nov 1984	25	53	20	0	*	0	2	100
Nov 1985[1]	27	32	30	-	0	2	9	100
Nov 1986[1]	30	34	25	-	0	3	8	100
Nov 1987[1]	27	33	33	-	0	2	6	100
Nov 1988[1]	21	58	12	-	0	1	9	100
Women aged 55-64								
Nov 1974	2	19	62	14	1	2	1	100
Mar 1976	15	17	53	12	0	3	1	100
Nov 1976	17	16	59	7	0	0	1	100
Nov/Dec 1977	25	11	52	5	0	3	6	100
Nov/Dec 1978	22	8	52	7	1	2	7	100
Nov/Dec 1979	24	7	61	0	*	2	6	100
Nov 1980	33	16	48	0	*	1	2	100
Nov 1982	27	19	43	0	*	1	10	100
Nov 1983	23	41	27	0	*	0	9	100
Nov 1984	42	28	23	0	*	0	6	100
Nov 1985[1]	23	35	32	-	0	3	8	100
Nov 1986[1]	35	39	16	-	0	5	5	100
Nov 1987[1]	25	41	28	-	0	3	4	100
Nov 1988[1]	35	45	15	-	0	3	1	100
Women aged 65+								
Nov 1974	3	6	71	15	0	1	4	100
Mar 1976	11	6	64	14	0	1	4	100
Nov 1976	9	21	61	6	1	1	0	100
Nov/Dec 1977	18	14	56	8	0	3	1	100
Nov/Dec 1978	20	11	57	7	0	0	4	100
Nov/Dec 1979	19	12	68	0	*	0	1	100
Nov/Dec 1980	21	15	55	0	*	2	7	100
Nov 1982	21	33	37	0	*	3	5	100
Nov 1983	30	42	21	0	*	3	4	100
Nov 1984	37	44	12	0	*	1	5	100
Nov 1985[1]	37	20	38	-	0	0	5	100
Nov 1986[1]	33	37	20	-	0	2	8	100
Nov 1987[1]	22	45	24	-	0	0	10	100
Nov 1988[1]	34	45	10	-	0	0	11	100

* Cigarettes with this tar yield no longer on the market
1 The definitions of the tar bands altered in 1985:

	1972-1984	1985-
Low	0-10 mg tar/cigarette	0- 9.99 mg tar/cigarette
Low/middle	11-16 mg tar/cigarette	10.0-14.99 mg tar/cigarette
Middle	17-22 mg tar/cigarette	15.0-17.99 mg tar/cigarette
Middle/high	23-28 mg tar/cigarette	no middle/high band
High	29+ mg tar/cigarette	18.0+ mg tar/cigarette
	(data rounded)	(data truncated)

Source: NOP

Fig. 9.4 Percentages of cigarette smokers: by age, and tar yield of brand of cigarette usually smoked, 1988
Cigarette smokers, men and women aged 16 and over, Great Britain. *Source*: NOP
Note: percentages may not total 100 due to 'Other/don't know' replies

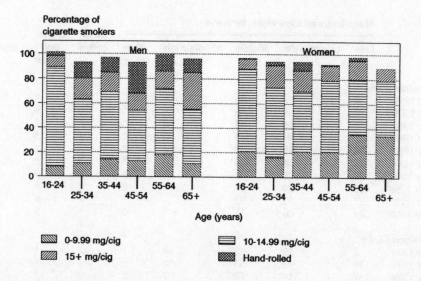

Table 9.11.1 Percentage of cigarette smokers: by social class, and tar yield of brand of cigarette usually smoked, 1974-1988
Cigarette smokers, men aged 16 and over, Great Britain

Survey date	Manufactured cigarettes, tar band					Hand-rolled	Other/ don't know	All cigarettes
	Low	Low/middle	Middle	Middle/high	High			
Men: social class AB								
Nov 1974	1	11	77	8	0	3	1	100
Mar 1976	8	12	69	6	2	1	1	100
Nov 1976	15	6	63	7	1	7	0	100
Nov/Dec 1977	21	8	50	7	0	10	4	100
Nov/Dec 1978	13	7	66	6	0	4	3	100
Nov/Dec 1979	13	4	74	2	*	3	4	100
Nov/Dec 1980	14	14	63	0	*	3	6	100
Nov 1982	13	12	67	0	*	2	5	100
Nov 1983	13	47	30	0	*	4	6	100
Nov 1984	16	57	24	0	*	2	2	100
Nov 1985[1]	20	41	33	-	0	4	2	100
Nov 1986[1]	29	30	30	-	0	8	2	100
Nov 1987[1]	12	40	40	-	4	0	3	100
Nov 1988[1]	36	29	18	-	3	9	6	100
Men: social class C1								
Nov 1974	2	6	70	13	1	7	1	100
Mar 1976	5	8	65	6	1	11	3	100
Nov 1976	11	7	64	8	1	10	0	100
Nov/Dec 1977	11	9	63	7	0	8	3	100
Nov/Dec 1978	18	4	63	7	0	2	4	100
Nov/Dec 1979	14	8	73	0	*	3	2	100

Survey date	Manufactured cigarettes, tar band					Hand-rolled	Other/don't know	All cigarettes
	Low	Low/middle	Middle	Middle/high	High			
Men: social class C1								
Nov/Dec 1980	9	11	63	1	*	11	4	100
Nov 1982	7	39	40	0	*	11	3	100
Nov 1983	14	43	26	1	*	10	6	100
Nov 1984	10	47	25	0	*	9	8	100
Nov 1985[1]	12	30	48	-	1	6	4	100
Nov 1986[1]	11	44	29	-	0	13	4	100
Nov 1987[1]	20	34	32	-	0	12	2	100
Nov 1988[1]	15	53	15	-	0	14	4	100
Men: social class C2								
Nov 1974	1	4	66	16	1	11	2	100
Mar 1976	3	4	64	14	1	13	2	100
Nov 1976	6	5	63	10	0	16	0	100
Nov/Dec 1977	7	4	60	13	0	14	1	100
Nov/Dec 1978	7	4	64	6	1	16	2	100
Nov/Dec 1979	7	6	68	0	*	15	4	100
Nov/Dec 1980	10	6	67	0	*	14	3	100
Nov 1982	7	18	53	1	*	18	4	100
Nov 1983	9	41	30	0	*	16	4	100
Nov 1984	7	43	29	0	*	17	3	100
Nov 1985[1]	4	33	39	-	0	21	3	100
Nov 1986[1]	10	33	33	-	0	19	4	100
Nov 1987[1]	8	39	33	-	0	13	6	100
Nov 1988[1]	11	65	14	-	0	8	2	100
Men: social class DE								
Nov 1974	0	4	60	22	0	13	2	100
Mar 1976	1	3	60	19	1	14	1	100
Nov 1976	4	3	60	17	2	15	0	100
Nov/Dec 1977	5	6	53	20	1	13	1	100
Nov 1978	5	2	63	12	0	13	5	100
Nov/Dec 1979	3	4	74	0	*	16	3	100
Nov/Dec 1980	8	6	64	0	*	16	5	100
Nov 1982	5	13	57	2	*	20	3	100
Nov 1983	6	42	26	1	*	21	5	100
Nov 1984	6	43	24	0	*	20	6	100
Nov 1985[1]	7	22	45	-	0	19	8	100
Nov 1986[1]	8	26	39	-	2	22	3	100
Nov 1987[1]	16	40	26	-	0	15	3	100
Nov 1988[1]	5	57	17	-	0	17	4	100

* Cigarettes with this tar yield no longer on the market
1 The definitions of the tar bands altered in 1985:

	1972-1984	1985-
Low	0-10 mg tar/cigarette	0- 9.99 mg tar/cigarette
Low/middle	11-16 mg tar/cigarette	10.0-14.99 mg tar/cigarette
Middle	17-22 mg tar/cigarette	15.0-17.99 mg tar/cigarette
Middle/high	23-28 mg tar/cigarette	no middle/high band
High	29+ mg tar/cigarette	18.0+ mg tar/cigarette
	(data rounded)	(data truncated)

Source: NOP

Table 9.11.2 Percentage of cigarette smokers: by social class, and tar yield of brand of cigarette usually smoked, 1974-1988
Cigarette smokers, women aged 16 and over, Great Britain

| Survey date | Manufactured cigarettes, tar band | | | | | Hand-rolled | Other/ don't know | All cigarettes |
	Low	Low/middle	Middle	Middle/high	High			
Women: social class AB								
Nov 1974	6	20	68	5	0	1	1	100
Mar 1976	15	19	61	3	0	3	1	100
Nov 1976	18	21	56	4	0	0	1	100
Nov/Dec 1977	34	14	44	0	0	3	4	100
Nov/Dec 1978	19	6	66	2	0	2	8	100
Nov/Dec 1979	21	12	59	0	*	1	8	100
Nov/Dec 1980	23	13	52	0	*	1	11	100
Nov 1982	40	25	33	0	*	0	3	100
Nov 1983	33	37	20	1	*	2	8	100
Nov 1984	35	45	15	0	*	1	4	100
Nov 1985[1]	41	24	31	-	0	2	2	100
Nov 1986[1]	41	39	15	-	0	2	3	100
Nov 1987[1]	33	45	14	-	0	4	4	100
Nov 1988[1]	28	62	7	-	0	0	3	100
Women: social class C1								
Nov 1974	1	19	67	5	0	2	6	100
Mar 1976	9	14	74	3	0	0	1	100
Nov 1976	20	15	56	6	0	3	0	100
Nov/Dec 1977	25	11	55	2	0	4	2	100
Nov/Dec 1978	21	9	61	3	1	1	5	100
Nov/Dec 1979	20	13	63	0	*	0	4	100
Nov/Dec 1980	25	18	53	0	*	0	4	100
Nov 1982	24	25	44	0	*	1	7	100
Nov 1983	38	36	19	0	*	0	7	100
Nov 1984	21	51	25	0	*	0	3	100
Nov 1985[1]	31	32	35	-	0	0	3	100
Nov 1986[1]	35	34	21	-	0	3	7	100
Nov 1987[1]	24	33	37	-	0	1	5	100
Nov 1988[1]	25	55	14	-	0	2	4	100
Women: social class C2								
Nov 1974	2	16	75	6	1	0	0	100
Mar 1976	9	9	72	5	0	1	3	100
Nov 1976	10	15	70	3	0	1	1	100
Nov/Dec 1977	16	13	66	1	0	1	3	100
Nov/Dec 1978	21	7	66	3	0	1	3	100
Nov/Dec 1979	18	6	69	0	*	0	7	100
Nov/Dec 1980	20	15	61	0	*	1	4	100
Nov 1982	19	22	49	0	*	2	7	100
Nov 1983	13	52	30	0	*	1	3	100
Nov 1984	25	46	23	0	*	1	6	100
Nov 1985[1]	16	34	39	-	0	1	9	100
Nov 1986[1]	21	42	27	-	0	2	7	100
Nov 1987[1]	19	51	27	-	0	0	3	100
Nov 1988[1]	25	53	13	-	0	4	6	100
Women: social class DE								
Nov 1974	0	10	73	12	0	0	4	100
Mar 1976	9	7	69	12	0	0	1	100
Nov 1976	10	9	73	6	1	1	1	100
Nov/Dec 1977	13	13	63	4	1	2	4	100
Nov/Dec 1978	15	7	68	6	0	2	3	100
Nov/Dec 1979	18	7	67	0	*	2	6	100

Table 9.11.2 (*continued*) Percentage of cigarette smokers: by social class, and tar yield of brand of cigarette usually smoked, 1974-1988
Cigarette smokers, women aged 16 and over, Great Britain

| Survey date | Manufactured cigarettes, tar band | | | | | Hand-rolled | Other/ don't know | All cigarettes |
	Low	Low/middle	Middle	Middle/high	High			
Women: social class DE								
Nov/Dec 1980	17	13	65	0	*	1	4	100
Nov 1982	14	24	55	0	*	3	5	100
Nov 1983	12	47	33	1	*	2	5	100
Nov 1984	19	48	25	0	*	2	6	100
Nov 1985[1]	16	32	41	-	0	3	8	100
Nov 1986[1]	24	44	26	-	0	1	4	100
Nov 1987[1]	15	48	29	-	0	2	6	100
Nov 1988[1]	21	55	15	-	0	2	7	100

* Cigarettes with this tar yield no longer on the market
1 The definitions of the tar bands altered in 1985:

	1972-1984	1985-
Low	0-10 mg tar/cigarette	0- 9.99 mg tar/cigarette
Low/middle	11-16 mg tar/cigarette	10.0-14.99 mg tar/cigarette
Middle	17-22 mg tar/cigarette	15.0-17.99 mg tar/cigarette
Middle/high	23-28 mg tar/cigarette	no middle/high band
High	29+ mg tar/cigarette	18.0+ mg tar/cigarette
	(data rounded)	(data truncated)

Fig. 9.5 Percentages of cigarette smokers: by social class, and tar yield of brand of cigarette usually smoked, 1988
Cigarette smokers, men and women aged 16 and over, Great Britain. *Source*: NOP
Note: percentages may not total 100 due to 'Other/don't know' replies

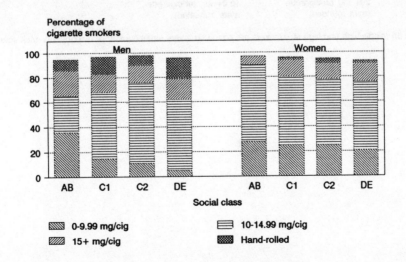

Table 9.12 Average number of manufactured cigarettes smoked yesterday: by tar yield of brand of cigarette usually smoked, 1979-1988
Manufactured cigarette smokers, men and women aged 16 and over, Great Britain

Survey date	Manufactured cigarettes, tar band				Hand-rolled	Other	Don't know	All cigarettes
	Low	Low/middle	Middle	Middle/high or high				
Men								
Nov/Dec 1979	18.0	16.9	18.7	15.8	..	17.2	8.9	18.4
Nov/Dec 1980	18.8	14.8	18.1	21.8	..	..	8.5	17.7
Nov 1982	15.6	18.0	19.0	13.2	2.5	23.4	6.6	18.2
Nov 1983	16.8	19.2	18.5	30.4	6.2	21.1	24.3	18.8
Nov 1984	16.1	19.4	16.9	..	..	19.6	12.4	18.1
Nov 1985[1]	21.1	19.6	17.8	34.5	..	14.3	19.5	18.7
Nov 1986[1]	19.8	17.2	16.8	22.8	0.0	18.0	4.5	17.4
Nov 1987[1]	18.1	17.6	16.0	24.5	0.0	21.5	9.1	17.0
Nov 1988[1]	16.2	16.8	17.6	5.0	0.0	24.5	10.8	16.8
Women								
Nov/Dec 1979	15.0	16.5	15.5	..	50.0	16.0	25.3	15.6
Nov/Dec 1980	13.5	15.3	15.1	..	..	10.9	7.8	14.7
Nov 1982	15.9	15.7	15.6	..	..	16.9	20.4	15.8
Nov 1983	15.1	16.8	14.8	8.1	..	14.4	6.2	15.7
Nov 1984	14.7	15.6	16.2	..	..	14.6	21.9	15.5
Nov 1985[1]	14.2	16.8	15.9	..	..	14.1	23.2	15.8
Nov 1986[1]	14.8	16.0	15.5	0.0	0.0	14.8	8.8	15.4
Nov 1987[1]	14.0	14.9	13.9	0.0	0.0	22.4	12.2	14.5
Nov 1988[1]	14.0	16.2	16.8	0.0	0.0	16.9	3.6	15.6

1 The definitions of the tar bands altered in 1985:

	1972-1984	1985-
Low	0-10 mg tar/cigarette	0- 9.99 mg tar/cigarette
Low/middle	11-16 mg tar/cigarette	10.0-14.99 mg tar/cigarette
Middle	17-22 mg tar/cigarette	15.0-17.99 mg tar/cigarette
Middle/high	23-28 mg tar/cigarette	no middle/high band
High	29+ mg tar/cigarette	18.0+ mg tar/cigarette
	(data rounded)	(data truncated)

Note that data on middle/high and high tar smokers are based on a very small number of respondents each year

Source: NOP

Table 9.13.1 Number of manufactured cigarettes smoked yesterday: by tar yield of brand of cigarette usually smoked, 1979-1988
Manufactured cigarette smokers, men aged 16 and over, Great Britain

Tar band	Survey date	Number of cigarettes smoked yesterday						Don't know	All smokers
		None	1-9	10-19	20-29	30-39	40+		
		Percentage of manufactured cigarette smokers							
Low	Nov/Dec 1979	4	12	31	41	4	8	0	100
	Nov/Dec 1980	2	13	23	44	12	6	1	100
	Nov 1982	7	23	38	23	5	4	0	100
	Nov 1983	4	21	33	35	7	0	0	100
	Nov 1984	2	32	25	27	11	0	2	100
	Nov 1985[1]	0	16	25	40	12	7	0	100
	Nov 1986[1]	0	23	25	36	4	10	0	100
	Nov 1987[1]	1	19	33	39	4	4	0	100
	Nov 1988[1]	5	22	40	24	0	8	0	100
Low/middle	Nov/Dec 1979	5	15	29	34	10	3	3	100
	Nov/Dec 1980	2	22	36	29	6	2	1	100
	Nov 1982	1	23	33	29	5	8	1	100
	Nov 1983	4	15	34	29	12	5	0	100
	Nov 1984	2	17	30	38	8	5	0	100
	Nov 1985[1]	1	14	35	36	7	6	1	100
	Nov 1986[1]	2	23	33	31	7	3	1	100
	Nov 1987[1]	5	23	28	33	7	5	0	100
	Nov 1988[1]	4	24	31	30	4	5	1	100
Middle	Nov/Dec 1979	2	18	25	33	12	9	2	100
	Nov/Dec 1980	2	15	31	35	9	7	1	100
	Nov 1982	1	18	31	36	7	6	1	100
	Nov 1983	4	14	37	32	8	4	0	100
	Nov 1984	5	25	31	25	7	6	0	100
	Nov 1985[1]	2	23	31	30	7	5	2	100
	Nov 1986[1]	2	21	44	23	5	5	0	100
	Nov 1987[1]	5	27	31	29	2	5	1	100
	Nov 1988[1]	0	22	41	25	7	5	0	100
Middle/ high or high	Nov/Dec 1979	0	0	56	44	0	0	0	100
	Nov/Dec 1980	0	0	43	57	0	0	0	100
	Nov 1982	0	14	86	0	0	0	0	100
	Nov 1983	0	0	0	41	59	0	0	100
	Nov 1984	..	..	..	..	..	..	..	100
	Nov 1985[1]	0	0	0	0	100	0	0	100
	Nov 1986[1]	0	12	27	39	0	1	0	100
	Nov 1987[1]	0	0	0	100	0	0	0	100
	Nov 1988[1]	0	100	0	0	0	0	0	100

1 The definitions of the tar bands altered in 1985:

	1972-1984	1985-
Low	0-10 mg tar/cigarette	0- 9.99 mg tar/cigarette
Low/middle	11-16 mg tar/cigarette	10.0-14.99 mg tar/cigarette
Middle	17-22 mg tar/cigarette	15.0-17.99 mg tar/cigarette
Middle/high	23-28 mg tar/cigarette	no middle/high band
High	29+ mg tar/cigarette	18.0+ mg tar/cigarette
	(data rounded)	(data truncated)

Note that data on middle/high and high tar smokers are based on a very small number of respondents each year

Source: NOP

Table 9.13.2 Number of manufactured cigarettes smoked yesterday: by tar yield of brand of cigarette usually smoked, 1979-1988
Manufactured cigarette smokers, women aged 16 and over, Great Britain

Tar band	Survey date	Number of cigarettes smoked yesterday						Don't know	All smokers
		None	1-9	10-19	20-29	30-39	40+		
		Percentage of manufactured cigarette smokers							
Low	Nov/Dec 1979	3	26	33	26	8	3	1	100
	Nov/Dec 1980	3	30	35	24	8	1	0	100
	Nov 1982	2	27	37	25	6	2	1	100
	Nov 1983	4	27	37	25	5	1	1	100
	Nov 1984	2	31	41	20	3	3	0	100
	Nov 1985[1]	6	27	39	24	3	1	0	100
	Nov 1986[1]	6	24	44	20	3	3	0	100
	Nov 1987[1]	6	25	47	17	2	2	0	100
	Nov 1988[1]	0	35	39	19	3	1	1	100
Low/middle	Nov/Dec 1979	2	19	32	32	3	7	5	100
	Nov/Dec 1980	2	31	25	29	7	6	1	100
	Nov 1982	6	18	42	30	1	2	1	100
	Nov 1983	2	26	32	33	5	3	0	100
	Nov 1984	3	28	38	23	4	4	0	100
	Nov 1985[1]	2	25	31	34	4	2	2	100
	Nov 1986[1]	5	20	41	29	2	3	0	100
	Nov 1987[1]	4	27	39	26	4	1	0	100
	Nov 1988[1]	2	24	39	29	3	3	0	100
Middle	Nov/Dec 1979	3	22	33	30	6	4	2	100
	Nov/Dec 1980	3	22	34	31	6	3	0	100
	Nov 1982	3	24	43	25	3	2	0	100
	Nov 1983	5	27	34	30	1	2	1	100
	Nov 1984	5	23	36	27	5	3	0	100
	Nov 1985[1]	2	24	36	30	2	2	4	100
	Nov 1986[1]	3	30	33	28	2	4	0	100
	Nov 1987[1]	3	39	28	27	2	2	0	100
	Nov 1988[1]	1	26	38	22	9	4	0	100
Middle/ high or high	Nov/Dec 1979	..	..	..	..	..	..	..	100
	Nov/Dec 1980	..	..	..	..	..	..	..	100
	Nov 1982	..	..	..	..	..	..	..	100
	Nov 1983	0	67	33	0	0	0	0	100
	Nov 1984	..	..	..	..	..	..	..	100
	Nov 1985[1]	..	..	..	..	..	..	..	100
	Nov 1986[1]	0	0	0	0	0	0	0	100
	Nov 1987[1]	0	0	0	0	0	0	0	100
	Nov 1988[1]	0	0	0	0	0	0	0	100

1 The definitions of the tar bands altered in 1985:

	1972-1984	1985-
Low	0-10 mg tar/cigarette	0- 9.99 mg tar/cigarette
Low/middle	11-16 mg tar/cigarette	10.0-14.99 mg tar/cigarette
Middle	17-22 mg tar/cigarette	15.0-17.99 mg tar/cigarette
Middle/high	23-28 mg tar/cigarette	no middle/high band
High	29+ mg tar/cigarette	18.0+ mg tar/cigarette
	(data rounded)	(data truncated)

Note that data on middle/high and high tar smokers are based on a very small number of respondents each year

Source: NOP

Smoking habits: by region

In this section, TAC data on the consumption of all tobacco products per person and per smoker in England and Wales and in Scotland between 1956 and 1981 are presented. Also included is the prevalence of cigarette smoking by region between 1974 and 1988 from the GHS.

TAC data show higher average annual consumption of all tobacco products between 1956 and 1981 for both men and women in Scotland than in England and Wales. Among men, consumption of all tobacco products by weight per adult and per smoker rose to a peak around 1962 and fell thereafter in both England and Wales, and Scotland. In England and Wales, consumption per smoker for men was slightly lower in 1981 than in 1956, but in Scotland it was higher. Tobacco consumption per person among women reached a peak in the mid-1970s in both England and Wales, and Scotland, and declined only slightly by 1981. Tobacco consumption per smoker among women rose steadily in England and Wales between 1956 and 1980, while in Scotland it reached a peak in 1978.

Data from the GHS show that the prevalence of cigarette smoking in Great Britain in 1988 ranged from 28 per cent in the South-east and the South-west, to 37 per cent in Scotland. In all regions a decrease was shown in the percentage of the population who smoke between 1974 and 1988. This data is not standardized, and therefore does not take acount of differences in age structure between the regions.

Table 10.1 Annual consumption (weight) of all tobacco products per person and per smoker for the United Kingdom, England and Wales, and Scotland, 1956-1981
Men and women aged 16 and over

	kg/person			kg/smoker		
	UK	England and Wales	Scotland	UK	England and Wales	Scotland
Men						
1956	4.6	4.6	4.8	6.1	6.2	6.3
1958	4.7	4.7	4.9	6.5	6.6	6.9
1961	4.9	4.9	5.1	6.7	6.8	7.1
1963	4.6	4.5	5.3	6.7	6.7	7.8
1965	4.1	4.1	4.9	6.1	6.0	7.2
1966	4.1	4.0	4.7	5.9	5.9	6.8
1967	4.1	4.0	4.8	5.9	5.9	6.9
1968	4.1	4.0	4.9	5.9	5.8	7.0
1969	3.9	3.8	4.6	5.6	5.5	6.6
1970	3.9	3.8	4.6	5.6	5.5	6.7
1971	3.7	3.6	4.6	5.6	5.5	7.0
1972	3.9	3.8	4.7	5.9	5.7	7.1
1973	3.9	3.8	4.9	5.9	5.8	7.5
1974	3.8	3.6	4.8	5.9	5.7	7.4
1975	3.6	3.4	4.7	5.8	5.6	7.6
1976	3.4	3.3	4.2	5.7	5.5	7.1
1977	3.2	3.1	4.0	5.5	5.3	6.8
1978	3.4	3.3	4.2	6.2	6.0	7.6
1979	3.4	3.2	4.0	6.1	5.9	7.4
1980	3.3	3.2	3.6	5.9	5.9	6.6
1981	2.9	2.9	3.6	5.9	5.8	7.3
Women						
1956	1.5	1.5	1.5	3.4	3.4	3.5
1958	1.5	1.5	1.6	3.9	3.9	4.1
1961	1.7	1.7	1.8	3.9	3.9	4.1
1963	1.7	1.7	2.0	4.0	3.9	4.5
1965	1.6	1.6	1.9	3.9	3.8	4.4
1966	1.7	1.7	2.0	3.8	3.8	4.3
1967	1.7	1.6	1.9	3.8	3.8	4.3
1968	1.6	1.6	1.9	3.8	3.7	4.4
1969	1.7	1.7	2.0	3.9	3.8	4.4
1970	1.7	1.7	2.0	3.8	3.8	4.4
1971	1.6	1.6	2.0	3.8	4.2	4.6
1972	1.7	1.7	2.0	4.0	4.0	4.7
1973	1.9	1.8	2.4	4.4	4.2	5.6
1974	1.9	1.9	2.4	4.4	4.2	5.4
1975	1.8	1.7	2.4	4.2	4.0	5.5
1976	1.9	1.8	2.4	4.4	4.2	5.6
1977	1.8	1.8	2.2	4.4	4.2	5.3
1978	2.0	1.9	2.4	4.9	4.8	5.9
1979	2.0	1.9	2.3	4.9	4.8	5.8
1980	1.9	1.9	2.0	4.9	4.9	5.2
1981	1.9	1.8	2.2	5.0	4.9	5.1

Table 10.1 (*continued*) Annual consumption (weight) of all tobacco products per person and per smoker for the United Kingdom, England and Wales, and Scotland, 1956-1981
Men and women aged 16 and over

	kg/person			kg/smoker		
	UK	England and Wales	Scotland	UK	England and Wales	Scotland
Men and women						
1956	2.9	2.9	3.0	5.1	5.1	5.3
1958	3.0	3.0	3.2	5.5	5.6	5.9
1961	3.2	3.2	3.4	5.6	5.6	5.9
1963	3.1	3.0	3.5	5.6	5.6	6.4
1965	2.9	2.8	3.3	5.2	5.1	6.0
1966	2.9	2.8	3.3	5.0	5.0	5.7
1967	2.8	2.8	3.2	5.1	5.0	5.8
1968	2.8	2.8	3.3	5.0	4.9	5.9
1969	2.8	2.7	3.2	4.9	4.8	5.6
1970	2.7	2.7	3.2	4.9	4.8	5.7
1971	2.6	2.5	3.2	4.9	4.8	6.0
1972	2.7	2.7	3.2	5.1	5.0	6.1
1973	2.9	2.8	3.6	5.3	5.1	6.7
1974	2.8	2.7	3.5	5.2	5.1	6.5
1975	2.6	2.5	3.4	5.1	4.9	6.6
1976	2.5	2.5	3.2	5.1	4.9	6.4
1977	2.4	2.4	3.0	5.0	4.9	6.1
1978	2.6	2.6	3.2	5.7	5.5	6.8
1979	2.6	2.5	3.1	5.6	5.4	6.7
1980	2.5	2.5	2.8	5.4	5.4	6.0
1981	2.4	2.3	2.9	5.5	5.4	6.2

Source: TAC

Table 10.2 Percentage of population who smoke cigarettes (manufactured and hand-rolled):
by region, 1974-1988
Adults aged 16 and over, Great Britain

Region	1974	1976	1978	1980	1982	1984	1986	1988
England								
North	46	45	41	41	41	36	35	36
Yorkshire and Humberside	43	40	39	40	35	39	34	32
North-west	48	46	43	43	36	35	35	33
East Midlands	44	41	39	39	33	31	31	32
West Midlands	45	43	39	37	35	33	34	29
East Anglia	39	39	38	36	30	24	31	29
Greater London	..	..	..	40	36	37	33	34
South-east	..	..	..	39	33	31	30	28
South-west	41	40	39	34	34	30	29	28
Wales	46	41	40	42	35	37	31	31
Scotland	48	46	45	44	42	39	36	37
Great Britain	45	42	40	39	35	34	33	32

Note: the data have not been standardized to take account of differences in age structure between the regions

Source: GHS

This section contains tables of the rates of duty on tobacco, and total receipts from duty and taxes on tobacco from 1900 to 1988.

Duties on tobacco appeared on the statute book in 1660; preferential rates were allowed to the Colonies and, after 1787, to the United States of America as well. In 1789 the duties were subdivided into two portions, Customs and Excise. In 1825 the Customs and Excise duties were consolidated into a single Customs duty, and the following year the differential duty on foreign tobacco was abolished. No distinction was made between raw and manufactured tobacco until 1823, when foreign cigars and manufactured tobacco were dutied separately. From 1863 the rate for raw tobacco was graduated according to the moisture content. From 1904, imported manufactured cigarettes were rated for duty separately.

The growing of tobacco in England and Ireland was prohibited during the seventeenth century, and in Scotland during the eighteenth century. This prohibition was lifted in Ireland in 1907, and in England and Scotland in 1910. Receipts from excise duty on home-grown raw tobacco have always been very small.

From 1904 to 1977 the revenue from tobacco duty was obtained mainly from duty on the weight of imported unmanufactured tobacco; revenue was also obtained from duty on imported manufactured tobacco, and from duty on home-grown unmanufactured tobacco (to a very small extent). Purchase tax was never levied on tobacco products.

In 1973 tobacco products became liable to VAT at the standard rate. During 1976-1977 tobacco duty was phased out in favour of tobacco-products duty which was introduced in May 1976. Tobacco-products duty is a duty on the final tobacco product rather than on unmanufactured tobacco, and applies equally to imported and home-manufactured tobacco products. Tobacco-products duty carries a different rate of duty for each product. For manufactured cigarettes, this duty is calculated on the number of items sold, as well as a percentage of the retail price. For all other tobacco products, the duty is charged on the weight of manufactured tobacco, i.e. the finished product. Since January 1978 tobacco, both unmanufactured and manufactured, imported from outside the European Community (EC) has been subject to a protective Common Customs Tariff of the EC.

Also tabulated in this section are the retail price of a pack of 20 cigarettes, the duty per pack, and the percentage of the retail price that is paid in duty and VAT. The type of cigarette chosen is that most commonly smoked, i.e. plain cigarettes from 1956-1967, standard size filter cigarettes from 1967-1978, and king size filter cigarettes from 1978-1988. In 1956 and 1989 the percentage of the retail price of 20 cigarettes that is paid in taxes stood at 75 per cent and 74 per cent, respectively, and ranged from 64 to 77 per cent in the intervening years.

Extracts from *Hansard* show that the ratio of the average price of a packet of 20 cigarettes to the average weekly wage fell from 1.1 per cent in 1959-1960 to 0.6 per cent in

1988-1989. Tobacco expenditure as a percentage of household expenditure fell from 4.5 per cent in 1972 to 2.8 per cent in 1988.

The retail price index for cigarettes was higher than the Retail Price Index (all items) between 1965 and 1969 and between 1984 and 1989 (see Table 11.10).

Figure 11.2 shows that the real price of cigarettes varied approximately inversely with the annual sales of manufactured cigarettes.

Table 11.1 Rates of tobacco duty on unmanufactured tobacco, 1900-1978
United Kingdom

Date of duty change	Full duty per lb[1,2] £	Imperial preference duty per lb[1,2] £
Apr 1900	0.150	
Apr 1909	0.183	
22 Sept 1915	0.275	
3 May 1917	0.367	1 Sept 1919 - 30 June 1925 1/6th preference
16 July 1917	0.321	1 July 1925 - 11 Apr 1927 1/4th preference
23 Apr 1918	0.408	
12 Apr 1927	0.442	0.340
11 Sept 1931	0.475	0.373
26 Apr 1939	0.575	0.473
28 Sept 1939	0.675	0.573
24 Apr 1940	0.875	0.773
24 July 1940	0.975	0.873
15 Apr 1942	1.475	1.373
13 Apr 1943	1.775	1.698
16 Apr 1947	2.742	2.665
7 Apr 1948	2.908	2.831
18 Apr 1956	3.058	2.981
5 Apr 1960	3.225	3.148
26 July 1961	3.544	3.467
15 Apr 1964	3.869	3.792
7 Apr 1965	4.369	4.292
20 Mar 1968	4.585	4.508
23 Nov 1968	5.042	4.965
15 Feb 1971	5.041	4.964
1 Apr 1973[3]	4.305	4.228

Date of duty change	Full duty per lb[1] £	Preference duties per lb[1]			
		Irish Republic £	Other EC £	Commonwealth preference area £	Commonwealth preference standstill area £
1 Jan 1974	4.2710 + 6%	4.2248	4.2710	4.2248 + 6%	4.2280
27 Mar 1974	5.6710 + 6%	5.6248	5.6710	5.6248 + 6%	5.6280
1 Jan 1975	5.6540 + 8.4%	5.6232	5.6540	5.6232 + 8.4%	5.6280
16 Apr 1975	7.7040 + 8.4%	7.6732	7.7040	7.6732 + 8.4%	7.6780
1 Jan 1976	7.6870 + 11.2%	7.6716	7.6870	7.6716 + 11.2%	7.6780
10 May 1976[4]	5.8320 + 11.2%	5.8166	5.8320	5.8166 + 11.2%	5.8230
16 Dec 1976	6.4152 + 12.32%	6.39826	6.4152	6.39826 + 12.32%	6.4053
30 Mar 1977	6.4170+ 11.2%	6.4016	6.4170	6.4016 + 11.2%	6.4080

1 July 1977	Full duty per lb = £6.4 + whichever is the less of 14% or .2041 Unit of Account Members of the EC subject only to duty of £6.4 per lb
1 Jan 1978	Imported unmanufactured tobacco subject only to duty imposed by the EC Common Customs Tariff

1 Duty on imported, unmanufactured, unstemmed tobacco, containing 10 per cent, or more of moisture
2 Duties before 1971 have been converted from shillings and pence to pounds and new pence using 240d=100p
3 Concurrently with the reduction of the rate of revenue duty on 1 Apr 1973 tobacco became liable to
Value Added Tax at the standard rate
4 The basic rate of duty was reduced on 10 May 1976 to allow for the introduction of tobacco-products duty
1 lb = 0.4536 kg

Source: HM Customs and Excise

Table 11.2 Rates of tobacco products duty[1], 1976-1990
United Kingdom

Date of duty change	Cigarette duty	Cigar duty per lb £	Hand-rolling tobacco duty per lb £	Other manufactured tobacco duty per lb £
10 May 1976[2]	20%[3]	2.765	2.400	1.550
4 Apr 1977	22% + £1.41/1000[4]	3.0415	3.825	1.705
1 Jan 1978	30% + £9.00/1000[5]	9.50	9.20	7.30
13 Aug 1979	21% +£11.77/1000			
		per kg	per kg	per kg
1 Jan 1980	21% + £11.77/1000	20.94	20.28	16.09
29 Mar 1980	21% + £13.42/1000	25.60	22.60	17.40
14 Mar 1981	21% + £18.04/1000	34.29	29.56	21.92
8 July 1981	21% + £19.03/1000	35.91	30.96	22.96
12 Mar 1982	21% + £20.68/1000	39.00	33.65	24.95
18 Mar 1983	21% + £21.67/1000	40.85	35.40	24.95
16 Mar 1984	21% + £24.97/1000	47.05	40.60	24.95
22 Mar 1985	21% + £26.95/1000	47.05	43.73	24.95
21 Mar 1986	21% + £30.61/1000	47.05	49.64	24.95
18 Mar 1988	21% + £31.74/1000	48.79	51.48	24.95
23 Mar 1990	21% + £34.91/1000	53.67	56.63	24.95

1 Tobacco products excise duty applies equally to imported manufactured and home-manufactured tobacco products
2 All duties subject to a 10% increase from 1 Jan 1977 to 3 Apr 1977
3 The percentage rates are percentages of the retail price. Retail price includes all duties and taxes, and is normally the retail price recommended by the manufacturer or importer
4 An amount per thousand manufactured cigarettes
5 From 4 Sep 1978 to 13 Mar 1981, cigarettes yielding 20 mg or more of tar were subject to an additional rate of tobacco products duty of £2.25 per thousand cigarettes

Source: HM Customs and Excise

Table 11.3 Receipts from tobacco duty, 1904-1976
United Kingdom

Year ended 31 Mar	Imported unmanufactured tobacco £ thousands	Imported manufactured tobacco £ thousands	Home-grown unmanufactured tobacco £ thousands	Total receipts £ thousands	Total receipts at constant 1913-14 prices[1] £ thousands
1903-04	11 946	681	..	12 627	14 030
1904-05	12 508	676	..	13 185	14 650
1905-06	12 713	668	1	13 382	14 705
1906-07	12 667	629	2	13 298	14 147
1907-08	13 173	566	7	13 746	14 171
1908-09	13 250	574	5	13 829	15 032
1909-10	15 104	577	7	15 688	17 240
1910-11	16 562	608	12	17 182	17 898
1911-12	16 749	594	10	17 352	17 889
1912-13	16 655	599	24	17 278	17 107
1913-14	17 651	612	20	18 284	18 103
1914-19	..	..	..	..	..
1919-20	59 270	1 588	13	60 871	..[2]

Year ended 31 Mar	Imported unmanufactured tobacco £ thousands	Imported manufactured tobacco £ thousands	Home-grown unmanufactured tobacco £ thousands	Total receipts £ thousands	Total receipts at constant 1913-14 prices[1] £ thousands
1920-21	55 002	518	11	55 532	21 441
1921-22	54 585	613	11	55 208	23 197
1922-23	52 763	628	4	53 396	26 303
1923-24	51 216	665	1	51 882	25 407
1924-25	51 267	643	3	51 913	27 323
1925-26	52 840	653	4	53 498	28 157
1926-27	53 233	625	2	53 859	28 347
1927-28	57 486	617	2	58 104	31 578
1928-29	58 439	647	1	59 087	32 113
1929-30	62 155	638	1	62 794	34 314
1930-31	63 511	565	1	64 077	35 998
1931-32	62 804	492	2	63 298	37 454
1932-33	66 869	359	2	67 229	40 499
1933-34	67 089	433	1	67 523	41 681
1934-35	70 162	498	1	70 661	43 618
1935-36	74 494	499	1	74 994	46 293
1936-37	76 766	570	1	77 336	47 156
1937-38	82 284	536	1	82 821	49 007
1938-39	84 284	529	5	84 818	49 313
1939-40	117 177	537	4	117 718	66 134
1940-41	172 591	196	9	172 796	85 542
1941-42	220 497	463	15	220 975	99 538
1942-43	329 746	1 020	11	330 777	140 160
1943-44	386 858	1 441	1	388 300	158 490
1944-45	380 443	2 267	3	382 713	153 085
1945-46	410 062	6 362	1	416 425	163 304
1946-47	443 911	2 395	1	446 308	157 706
1947-48	568 527	2 157	1	567 809	188 016
1948-49	608 774	1 334	0	604 248	185 352
1949-50	609 713	1 268	0	600 943	179 923
1950-51	613 945	1 401	0	604 260	175 148
1951-52	623 924	1 563	2	613 473	164 912
1952-53	628 026	1 599	1	616 760	156 142
1953-54	639 200	1 602	0	627 043	155 981
1954-55	662 648	1 828	0	649 880	158 895
1955-56	681 940	1 998	0	668 526	158 418
1956-57	715 831	2 262	0	701 829	159 145
1957-58	725 006	2 466	0	712 504	157 286
1958-59	733 662	2 549	..	736 161	157 974
1959-60	785 735	2 798	..	788 533	168 851
1960-61	821 689	3 529	..	825 218	172 423
1961-62	866 191	3 422	..	869 613	175 608
1962-63	874 025	4 132	..	878 157	170 185
1963-64	887 306	4 806	..	892 112	169 474
1964-65	977 562	6 094	..	983 656	180 852
1965-66	1 006 498	7 685	..	1 014 182	178 145
1966-67	1 016 759	7 731	..	1 024 579	173 159
1967-68	1 034 639	8 463	..	1 043 390	172 091
1968-69	1 089 100	14 407	..	1 103 655	173 667
1969-70	1 117 000	24 360	..	1 141 543	170 456

Table 11.3 (*continued*) Receipts from tobacco duty, 1904-1976
United Kingdom

Year ended 31 Mar	Imported unmanufactured tobacco £ thousands	Imported manufactured tobacco £ thousands	Home-grown unmanufactured tobacco £ thousands	Total receipts £ thousands	Total receipts at constant 1913-14 prices[1] £ thousands
1970-71	1 104 600	37 770	..	1 142 364	160 332
1971-72	1 067 600	57 640	..	1 125 252	144 300
1972-73	1 098 200	86 435	..	1 184 664	141 808
1973-74	993 700	92 845	..	1 086 536	119 216
1974-75	1 220 000	119 652	..	1 339 646	126 668
1975-76	1 515 500	163 925	..	1 679 455	127 822

1 Price index used to deflate receipts to 1913-14 prices was derived from the London and Cambridge Economic Service retail price index 'Bulletin, Times Review Of Industry', June 1960, the retail price index in A.L.Bowley, *Wages and Income Since 1860*, 1937, pp. 121-2, as used by Deane and Cole, *British Economic Growth, 1688-1959*, 1967, pp. 329-31, and from the Department of Employment Gazette
2 No retail price index data available for 1915-19

Note: small discrepancies between total receipts and sum of first three columns for years 1947-48 to 1958-59 due to Old Age Pensioner tobacco duty relief and excise duty on tobacco stocks; discrepancies for years 1966-67 to 1969-70 due to receipts from baggage etc.

Source: HM Customs and Excise

Table 11.4 Receipts from tobacco products duty[1], 1977-1990
United Kingdom

Year ended 31 Mar	Cigarette £ thousands	Cigars £ thousands	Hand-rolling tobacco £ thousands	Other manufactured tobacco £ thousands	Total £ thousands	Total receipts at constant prices 15 Jan 1974=100[2] £ thousands
1976-77					1 874 741	1 193 342
1977-78					2 057 103	1 130 276
1978-79	2 194 755	66 370	122 321	68 670	2 448 635	1 242 331
1979-80	2 327 903	71 295	117 938	65 490	2 582 625	1 155 537
1980-81	2 544 645	79 132	132 380	64 405	2 820 562	1 069 610
1981-82	3 052 137	99 762	189 560	78 969	3 420 428	1 159 467
1982-83	3 057 565	101 917	206 262	80 061	3 445 805	1 075 470
1983-84	3 403 308	110 741	211 795	79 674	3 805 518	1 135 637
1984-85	3 727 910	117 346	219 322	75 403	4 139 981	1 176 800
1985-86	4 051 498	115 541	221 423	70 959	4 459 421	1 194 915
1986-87	4 331 986	118 969	235 918	67 944	4 754 817	1 232 137
1987-88	4 346 828	118 762	236 452	64 569	4 766 611	1 185 724
1988-89	4 582 951	120 078	225 654	61 451	4 990 134	1 183 338
1989-90	4 637 396	119 313	222 448	56 136	5 035 293	1 107 875

1 Tobacco products excise duty applies equally to imported and home-manufactured tobacco products. From 10 May 1976 to 31 Dec 1977 customs revenue duty was charged on unmanufactured tobacco and has been included in receipts. From 1 Jan 1978 duty on unmanufactured tobacco imposed by the EC Common Customs Tariff has been a separate duty and is not included in receipts
2 General Index of Retail Prices: All Items Index used to deflate receipts. Source: Central Statistical Office

Source: HM Customs and Excise

Year	Total receipts £ millions	Total receipts at constant prices 15 Jan 1974=100[1] £ millions	
1973	135	144	VAT introduced at standard rate of 10% on 1 Apr 1973
1974	185	171	Standard rate reduced to 8% on 29 July 1974
1975	205	152	
1976	230	146	
1977	270	148	
1978	290	147	
1979	450	201	Standard rate raised to 15% on 18 June 1979
1980	630	239	
1981	720	244	
1982	765	239	
1983	810	242	
1984	865	246	
1985	915	245	
1986	975	253	
1987	1000	249	
1988	1035	246	

1 General Index of Retail Prices: All Items Index used to deflate receipts. Source: Central Statistical Office

Source: HM Customs and Excise, unpublished

Table 11.6 Rate of duty on unmanufactured tobacco imposed by the European Community Common Customs Tariff (CCT), 1978-1990
United Kingdom

Date of duty change	Duty[1]
5 Jan 1978	14% with a maximum of 45 tua per 100 kg
1 Jan 1979	23% subject to a minimum of 28 EUA and a maximum of 30 EUA per 100 kg
1 Jan 1980	23% subject to a minimum of 28 ECU and a maximum of 30 ECU per 100 kg

1 The duty listed is that imposed on flue cured Virginia type and light air cured Burley type tobacco

tua: transiting European unit of account
EUA: European Unit of Account
ECU: European Currency Unit

Note: (i) There was no change in CCT on unmanufactured tobacco from 1980 through to 1990
(ii) Receipts from CCT on unmanufactured tobacco not available from HM Customs and Excise

Source: HM Customs and Excise

Table 11.7 Retail price, tobacco duty, and Value Added Tax on 20 cigarettes, 1956-1990
United Kingdom

Year	Retail price[1] of 20 most commonly smoked plain cigarettes pence	Date of duty change	Approximate duty[1] per 20 standard cigarettes pence	Duty as a percentage of the retail price %
1956	19.2	18 Apr 1956	14.4	75
1957	19.6			
1958	19.6			
1959	19.6			
1960	20.4	5 Apr 1960	15.2	75
1961	20.8			
	22.5	26 July 1961	16.7	74
1962	22.5			
1963	22.5			
1964	24.2			
	24.6	15 Apr 1964	18.5	75
1965	27.1	7 Apr 1965	20.8	77
1966	27.1			
1967	27.1			

Year	Retail price[1] of 20 most commonly smoked filter cigarettes pence	Date of duty change	Approximate duty[1] per 20 standard cigarettes pence	VAT pence	Duty (and VAT) as a percentage of the retail price %
1967	22.9		15.8		69
1968	23.8	20 Mar 1968	16.7		70
	24.2	23 Nov 1968	18.3		76
1969	25.8		18.3		71
1970	25.8		18.3		71
1971	26.0		17.5		67
1972	26.5		17.5		66
1973	26.5	1 Apr 1973	14.5	2.4	64
1974	32.0	27 Mar 1974	19.5	2.9	70
1975	42.0	16 Apr 1975	26.0	3.1	69
1976	45.0	10 May 1976	28.0	3.3	70
1977	49.0	1 Jan 1977	31.5	3.6	72

Table 11.7 (*continued*) Retail price, tobacco duty, and Value Added Tax on 20 cigarettes, 1956-1990 United Kingdom

Year	Retail price of 20 most commonly smoked king size cigarettes pence	Date of duty change	Duty and VAT per 20 king size cigarettes				Duty and VAT as a percentage of the retail price %
			Specific duty pence	Ad valorem duty pence	VAT pence	Total duty + VAT pence	
1978	55	1 Jan 1978	18.0	16.5	4.1	38.6	70
1979	57	18 June 1969	18.0	17.1	4.2	39.3	69
	66	13 Aug 1979	23.5	13.9	8.6	46.0	70
1980	73	29 Mar 1980	26.8	15.3	9.5	51.6	71
1981	91	14 Mar 1981	36.1	19.1	11.9	67.1	74
	95	8 July 1981	38.1	20.0	12.4	70.5	74
1982	102	12 Mar 1982	41.4	21.4	13.3	76.1	75
1983	109	18 Mar 1983	43.3	22.9	14.2	80.4	74
1984	123	16 Mar 1984	49.9	25.8	16.0	91.8	75
1985	133	22 Mar 1985	53.9	27.9	17.3	99.2	75
1986	148	21 Mar 1986	61.2	31.3	19.3	111.6	75
1987	152	18 Mar 1988	61.2	31.9	19.8	112.9	74
1988	155	18 Mar 1988	63.5	32.6	20.2	116.3	75
1989	161	18 Mar 1989	63.5	33.8	21.0	118.3	74
1990	175	23 Mar 1990	69.8	36.8	22.8	129.4	74

1 Price and duty from 1956 to 1970 have been converted from shillings and pence to new pence, using 240d=100p

Source: HM Customs and Excise

Table 11.8 Ratio of the average price of a packet of 20 cigarettes to the average weekly wage, 1959-60 to 1988-89
Extract from *Hansard*, 13 March 1989

Mr. Amos asked the Chancellor of the Exchequer if he will publish in the Official Report a table showing in real terms the ratio of the price of an average priced packet of 20 cigarettes to the average weekly wage in each of (a)1959, (b)1969, (c)1979 and the latest year for which figures are available; and if he will make a statement.
Mr. Lilley: The ratio of the average price of a packet of 20 cigarettes to the average weekly wage in the relevant financial years is shown below:

Year	Ratio %
1959-60	1.1
1969-70	1.0
1979-80	0.6
1988-89	0.6

Source: Hansard

Table 11.9   Tobacco expenditure as a percentage of household expenditure, 1972-1988
Extract from *Hansard*, 21 February 1989

Mr. Jessel asked the Secretary of State for Health if he will provide figures to show changes in the proportion of smokers and non-smokers and the average daily number of cigarette expenditure per person and per household as a proportion of income in the last 30 years.

Mr. Mellor (holding answer 20 February 1989): The information available centrally is given in the table.

Year	Percentage of population who smoke cigarettes (16+ years)		Cigarettes smoked per day (16+ years)		Tobacco expenditure as a percentage of household expenditure
	Males	Females	Males	Females	
1972	52	41	17.1	12.4	4.5
1974	51	41	17.9	13.4	4.3
1976	46	38	18.4	14.4	4.2
1978	45	37	18.1	14.4	3.9
1980	42	37	17.7	14.6	3.5
1982	38	33	17.3	14.0	3.6
1984	36	32	16.4	13.7	3.4
1986	35	31	16.4	13.9	3.2
1988[1]	33	30	17.1	14.1	2.8

1 The 1988 figures were not originally included in this table at the time of publication
Note: the figures on smoking exclude cigar and pipe smoking. In 1986 9 per cent of men smoked a pipe or cigars
(in 1988 7 per cent of men smoked a pipe or cigars)
Source: General Household Survey

Source: Hansard

Fig. 11.1   The Retail Price Index (RPI) and the retail price index for cigarettes, 1962-1989 (prices in January 1962=100) United Kingdom. *Source*: Central Statistical Office

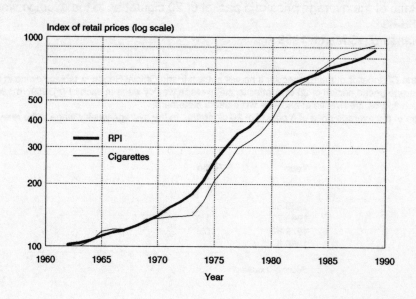

Table 11.10 The retail price index for cigarettes[1], the Retail Price Index (RPI), the increase in the price of cigarettes allowing for inflation, and the real price of cigarettes, 1962-1989
United Kingdom

Year	Retail price index for cigarettes[1] Jan 1962=100[2]		Retail Price Index Jan 1962=100[2]		Percentage change from previous year in price of cigarettes relative to RPI	Real price of cigarettes[1] 1962=100
1962	100.0		101.6		—	100.0
1963	100.0		103.6		-1.9	98.1
1964	105.8		107.0		2.4	100.5
1965	118.0		112.1		1.3	106.9
1966	120.8		116.5		-1.4	105.4
1967	120.8		119.4		-2.5	102.8
1968	125.5		125.0		-0.8	102.0
1969	135.5		131.8		2.5	104.5
1970	136.3		140.2		-5.5	98.8
1971	138.5		153.4		-7.2	91.7
1972	139.5		164.3		-5.9	86.3
1973	141.2		179.4		-7.3	80.0
1974	164.5	(115.7)	208.1	(108.5)	0.4	80.3
1975	209.0	(147.0)	258.5	(134.8)	2.2	82.1
1976	242.6	(170.6)	301.3	(157.1)	-0.4	81.8
1977	297.2	(209.0)	349.1	(182.0)	5.7	86.5
1978	320.8	(225.6)	378.0	(197.1)	-0.3	86.2
1979	351.8	(247.4)	428.7	(223.5)	-3.2	83.4
1980	412.9	(290.4)	505.8	(263.7)	-0.6	82.9
1981	516.0	(362.9)	565.8	(295.0)	11.8	92.7
1982	588.7	(414.0)	614.5	(320.4)	5.0	97.3
1983	627.7	(441.4)	642.7	(335.1)	2.0	99.2
1984	697.1	(490.2)	674.8	(351.8)	5.8	105.0
1985	760.1	(534.5)	715.8	(373.2)	2.8	107.9
1986	834.4	(589.6)	740.2	(385.9)	6.1	114.5
1987	866.6	(100.2)	771.0	(101.9)	-0.3	114.2
1988	896.9	(103.7)	808.9	(106.9)	-1.3	112.7
1989	921.9	(106.6)	871.7	(115.2)	-4.6	107.5

1 Includes other tobacco products in addition to cigarettes before 1974 (no separate index for cigarettes and tobacco was available at that time)
2 The index was rebased in 1962, in 1974, and in 1987 (January=100 for each year) and the appropriate figures are given in brackets. The other figures show a continuation of the retail prices index as rebased in 1962 (Jan 1962=100). For cigarettes the link between the series is 142.2 and 608.2, and for the RPI 191.8 and 394.5, respectively for January 1974 and January 1987

Note: annual averages are shown

Source: Central Statistical Office

(i)

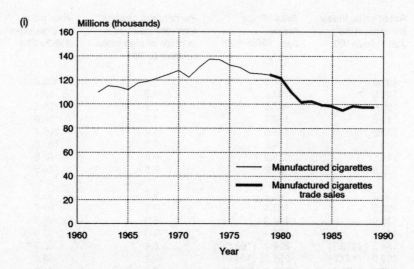

(ii)

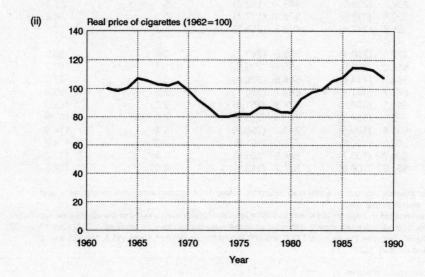

Children and smoking

Data on the smoking habits of children are available from different surveys from 1966 to 1988 and the results are summarized in this section.

As one would expect, the adoption of smoking increases steadily as children progress through secondary school. In the 1960s and 1970s, the prevalence of regular smoking (defined as smoking one cigarette or more a week in most surveys) was higher among boys than girls. In the late 1980s the proportion of children smoking was lower than in the early 1980s. Smoking declined more markedly among boys and by 1988 smoking was more prevalent among girls than boys.

McKennell (1980) found that the prevalence of smoking regularly was higher (i) when the questionnaire was self-administered rather than completed by an interviewer, (ii) when the answers were obtained in school rather than at home, and (iii) in school when the children completed the questionnaire together in a group or classroom setting rather than individually. These differences were greater for boys than for girls and were statistically significant only for boys.

In a study conducted by OPCS in 1988 (Goddard, 1989) among secondary school children, saliva specimens were obtained from half the sample and were tested for the presence of cotinine (a metabolite of nicotine). The saliva specimens were taken in addition to the collection of smoking information from pupils using self-completion questionnaires, in order to encourage honest reporting as children tend to under-report their smoking. The pupils who gave saliva specimens were aware of the purpose of the procedure. As expected, the reported prevalence of cigarette smoking increased among those who were tested compared to those who were not, from 6 to 8 per cent for boys and from 6 to 11 per cent for girls. Another finding of this study was that, of all children, 20 per cent had tried smoking by the age of 11 and 46 per cent by the age of 15. About 20 per cent of 15-year-olds were regular smokers, 17 per cent of boys and 22 per cent of girls. About half of the children who were regular smokers smoked more than 70 cigarettes a week.

Table 12.1 Percentages of boys and girls smoking cigarettes regularly: summary of some British studies, 1965-1988

Study	Year	Sample	Boys 11	12	13	14	15	16	Girls 11	12	13	14	15	16
Bynner[1]	1966	Random sample of 5 601 boys in 1st-4th years in England and Wales	4	9	17	27	38							
Tobacco Research Council[2]	1965-66	Random sample of 1 944 boys aged 10-15	5	4	5	16	22							
Holland and Elliott[3]	1965	Sample of 9 786 boys and girls in South East England	← 19 →		← 27 →				← 5 →		← 18 →			
	1966		← 17 →		← 29 →				← 4 →		← 20 →			
Rawbone, Keeling, Jenkins, and Guz[4]	1975	10 498 boys and girls in Hounslow schools	5	8	15	19	26	24	3	5	11	20	23	22
	1979		4	4	9	16	21	22	3	5	12	17	23	19
Aitken[5]	1976	384 boys and girls aged 10, 12, and 14 in central Scotland		2		11				2		11		
		(boys and girls analysed together)												
Murray, Swan, Bewley, and Johnson[6]	1974-78	Cohort of 6 000 boys and girls starting at secondary schools in Derbyshire in 1974		6	9	16	21	26		2.5	6	13	19	23
McKennell[7]	1980	Methodological study using 4 000 boys and girls in British secondary schools	9	10	29	21	33	28	5	13	16	16	26	22
		(classroom questionnaire)												
			6	0	5	8	23	17	0	0	9	14	20	18
		(oral interview at home)												
Ledwith and Osman[8]	1981	2 045 boys and girls in schools in Lothian, Scotland		7	7	24	24	23		5	9	37	35	38
Dobbs and Marsh[9]	1982	Random sample of 2 979 boys and girls from 105 schools in England and Wales	1	2	8	18	24	26	0	1	6	14	25	25
		Random sample of 2 287 boys and girls from 71 schools in Scotland	3	6	8	21	29	..	0	5	10	21	26	..
Dobbs and Marsh[10]	1984	Random sample of 3 658 boys and girls from 144 schools in England and Wales	0	2	10	16	28	29	1	2	9	19	28	30
		Random sample of 2 798 boys and girls from 96 schools in Scotland	4	8	10	22	29	..	3	3	12	22	34	..
Goddard and Ikin[11]	1986	Random sample of 3 189 boys and girls from 119 schools in England and Wales	0	2	5	6	18*	..	0	2	5	16	27*	..
		Random sample of 2 365 boys and girls from 81 schools in Scotland	..	2§	7	11	24	..	..	3§	8	21	26	..

Table 12.1 (*continued*) Percentages of boys and girls smoking cigarettes regularly: summary of some British studies, 1965-1988

			Age (years)											
			11	12	13	14	15	16	11	12	13	14	15	16
Study	Year	Sample	Boys						Girls					
Balding[12]	1985	Opportunity sample of 12 488 boys and girls from 87 schools in Britain[¶,+]	3	10	15	21	30	..	2	11	17	25	29	..
Balding[13]	1986	Opportunity sample of 17 678 boys and girls from 88 schools in Britain[¶,+]	2	5	12	18	24	..	2	6	16	25	25	..
Balding[14]	1987	Opportunity sample of 16 663 boys and girls from 121 schools in Britain[¶,+]	3	4	8	15	25	..	2	4	13	20	25	..
Balding[15]	1988	Opportunity sample of 33 459 boys and girls from 188 schools in England[¶]	2	4	9	13	19	..	2	5	12	20	25	..
Goddard[16]	1988	Random sample of 3 378 boys and girls from 137 schools in England	0	2	5	8	17*	..	0	0	4	12	22*	..

Note: in most studies, the definition of smoking regularly was smoking one cigarette or more per week

¶ The figures shown are for five school year groups; the first school year includes 11 and 12-year-olds, the second 12 and 13-year-olds, etc.
+ Britain includes Scotland, Wales, England, and Ireland
* Figures are not shown separately for 16-year-olds
§ Figures are not shown separately for 11-year-olds

1 Bynner, J.M. The Young Smoker, HMSO, 1969
2 Todd, G.F.(ed) Statistics of smoking in the United Kingdom (Research Paper 1), 4th edition. London: Tobacco Research Council, 1966
3 Holland, W.W. and Elliott, A. Cigarette smoking, respiratory symptoms, and anti-smoking propaganda. *Lancet*, 1968; **1**:41-3
4 Rawbone, R.G., Keeling, C.A., Jenkins, A., and·Guz, A. Cigarette smoking among secondary schoolchildren in 1975. *Journal of Epidemiology and Community Health*, 1978;**32**:53-8, and *Health Education Journal*, 1979; **38**:92-9
5 Aitken, P.P. Peer group pressures, parental controls and cigarette smoking among 10 to 14 year-olds. *British Journal of Social and Clinical Psychology*, 1980; **19**:141-6. N.B. The percentages are for boys and girls combined
6 Murray, M., Swan, A.V., Bewley, B.R., and Johnson, M.R.D. The development of smoking during adolescence - The MRC/Derbyshire Smoking Study. *International Journal of Epidemiology*, 1983; **12**:185-92
7 McKennell, A.C. Bias in the reported incidence of smoking by children. *International Journal of Epidemiology*, 1980; **9**:167-77
8 Ledwith, F. and Osman, L. The concomitance of smoking in primary and secondary school children in Scotland. In: *Health Education and Youth*. London: Falmer Press, 1984
9 Dobbs, J. and Marsh, A. Smoking among secondary school children. HMSO, 1983
10 Dobbs, J. and Marsh, A. Smoking among secondary school children in 1984. HMSO, 1985
11 Goddard, E. and Ikin, C. Smoking among secondary school children in 1986. HMSO, 1987
12 Balding, J. Teenage smoking: the levels are falling at last! *Education and Health*, 1986; **6(3)**:68-70
13 Balding, J. Young People in 1986. HEA Schools Health Education Unit, 1987
14 Balding, J. Young People in 1987. HEA Schools Health Education Unit, 1988
15 Balding, J. Young People in 1988. HEA Schools Health Education Unit, 1989
16 Goddard, E. Smoking among secondary school children in England in 1988. HMSO, 1989

Table 12.2 Percentages of boys and girls with various smoking habits: by age, 1988

Smoking habit		Age in years									
		11		**12**		**13**		**14**		**15**	
		Boys	Girls	Boys	Girls	Boys	Girls	Boys	Girls	Boys	Girls
England											
Has never smoked	All[1]	86	90	75	78	56	59	47	46	36	34
	Test	87	85	76	72	62	49	44	45	35	29
	Control	85	93	75	83	50	68	51	48	37	40
Tried smoking once	All[1]	12	8	19	18	25	24	28	20	27	19
	Test	10	12	17	22	17	26	26	18	28	19
	Control	12	6	20	14	33	23	30	22	27	19
Used to smoke	All[1]	1	0	1	3	9	8	10	14	13	16
	Test	2	1	2	3	12	12	14	14	12	16
	Control	1	0	1	2	7	3	5	13	14	17
Smokes occasionally[2]	All[1]	1	1	2	1	5	5	7	7	7	9
	Test	1	2	3	1	5	7	6	9	8	10
	Control	1	1	2	1	4	3	7	5	7	8
Smokes regularly[3]	All[1]	0	0	2	0	5	4	8	12	17	22
	Test	1	0	2	1	4	7	9	14	18	27
	Control	0	0	2	0	6	2	6	11	16	17
Number of pupils (=100%)		229	226	280	315	318	297	311	315	350	376

(Crown Copyright reserved in respect of data included in this table)

1 From half of the sample (test sample) a saliva specimen was obtained and was tested for the presence of cotinine, a metabolite of nicotine. No saliva specimen was obtained from the other half of the sample (control sample)

2 Occasional smokers claim to smoke sometimes but not usually as much as one cigarette a week

3 Regular smokers smoke at least one cigarette a week

Source: Goddard, E. Smoking among secondary school children in England in 1988. HMSO, 1989

Fig. 12.1 Percentages of boys and girls who smoke cigarettes regularly: by age, 1988
Boys and girls aged 12-15 years, England. *Source*: Goddard, 1989

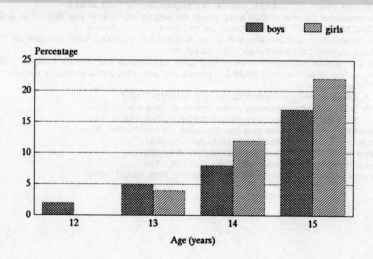

Number of cigarettes smoked per week (recorded in diary)	Occasional smokers[1] %		Regular smokers[2] %		All smokers %	
	Boys	Girls	Boys	Girls	Boys	Girls
England						
None	41	38	3	3	18	16
1- 6	41	47	9	12	22	25
7-70	16	13	58	71	41	50
71 or more	1	1	30	15	19	10
Mean number	8	4	52	41	35	28
Median number	1	1	49	38	16	15
Number of pupils (=100%)	70	76	107	136	177	212

(Crown Copyright reserved in respect of data included in this table)
1 Occasional smokers claim to smoke sometimes but not usually as much as one cigarette a week
2 Regular smokers smoke at least one cigarette a week

Source: Goddard, E. Smoking among secondary school children in England in 1988. HMSO, 1989

Pregnant women and smoking

This section provides a summary of the smoking habits among pregnant women found in the major British surveys conducted between 1959 and 1989.

The percentage of women who stopped smoking at some point during the pregnancy ranged from 6 to 9 per cent, or between 13 and 24 per cent of smokers. For most studies the percentage of women who smoke before pregnancy was comparable to the percentage of women who smoke as reported by the TAC or GHS for the relevant age group and the year in which the data was collected.

A study conducted by OPCS in 1985 (Martin and White, 1988) looked at the smoking habits of pregnant women by social class. In this study, about half of the smokers in social class I stopped smoking during pregnancy, while only 13% of smokers in social class V gave up the habit during pregnancy.

One study has investigated the proportion of smokers who stopped smoking in pregnancy and remained non-smokers after their pregnancy; nearly all do. The same study (see Table 13.3) showed that the proportion of women who said they stopped smoking was about twice as great (about 20 per cent instead of 10 per cent) when advice was given on the health effects of smoking.

Table 13.1 Percentage of women who (i) smoked throughout pregnancy; (ii) stopped smoking during pregnancy, and (iii) both stopped and restarted smoking during pregnancy: summary of some British studies, 1959-1989

Study	Year	Sample	Smoked throughout pregnancy	Stopped during pregnancy	Stopped and restarted	Non-smokers (including ex-smokers)	All
Lowe[1]	1958	2 042 women in six Birmingham hospitals	33	9	2	56	100
Butler, Goldstein, and Ross[2]	1958	21 671 women in England, Wales, and Scotland (British Perinatal Mortality Survey)	31	7	..	62	100
Andrews and McGarry[3]	1965-68	15 723 women in Cardiff (Cardiffs Births Survey)	41	6	..	52	100
Rush and Cassano[4]	1970	16 688 women in Britain (British birth cohort)	41	6	..	53	100
Martin and White[5]	1985	Random sample of 5 233 women in England, Wales, and Scotland	30	9		61	100
MacArthur and Knox[6]	1981-82	4 341 white European women at a West Midlands hospital	21	6	1	72	100
Waterson and Murray-Lyon[7]	1982-83	Cohort of 2 266 women at an antenatal clinic in London	23	6	..	71	100
Madeley, Gillies, Lindsay Power, and Symonds[8]	1986	3 483 women in two antenatal clinics in Nottingham	31	7	..	62	100
Anderson, Bland, and Peacock[9]	1982-84	1 513 white women at a district hospital in London	32	9	..	59	100

1 Lowe, C.R. Effect of mothers' smoking habits on birth weight of their children. *British Medical Journal*, 1959; **ii**: 673-6
2 Butler, N.R., Goldstein, H., and Ross, E.M. Cigarette smoking in pregnancy: its influence on birth weight and perinatal mortality. *British Medical Journal*, 1972; **ii**: 127-30
3 Andrews, J. and McGarry, J.M. A community study of smoking in pregnancy. *The Journal of Obstetrics and Gynaecology of the British Commonwealth*, 1972; **79**: 1057-73
4 Rush, D. and Cassano, P. Relationship of cigarette smoking and social class to birth weight and perinatal mortality among all births in Britain, 5-11 April 1970. *Journal of Epidemiology and Community Health*, 1983; **37**: 249-255
5 Martin, J. and White, A. Infant feeding 1985. HMSO, 1988
6 MacArthur, Ch. and Knox, E.G. Smoking in pregnancy: effects of stopping at different stages. *British Journal of Obstetrics and Gynaecology*, 1988; **95**: 551-5
7 Waterson, E.J. and Murray-Lyon, I.M. Drinking and smoking patterns amongst women attending an antenatal clinic — ii During pregnancy. *Alcohol and Alcoholism*, 1989; **24(2)**: 163-73
8 Madeley, R.J., Gillies, P.A., Lindsay Power, F., and Symonds, E.M. Nottingham Mothers Stop Smoking Project - baseline survey of smoking in pregnancy. *Community Medicine*, 1989; **11(2)**: 124-30
9 Anderson, H.R., Bland J.M., and Peacock, J.L. The effects of smoking on fetal growth: evidence for a threshold, the importance of brand of cigarette, and interaction with alcohol and caffeine consumption. Proceedings of the ISCSH Symposium on 'The effects of smoking on the fetus, neonate and child', 9-11 July 1990

Table 13.2 Percentage of women who (i) smoked before pregnancy, (ii) smoked throughout pregnancy, and (iii) who smoked before pregnancy but gave up: by social class, 1985

| Social class | Percentage of women who smoked | | Number of women | Percentage of women who smoked before pregnancy but gave up | Those who smoked before pregnancy |
	Before pregnancy %	Throughout pregnancy %	n	%	n
I	16	8	307	51	49
II	26	18	1 028	32	268
IIINM	28	19	436	35	124
IIIM	41	31	1 666	25	683
IV	41	32	738	23	303
V	53	46	247	13	130
Unclassified	45	38	207	15	93
No partner	64	53	595	17	381
Total	39	30	5 223	24	2 031

Source: Martin, J. and White, A. Infant feeding 1985. HMSO, 1988

Fig. 13.1 Percentage of women who smoked before and who smoked throughout pregnancy: by social class, 1985. *Source*: Martin and White, 1988

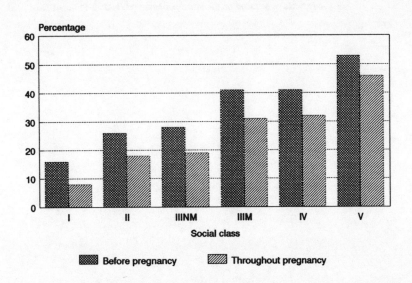

Table 13.3 Percentage of female smokers who stopped smoking during pregnancy and who remained non-smokers after their pregnancy, 1987-88

	Control[1] (n=296)	Intervention[2] (n=419)
Stopped smoking while pregnant and still stopped at delivery	9	22
Smoking at delivery	91	78
	(n=172)	(n=236)
Stopped smoking while pregnant and still stopped 6 months after delivery	11	18
Smoking 6 months after delivery	89	72

1 The Control group (matched control design where antenatal clinics matched) received routine health education advice to smoking women
2 Apart from routine health education advice to smoking women, the Intervention group received counselling, received a specially prepared booklet, and had the option to use a carbon monoxide monitor to check and record progress in stopping or giving up smoking

Note: the response rate just after delivery was high, 93 per cent for the Intervention group and 76 per cent for the Control group, but fell to 52 and 44 per cent, respectively, at six month follow-up

Source: Gillies, P. Anti-smoking intervention during pregnancy - impact on smoking behaviour and birthweight. Proceedings of the ISCSH Symposium on 'The effects of smoking on the fetus, neonate and child', 9-11 July 1990

APPENDIX I Size of surveys

The unweighted sample sizes of the surveys are given below. The numbers include all respondents, i.e., both smokers and non-smokers.

Tobacco Advisory Council (TAC)

Year	Men+women	Year	Men	Women	Year	Men	Women	Year	Men	Women
1948	10 000	1957	4 721	5 262	1971	4 997	5 358	1980	4 256	4 548
1949	10 000	1958	4 952	5 549	1972	4 955	5 220	1981	4 240	4 556
		1959	4 739	5 267	1973	4 921	5 200	1982	4 283	4 542
1950	10 000				1974	4 915	5 262	1983	4 321	4 580
1951	13 000	1960	4 765	5 235	1975	4 910	5 151	1984	4 282	4 524
1952	13 000	1961	4 901	5 387	1976	4 019	5 278	1985	4 292	4 565
1953	22 000	1963	4 859	5 275	1977	4 866	5 193	1986	4 337	4 580
1954	25 000	1965	4 838	5 178	1978	4 218	4 496	1987	4 324	4 526
1955	22 000	1968	4 842	5 169	1979	4 253	4 520			
1956	10 000									

Sample sizes for 1948-56 are approximate
Until 1977 men and women in the age group 16-34 years were sampled at twice the rate of other age groups
Subsequently, this over-sampling has only been applied to men and women in the age group 16-24 years

General Household Survey (GHS)

Year	Men	Women
1972	10 351	12 143
1974	9 852	11 480
1976	10 888	12 554
1978	10 480	12 156
1980	10 454	12 100
1982	9 199	10 641
1984	8 417	9 788
1986	8 874	10 304
1988	8 673	10 122

National Opinion Polls (NOP)

Date	Men+women	Date	Men	Women
Nov 1974	3 832	Nov/Dec 1980	1 705	2 105
Mar 1976	4 024	Nov 1982	1 635	2 036
Nov 1976	3 807	Nov 1983	1 681	2 091
Nov/Dec 1977	3 964	Nov 1984	1 650	2 098
Nov/Dec 1978	3 827	Nov 1985	1 514	1 816
Nov/Dec 1979	3 693	Nov 1986	1 554	1 691
		Nov 1987	1 472	1 853
		Nov 1988	1 390	1 805

'Tar and nicotine yields of cigarettes', 1972-1981

'Tar, carbon monoxide, and nicotine yields of cigarettes', 1981-1989

Surveys by the Laboratory of the Government Chemist; leaflets issued by the Health Departments of the United Kingdom.

Note that the data in surveys 1-21 are rounded, and the data in surveys 22-29 are truncated. Surveys 20 and 21 have not been previously published by the Health Departments due to the change in the tar bands. Surveys 24 and 26 have also not been previously published by the Health Departments.

(Crown Copyright reserved in respect of data included in this appendix; the leaflets were reproduced with the permission of the Controller of Her Majesty's Stationery Office.)

LGC Survey 1
Sampling period July 1972-December 1972

Tar yield mg/cig	Brand	Filter or plain	Nicotine yield mg/cig	Tar yield mg/cig	Brand	Filter or plain	Nicotine yield mg/cig
4	Silk Cut Extra Mild	F	under 0.3	21	Bachelor	F	1.5
7	Player's Mild De Luxe	F	under 0.3	21	Benson and Hedges Va Red	F	1.3
8	Bristol	F	0.4	21	Kensitas Tipped	F	1.4
8	Piccadilly Mild	F	0.4	21	Macdonald's Export 'A'	F	1.4
8	Player's Mild Milford	F	under 0.3	21	Nelson	F	1.3
11	Embassy Extra Mild	F	0.8	21	Park Drive Tipped	F	1.4
11	Ransom Multifilter	F	0.7	21	Player's Gold Leaf	F	1.5
11	Rothmans Masters	F	0.6	21	Slim Kings	F	1.4
11	Silk Cut KS	F	0.8	21	Solent	F	1.2
12	Player's No. 6 Extra Mild	F	0.8	21	Sotheby's	F	1.4
12	Silk Cut	F	0.8	21	Sterling	F	1.3
12	Silk Cut No. 3	F	0.8	21	Woodbine Filter	F	1.3
13	Buckingham	F	0.8	22	Du Maurier	F	1.4
13	Pall Mall Long Size	F	0.8	22	John Player Special	F	1.4
13	Player's Special Mild	F	0.8	22	Player's No. 6 Kings	F	1.4
13	Player's York Mild	F	1.0	22	Player's Perfectos	F	1.5
14	Consulate Menthol	F	0.8	23	Player's Filter Virginia	F	1.6
14	St Moritz	F	1.0	23	Richmond Filter	F	1.6
15	Craven 'A' Filter	F	1.0	24	Player's Mild Navy Cut	P	1.6
15	Everest Menthol	F	0.9	25	Player's No. 6 Plain	P	1.6
15	Kool	F	1.0	26	Gallaher's De Luxe Mild	P	1.6
15	Piccadilly No. 7	F	0.8	26	Weights Plain	P	1.6
15	Rembrandt Filter De Luxe	F	0.8	27	Craven 'A' Cork Tipped	P	1.6
16	Cambridge	F	1.0	27	Player's Medium Navy Cut	P	1.7
17	Olivier	F	1.0	27	Woodbine Plain	P	1.7
17	Peter Stuyvesant KS	F	1.0	28	Embassy Plain	P	1.5
18	Cadets	F	1.1	28	Gauloises Caporal Plain	P	1.8
18	Crown Filter	F	1.1	28	Park Drive Plain	P	1.9
18	Embassy Gold	F	1.2	28	Piccadilly No. 1	P	1.6
18	Embassy Regal	F	1.2	29	Kensitas Plain	P	1.8
18	Gitanes Caporal Filter	F	1.4	31	Churchmans No. 1	P	1.9
18	Piccadilly KS	F	1.1	31	Gallaher's De Luxe Medium	P	2.0
18	Sovereign	F	1.2	31	Richmond Plain	P	2.0
18	Three Castles Filter	F	1.2	31	Senior Service Plain	P	1.9
19	Albany	F	1.2	32	Capstan Medium	P	2.0
19	Cameron	F	1.2	32	Gold Flake	P	2.0
19	Dunhill International	F	1.4	32	Three Castles Plain	P	2.0
19	Gold Bond	F	1.2	33	Player's No. 3	P	2.1
19	Kensitas Club Filter	F	1.2	34	Passing Clouds	P	2.1
19	Kensitas Corsair	F	1.2	38	Capstan Full Strength	P	3.2
19	Kent	F	1.2				
19	Piccadilly Filter De Luxe	F	1.1				
19	Rothmans KS	F	1.4				
19	Senior Service Extra	F	1.2				
19	Silva Thins	F	1.2				
20	Benson and Hedges KS	F	1.4				
20	Benson and Hedges Va Blue	F	1.2				
20	Embassy Filter	F	1.3				
20	Embassy Kings	F	1.3				
20	Gauloises Disque Bleu	F	1.5				
20	Guards	F	1.3				
20	Hallmark	F	1.2				
20	Louis Rothmans Select	F	1.4				
20	Marlboro	F	1.7				
20	Park Drive Special	F	1.5				
20	Peter Stuyvesant Lux Length	F	1.2				
20	Player's No. 6 Filter	F	1.2				
20	Player's No. 10	F	1.3				
20	Senior Service Tipped	F	1.3				
20	Sobranie Virginia Intern	F	1.3				
20	Weights Filter	F	1.5				

New brands introduced during July to December 1972 but not yet analysed by the Government Chemist for a period of six months. Estimates by the manufacturers of the tar and nicotine yields for these brands are as follows:

Tar yield mg/cig	Brand	Filter or plain	Nicotine yield mg/cig
under 4	Embassy Ultra Mild	F	under 0.3
12	Benson and Hedges Vogue	F	0.8
12	Vogue Satin Tipped	F	0.8
14	Kensitas Mild	F	0.9
15	John Player Carlton KS	F	1.3
15	John Player Carlton Long Size	F	1.2
16	John Player Carlton Premium	F	1.3
17	Rothmans International	F	1.1
18	HB Crown	F	1.0
20	Gladstone Filter	F	1.5

Tar yield mg/cig	Brand	Filter or plain	Nicotine yield mg/cig
Low Tar			
under 4	Embassy Ultra Mild	F	under 0.3
under 4	Player's Mild De Luxe	F	under 0.3
under 4	Player's Mild Milford	F	under 0.3
under 4	Silk Cut Extra Mild	F	under 0.3
8	Bristol	F	0.3
8	Piccadilly Mild	F	0.5
8	Player's No. 6 Extra Mild	F	0.5
8	Rothmans Ransom	F	0.5
9	Silk Cut KS	F	0.7
10	Player's Special Mild	F	0.7
Low to Middle Tar			
11	Benson and Hedges Vogue	F	0.8
11	Buckingham	F	0.7
11	Embassy Extra Mild	F	0.8
11	Pall Mall Long Size	F	0.7
11	Silk Cut	F	0.7
11	Silk Cut No. 3	F	0.8
12	Player's York Mild	F	0.8
12	Rembrandt Filter De Luxe	F	0.7
13	Consulate Menthol	F	0.8
13	Gallia	F	0.5
13	Kensitas Mild	F	0.8
13	St Moritz	F	0.9
13	Vogue Satin Tipped	F	0.9
14	Belair Menthol Kings	F	0.8
14	Everest Menthol	F	0.9
14	Piccadilly No. 7	F	0.8
15	Cambridge	F	0.9
15	Kool	F	1.0
16	John Player Carlton Long Size	F	1.3
16	Kent	F	1.0
16	Peter Stuyvesant KS	F	1.1
16	Three Castles Filter	F	1.1
Middle Tar			
17	Crown Filter	F	1.0
17	Embassy Regal	F	1.1
17	HB Crown	F	0.9
17	Peter Stuyvesant Lux Length	F	1.2
17	Piccadilly Filter De Luxe	F	1.0
17	Rothmans International	F	1.2
18	Benson and Hedges Sovereign	F	1.1
18	Cadets	F	1.1
18	Embassy Gold	F	1.1
18	Gitanes Caporal Filter	F	1.3
18	John Player Carlton KS	F	1.5
18	John Player Carlton Premium	F	1.3
18	Kensitas Corsair	F	1.2
18	Player's No. 6 Filter	F	1.2
19	Benson and Hedges Gold Bond	F	1.2
19	Cameron	F	1.2
19	Dunhill International	F	1.4
19	Embassy Filter	F	1.2
19	Guards	F	1.2
19	Hallmark	F	1.1
19	Kensitas Tipped	F	1.2
19	Marlboro	F	1.4
19	Nelson	F	1.2
19	Park Drive Tipped	F	1.3

Tar yield mg/cig	Brand	Filter or plain	Nicotine yield mg/cig
19	Piccadilly KS	F	1.2
19	Player's Gold Leaf	F	1.3
19	Player's Gold Leaf KS	F	1.4
19	Player's No. 6 Kings	F	1.2
19	Player's No. 10	F	1.2
19	Rothmans KS	F	1.3
19	Silva Thins	F	1.2
19	Sobranie Virginia Intern	F	1.3
19	Weights Filter	F	1.5
19	Woodbine Filter	F	1.2
20	Benson and Hedges KS	F	1.3
20	Du Maurier	F	1.3
20	Embassy Kings	F	1.3
20	Embassy Plain	P	1.1
20	Gladstone Filter	F	1.4
20	Kensitas Club	F	1.2
20	Senior Service Tipped	F	1.2
20	Sterling	F	1.2
21	Gauloises Disque Bleu	F	1.2
21	Louis Rothmans Select	F	1.6
21	Park Drive Special	F	1.4
21	Player's Filter Virginia	F	1.4
21	Player's Mild Navy Cut	P	1.5
21	Player's Perfectos	F	1.4
21	Solent	F	1.2
21	Bachelor	F	1.4
22	Gauloises Caporal Filter	F	1.2
22	Slim Kings	F	1.4
Middle to High Tar			
23	Park Drive Plain	P	1.6
23	Senior Service Plain	P	1.4
24	Gallaher's De Luxe Mild	P	1.5
24	Player's No. 6 Plain	P	1.5
24	Richmond Filter	F	1.6
24	Weights Plain	P	1.5
25	Capstan Medium	P	1.6
25	Gitanes Caporal Plain	P	1.6
25	Kensitas Plain	P	1.6
25	Richmond Plain	P	1.6
26	Player's Medium Navy Cut	P	1.6
26	Woodbine Plain	P	1.6
27	Craven 'A' Cork Tipped	P	1.6
28	Piccadilly No. 1	P	1.7
High Tar			
29	Gallaher's De Luxe Medium	P	1.9
30	Churchmans No. 1	P	1.9
30	Player's No. 3	P	1.9
31	Gauloises Caporal Plain	P	1.6
32	Gold Flake	P	2.0
38	Capstan Full Strength	P	3.4

New brands introduced during June to November 1973 not yet analysed by the Government Chemist for a period of six months. Estimates by the manufacturers of the tar and nicotine yields for these brands are as follows:

Tar yield mg/cig	Brand	Filter or plain	Nicotine yield mg/cig
19	Ambassador Luxury Length	F	1.2
19	Player's No. 6 Classic	F	1.1
20	Kensitas KS	F	1.4
21	Benson and Hedges De Luxe Length	F	1.6

LGC Survey 3
Sampling period January 1974-June 1974

Tar yield mg/cig	Brand	Filter or plain	Nicotine yield mg/cig	Tar yield mg/cig	Brand	Filter or plain	Nicotine yield mg/cig
Low Tar				19	Gauloises Disque Bleu	F	1.1
under 4	Embassy Ultra Mild	F	under 0.3	19	Kensitas Club	F	1.2
under 4	Player's Mild De Luxe	F	under 0.3	19	Kensitas KS	F	1.3
under 4	Silk Cut Extra Mild	F	under 0.3	19	Kensitas Tipped	F	1.1
7	Piccadilly Mild	F	0.4	19	L and M Box Filter Tip	F	1.3
8	Player's No. 6 Extra Mild	F	0.5	19	Park Drive Tipped	F	1.3
9	Blend 75	F	0.5	19	Piccadilly KS	F	1.2
9	Player's Special Mild	F	0.6	19	Player's No. 6 Filter	F	1.3
9	Rothmans Ransom	F	0.5	19	Player's No. 6 Kings	F	1.1
9	Silk Cut KS	F	0.7	19	Player's No. 10	F	1.3
				19	Silva Thins	F	1.2
Low to Middle Tar				19	Sobranie Virginia Intern	F	1.3
11	Buckingham	F	0.6	19	Sterling	F	1.2
11	Embassy Extra Mild	F	0.8	19	Woodbine Filter	F	1.2
11	Pall Mall Long Size	F	0.8	20	Benson and Hedges De		
11	Rembrandt Filter De Luxe	F	0.7		Luxe Length	F	1.4
11	Silk Cut	F	0.8	20	Du Maurier	F	1.3
11	Silk Cut No. 3	F	0.8	20	Embassy Plain	P	1.1
12	Benson and Hedges Vogue	F	0.8	20	Hallmark	F	1.1
12	Gallia	F	0.5	20	Louis Rothmans Select	F	1.5
13	Belair Menthol Kings	F	0.8	20	Park Drive Special	F	1.3
13	Consulate Menthol	F	0.8	20	Player's Filter Virginia	F	1.4
13	Everest Menthol	F	0.8	20	Player's Gold Leaf	F	1.4
13	St Moritz	F	0.9	20	Player's Mild Navy Cut	P	1.5
13	Vogue Satin Tipped	F	0.9	20	Rothmans KS	F	1.3
14	Kensitas Mild	F	0.8	20	Senior Service Tipped	F	1.2
15	Embassy Mild	F	1.0	20	Slim Kings	F	1.3
15	Piccadilly No. 7	F	0.9	20	Solent	F	1.2
16	Cambridge	F	0.9	20	Weights Filter	F	1.5
16	John Player Carlton Long Size	F	1.3	21	John Player Special	F	1.3
16	John Player Carlton Premium	F	1.3	21	Pall Mall Filter	F	2.0
16	Kent	F	0.9	21	Player's Gold Leaf KS	F	1.5
16	Peter Stuyvesant KS	F	1.2	21	Player's Perfectos	F	1.5
16	Peter Stuyvesant Lux Length	F	1.2	22	Bachelor	F	1.5
16	Rothmans International	F	1.2				
16	Three Castles Filter	F	1.1	**Middle to High Tar**			
				23	Richmond Plain	P	1.5
Middle Tar				23	Weights Plain	P	1.5
17	Camel Filter Tip	F	1.0	24	Craven 'A' Cork Tipped	P	1.4
17	Embassy Regal	F	1.1	24	Kensitas Plain	P	1.6
17	John Player Carlton KS	F	1.3	24	Lucky Filters	F	2.1
17	Nelson	F	1.0	24	Park Drive Plain	P	1.7
18	Benson and Hedges Gold Bond	F	1.1	24	Piccadilly No. 1	P	1.4
18	Cadets	F	1.1	24	Player's No. 6 Plain	P	1.6
18	Crown Filter	F	1.0	24	Richmond Filter	F	1.7
18	Embassy Gold	F	1.2	25	Gallaher's De Luxe Mild	P	1.6
18	Gitanes Caporal Filter	F	1.2	25	Gitanes Caporal Plain	P	1.6
18	Guards	F	1.2	25	Capstan Medium	P	1.8
18	Kensitas Corsair	F	1.2	26	Player's Medium Navy Cut	P	1.8
18	Lark Filter Tip	F	1.3	26	Senior Service Plain	P	1.6
18	Marlboro	F	1.3	27	Woodbine Plain	P	1.7
18	Piccadilly Filter De Luxe	F	1.1				
18	Player's No. 6 Classic	F	1.2	**High Tar**			
19	Benson and Hedges KS	F	1.2	29	Gauloises Caporal Plain	P	1.5
19	Benson and Hedges Sovereign	F	1.2	30	Churchmans No. 1	P	1.9
19	Cameron	F	1.3	30	Gallaher's De Luxe Medium	P	2.0
19	Chesterfield Filter Tip	F	1.4	30	Player's No. 3	P	2.0
19	Dunhill International	F	1.3	32	Gold Flake	P	2.1
19	Embassy Filter	F	1.3	33	Lucky Strike Plain	P	2.8
19	Embassy Kings	F	1.3	36	Capstan Full Strength	P	3.2
19	Gauloises Caporal Filter	F	1.0				

LGC Survey 4
Sampling period August 1974-January 1975

Tar yield mg/cig	Brand	Filter or plain	Nicotine yield mg/cig
Low Tar			
under 4	Embassy Ultra Mild	F	under 0.3
under 4	Player's Mild De Luxe	F	under 0.3
under 4	Silk Cut Extra Mild	F	under 0.3
8	Piccadilly Mild	F	0.5
8	Silk Cut KS	F	0.6
9	Player's Special Mild	F	0.6
9	Rothmans Ransom	F	0.6
9	Silk Cut	F	0.6
9	Silk Cut No. 1	F	0.6
9	Silk Cut No. 3	F	0.6
10	Player's No. 6 Extra Mild	F	0.6
Low to Middle Tar			
11	Embassy Extra Mild	F	0.8
11	Embassy Extra Mild KS	F	0.7
11	Gallia	F	0.5
11	Pall Mall Long Size	F	0.9
11	Rembrandt Filter De Luxe	F	0.7
12	Belair Menthol Kings	F	0.7
12	Buckingham	F	0.7
13	Consulate Menthol	F	0.9
13	St Moritz	F	1.0
14	Everest Menthol	F	1.0
14	Kensitas Mild	F	0.9
14	Piccadilly No. 7	F	0.8
15	Kent	F	0.9
15	Three Castles Filter	F	1.0
16	John Player Carlton KS	F	1.3
16	John Player Carlton Long Size	F	1.2
16	John Player Carlton Premium	F	1.3
16	Marlboro	F	1.1
Middle Tar			
17	Cambridge	F	1.0
17	Camel Filter Tip	F	1.0
17	Gitanes Caporal Filter	F	1.0
17	Nelson	F	1.1
17	Peter Stuyvesant KS	F	1.4
18	Benson and Hedges Gold Bond	F	1.2
18	Benson and Hedges Sovereign	F	1.1
18	Cadets	F	1.1
18	Embassy Regal	F	1.1
18	Gauloises Caporal Filter	F	0.9
18	Gauloises Disque Bleu	F	0.9
18	Guards	F	1.2
18	Kensitas Club	F	1.2
18	Kensitas KS	F	1.2
18	Louis Rothmans Select	F	1.4
18	Peter Stuyvesant Lux Length	F	1.5
18	Piccadilly Filter De Luxe	F	1.1
18	Player's No. 6 Classic	F	1.3
18	Rothmans International	F	1.4
18	Sobranie Virginia Intern	F	1.2
18	Woodbine Filter	F	1.2
19	Benson and Hedges KS	F	1.2
19	Cameron	F	1.2
19	Chesterfield Filter Tip	F	1.5
19	Crown Filter	F	1.1
19	Du Maurier	F	1.2
19	Dunhill International	F	1.3
19	Embassy Filter	F	1.3
19	Embassy Kings	F	1.3
19	Hallmark	F	1.1
19	Kensitas Corsair	F	1.2
19	Kensitas Tipped	F	1.2
19	Lark Filter Tip	F	1.3
19	Park Drive Tipped	F	1.3
19	Player's No. 10	F	1.3
19	Senior Service Tipped	F	1.2
19	Sterling	F	1.2
19	Weights Filter	F	1.5
20	John Player Special	F	1.3
20	L and M Box Filter Tip	F	1.5
20	Piccadilly KS	F	1.2
20	Player's Gold Leaf	F	1.3
20	Player's No. 6 Filter	F	1.3
20	Player's No. 6 Kings	F	1.3
20	Player's Perfectos	F	1.4
20	Rothmans KS	F	1.3
20	Silva Thins	F	1.3
20	Slim Kings	F	1.3
21	Embassy Plain	P	1.2
21	Pall Mall Filter	F	2.0
21	Player's Filter Virginia	F	1.4
21	Player's Gold Leaf KS	F	1.5
21	Player's Mild Navy Cut	F	1.5
21	Solent	F	1.3
22	Bachelor	F	1.5
Middle to High Tar			
23	Craven 'A' Cork Tipped	P	1.3
23	Gitanes Caporal Plain	P	1.3
23	Piccadilly No. 1	P	1.3
23	Richmond Plain	P	1.5
23	St. Michel	F	1.1
24	Lucky Filters	F	2.2
24	Player's No. 6 Plain	P	1.6
24	Woodbine Plain	P	1.7
24	Kensitas Plain	P	1.6
25	Park Drive Plain	P	1.8
25	Richmond Filter	F	1.6
25	Weights Plain	P	1.6
26	Capstan Medium	P	1.7
26	Gallaher's De Luxe Mild	P	1.7
26	Senior Service Plain	P	1.7
27	Gauloises Caporal Plain	P	1.3
27	Player's Medium Navy Cut	P	1.7
High Tar			
29	Gold Flake	P	2.1
31	Churchmans No. 1	P	1.9
31	Gallaher's De Luxe Medium	P	2.1
31	Player's No. 3	P	2.0
35	Capstan Full Strength	P	3.2
36	Lucky Strike Plain	P	3.0
36	Pall Mall KS	P	3.3

Tar yield mg/cig	Brand	Nicotine yield mg/cig
Low Tar		
under 4	Embassy Ultra Mild	under 0.3
under 4	Player's Mild De Luxe	under 0.3
under 4	Silk Cut Extra Mild	under 0.3
8	Piccadilly Mild	0.5
8	Silk Cut	0.7
8	Silk Cut No. 3	0.7
9	Player's No. 6 Extra Mild	0.6
9	Player's Special Mild	0.7
9	Silk Cut KS	0.8
9	Silk Cut No. 1	0.7
10	Pall Mall Long Size	0.8
10	Rothmans Ransom	0.8
Low to Middle Tar		
11	Embassy Extra Mild KS	0.8
12	Embassy Extra Mild	0.9
12	St Moritz	0.9
13	Belair Menthol Kings	0.8
13	Consulate Menthol	0.8
13	Everest Menthol	0.9
13	Piccadilly No. 7	0.7
14	Kensitas Mild	0.9
15	Gauloises Caporal Filter	0.9
15	Gauloises Disque Bleu	0.9
15	John Player Carlton KS	1.4
15	John Player Carlton Premium	1.3
15	Kent	0.9
15	Peter Stuyvesant KS	1.2
15	Three Castles Filter	1.1
16	Gitanes Caporal Filter	1.0
16	Guards KS	1.0
16	John Player Carlton Long Size	1.4
16	Marlboro	1.2
Middle Tar		
17	Benson and Hedges Gold Bond	1.2
17	Cambridge	1.0
17	Camel Filter Tip	1.1
17	Embassy Regal	1.2
17	Guards	1.2
17	Kensitas KS	1.3
17	Louis Rothmans Select	1.3
17	Peter Stuyvesant Lux Length	1.3
17	Piccadilly Filter De Luxe	1.1
17	Rothmans International	1.4
17	Sobranie Virginia Intern	1.2
18	Benson and Hedges Sovereign	1.2
18	Cadets	1.2
18	Crown Filter	1.1
18	Dunhill International	1.3
18	Dunhill KS	1.3
18	Embassy Gold	1.2
18	Kent De Luxe Length	1.2
18	Lark Filter Tip	1.4
18	Nelson	1.3
18	Park Drive Tipped	1.3
18	Player's No. 6 Classic	1.3
18	Slim Kings	1.2
18	Woodbine Filter	1.2
19	Benson and Hedges KS	1.3
19	Cameron	1.3
19	Chesterfield Filter Tip	1.5
19	Du Maurier	1.4
19	Embassy Filter	1.3
19	Embassy Kings	1.4
19	John Player Special	1.3
19	Kensitas Club	1.3
19	Kensitas Corsair	1.3
19	Kensitas Tipped	1.3
19	L and M Box Filter Tip	1.5
19	Senior Service Tipped	1.3
19	Sterling	1.4
19	Weights Filter	1.5
20	Embassy Plain (P)	1.2
20	Lambert and Butler Intern Size	1.6
20	Piccadilly KS	1.4
20	Player's Gold Leaf	1.4
20	Player's Gold Leaf KS	1.5
20	Player's Mild Navy Cut (P)	1.6
20	Player's No. 6 Filter	1.3
20	Player's No. 6 Kings	1.3
20	Player's No. 10	1.4
20	Silva Thins	1.6
21	Bachelor	1.4
21	John Player Kings	1.4
21	Pall Mall Filter	2.2
21	Rothmans KS	1.5
22	Player's Filter Virginia	1.5
22	Player's Perfectos	1.6
22	St. Michel Filter	1.1
22	Solent	1.3
Middle to High Tar		
23	Craven 'A' Cork Tipped (P)	1.4
23	Gitanes Caporal Plain (P)	1.5
23	Kensitas Plain (P)	1.7
23	Lucky Filters	2.4
23	Richmond Plain (P)	1.6
24	Gallaher's De Luxe Mild (P)	1.7
24	Gauloises Caporal Plain (P)	1.4
24	Piccadilly No. 1 (P)	1.5
24	Player's No. 6 Plain (P)	1.7
24	Woodbine Plain (P)	1.8
25	Park Drive Plain (P)	2.0
25	Richmond Filter	1.8
25	Weights Plain (P)	1.7
26	Player's Medium Navy Cut (P)	1.9
26	Senior Service Plain (P)	1.9
27	Capstan Medium (P)	1.9
27	Gold Flake (P)	2.1
High Tar		
30	Gallaher's De Luxe Medium (P)	2.3
30	Lucky Strike Plain (P)	2.6
32	Churchmans No. 1 (P)	2.1
32	Player's No. 3 (P)	2.2
34	Capstan Full Strength (P)	3.4
35	Pall Mall KS (P)	3.2

(P) indicates plain cigarettes; all other brands have filters

LGC Survey 6
Sampling period October 1975-March 1976

Tar yield mg/cig	Brand	Nicotine yield mg/cig
Low Tar		
under 4	Embassy Ultra Mild	under 0.3
under 4	Player's Mild De Luxe	under 0.3
under 4	Silk Cut Extra Mild	under 0.3
7	Piccadilly Mild	0.4
8	Peter Stuyvesant Extra Mild	0.6
8	Silk Cut International	0.7
8	Silk Cut No. 1	0.7
9	Player's Special Mild	0.7
9	Rothmans Ransom	0.6
9	Silk Cut	0.8
9	Silk Cut KS	0.8
9	Silk Cut No. 3	0.7
10	Player's No. 6 Extra Mild	0.7
Low to Middle Tar		
11	Embassy Extra Mild	0.8
11	Pall Mall Long Size	0.8
12	Belair Menthol Kings	0.8
12	Consulate Menthol	0.8
12	Consulate No. 2	0.7
12	Embassy Extra Mild KS	0.8
12	Everest Menthol	0.8
12	St Moritz	0.9
13	Kensitas Club Mild	0.8
13	Kensitas Mild	0.8
13	Piccadilly No. 7	0.7
13	Player's No. 10 Extra Mild	0.7
14	Gauloises Caporal Filter	0.7
14	Gitanes Caporal Filter	0.8
14	Kent	0.9
15	Camel Filter Tip	0.9
15	Gauloises Disque Bleu	0.8
15	Marlboro	1.2
15	Peter Stuyvesant KS	1.2
15	Peter Stuyvesant Long Size	1.0
15	Three Castles Filter	1.1
16	Benson and Hedges Special Vending Size	1.1
16	Cambridge	0.9
16	Guards	1.0
16	Guards KS	1.0
16	John Player Carlton KS	1.4
16	John Player Carlton Long Size	1.4
16	John Player Carlton Premium	1.2
16	Lark Filter Tip	1.2
16	Louis Rothmans Select	1.1
16	Peter Stuyvesant Lux Length	1.2
Middle Tar		
17	Benson and Hedges Gold Bond	1.1
17	Dunhill KS	1.1
17	Embassy Regal	1.2
17	Piccadilly Filter De Luxe	1.0
17	Rothmans International	1.3
17	Slim Kings	1.1
17	Winston	1.2
18	Benson and Hedges KS	1.2
18	Benson and Hedges Sovereign	1.2
18	Cadets	1.1
18	Cameron	1.2
18	Chesterfield Filter Tip	1.4
18	Crown Filter	1.0
18	Dunhill Premium	1.2
18	Embassy American KS	1.3
18	Embassy Gold	1.2

Tar yield mg/cig	Brand	Nicotine yield mg/cig
18	Guards Select	1.1
18	Kensitas Club	1.2
18	Kensitas KS	1.3
18	Kent De Luxe Length	1.2
18	L and M Box Filter Tip	1.3
18	Nelson	1.2
18	Park Drive Tipped	1.2
18	Piccadilly No. 3	1.2
18	Player's No. 6 Classic	1.2
18	Sobranie Virginia Intern	1.2
18	Woodbine Filter	1.2
19	Du Maurier	1.3
19	Embassy American Regular	1.4
19	Embassy Filter	1.3
19	Embassy Kings	1.3
19	John Player Special	1.3
19	Kensitas Corsair	1.2
19	Kensitas Plain (P)	1.4
19	Kensitas Tipped	1.2
19	Piccadilly KS	1.2
19	Player's No. 6 Filter	1.2
19	Senior Service Tipped	1.2
19	Silva Thins	1.4
19	Sterling	1.2
20	Bachelor	1.3
20	Dunhill International	1.4
20	Gallaher's De Luxe Mild (P)	1.5
20	Lambert and Butler Intern Size	1.6
20	Pall Mall Filter	2.1
20	Player's Gold Leaf	1.4
20	Player's No. 6 KS	1.3
20	Player's No. 10	1.2
20	Weights Filter	1.3
21	Embassy Plain (P)	1.2
21	John Player Kings	1.4
21	Player's Filter virginia	1.4
21	Player's Mild Navy Cut (P)	1.7
21	Player's Perfectos	1.5
21	Rothmans KS	1.4
21	Solent	1.2
22	Gitanes Caporal Plain (P)	1.3
22	Piccadilly No. 1 (P)	1.3
22	Player's No. 6 Plain (P)	1.6
Middle to High Tar		
23	Craven 'A' Cork Tipped (P)	1.3
23	Gauloises Caporal Plain (P)	1.2
23	Lucky Filters	2.3
23	Lucky Strike Plain (P)	1.4
24	Richmond Filter	1.8
24	Richmond Plain (P)	1.7
24	Woodbine Plain (P)	1.8
25	Park Drive Plain (P)	1.9
25	Weights Plain (P)	1.7
26	Player's Medium Navy Cut (P)	1.8
26	Senior Service Plain (P)	1.8
27	Capstan Medium (P)	1.9
27	Gold Flake (P)	2.2
High Tar		
31	Gallaher's De Luxe Medium (P)	2.3
33	Churchmans No. 1 (P)	2.2
34	Capstan Full Strength (P)	3.5
34	Pall Mall KS (P)	3.3
34	Player's No. 3 (P)	2.3

(P) indicates plain cigarettes; all other brands have filters

LGC Survey 7
Sampling period May 1976-October 1976

Tar yield mg/cig	Brand	Nicotine yield mg/cig	Tar yield mg/cig	Brand	Nicotine yield mg/cig
Low Tar			18	Embassy Filter	1.4
under 4	Embassy Ultra Mild	under 0.3	18	John Player KS	1.4
under 4	Player's Mild De Luxe	under 0.3	18	John Player Special	1.4
under 4	Silk Cut Extra Mild	under 0.3	18	Kensitas Club	1.2
6	Piccadilly Mild	0.4	18	Kensitas Corsair	1.3
7	Peter Stuyvesant Extra Mild KS	0.6	18	Kensitas 2	1.3
8	Player's Special Mild	0.7	18	Nelson	1.3
8	Silk Cut	0.8	18	Park Drive Tipped	1.3
8	Silk Cut International	0.8	18	Piccadilly Filter De Luxe	1.1
8	Silk Cut KS	0.8	18	Player's No. 6 KS	1.4
8	Silk Cut No. 3	0.7	18	Sobranie Virginia Intern	1.4
8	Silk Cut No. 5	0.7	18	Weights Filter	1.3
9	Player's No. 6 Extra Mild	0.7	19	Bachelor	1.4
9	Rothmans Ransom	0.7	19	Benson and Hedges KS	1.4
9	Silk Cut No. 1	0.8	19	Du Maurier	1.3
			19	Dunhill International	1.4
Low to Middle Tar			19	Embassy American Regular	1.4
11	Consulate Menthol	0.7	19	Embassy Gold	1.3
11	Consulate No. 2	0.7	19	Embassy Kings	1.4
11	Embassy Extra Mild	0.9	19	Kensitas KS	1.4
11	Embassy Extra Mild KS	0.9	19	Kensitas Plain (P)	1.5
12	Belair Menthol Kings	0.8	19	Kensitas Tipped	1.3
12	Black Cat Filter	0.8	19	Piccadilly KS	1.3
12	Black Cat No. 9	0.7	19	Player's No. 6 Filter	1.3
12	Embassy Extra Mild No. 5	1.0	19	Player's No. 10	1.3
12	Everest Menthol	0.8	19	Senior Service Tipped	1.4
12	Piccadilly No. 7	0.7	19	Silva Thins	1.5
12	St Moritz	0.9	19	Sterling	1.3
13	Gauloises Caporal Filter	0.7	20	Embassy Plain (P)	1.2
13	Gauloises Disque Bleu	0.7	20	Gallaher's De Luxe Mild (P)	1.6
13	Gitanes Caporal Filter	0.9	20	Lambert and Butler Intern Size	1.7
13	Kent	1.0	20	More	1.6
13	Player's No. 10 Extra Mild	0.9	20	More Menthol	1.6
14	Benson and Hedges Sovereign Mild	1.3	20	Player's Filter Virginia	1.4
14	Guards Select	0.8	20	Player's Gold Leaf	1.5
14	Peter Stuyvesant KS	1.3	20	Player's Mild Navy Cut (P)	1.8
14	Philip Morris International	1.2	20	Rothmans KS	1.4
15	Cadets	1.0	20	Woodbine Filter	1.5
15	Cambridge	0.9	21	Pall Mall Filter	2.3
15	Camel Filter Tip	1.0	21	Player's No. 6 Plain (P)	1.6
15	Kensitas Club Mild	1.2	21	Solent	1.3
15	Kensitas Corsair Mild	1.3			
15	Lark Filter Tip	1.3	**Middle to High Tar**		
15	Marlboro	1.2	23	Craven 'A' Cork Tipped (P)	1.3
15	Three Castles Filter	1.2	23	Gauloises Caporal Plain (P)	1.3
16	Benson and Hedges Special Vending Size	1.3	23	Gitanes Caporal Plain (P)	1.5
16	Dunhill KS	1.2	23	Piccadilly No. 1 (P)	1.4
16	Embassy Envoy	1.2	23	Richmond Filter	1.9
16	Guards	1.1	24	Lucky Filters	2.4
16	John Player Carlton KS	1.5	24	Park Drive Plain (P)	1.9
16	John Player Carlton Long Size	1.4	24	Richmond Plain (P)	1.8
16	John Player Carlton Premium	1.3	24	Weights Plain (P)	1.7
16	Kensitas Mild	1.1	24	Woodbine Plain (P)	2.0
16	Peter Stuyvesant Long Size	1.0	25	Lucky Strike Plain (P)	1.6
			25	Senior Service Plain (P)	1.9
Middle Tar			27	Capstan Medium (P)	2.0
17	Benson and Hedges Gold Bond	1.2	27	Gold Flake (P)	2.2
17	Embassy Regal	1.3	27	Player's Medium Navy Cut (P)	2.0
17	L and M Box Filter Tip	1.4			
17	Piccadilly No. 3	1.0	**High Tar**		
17	Rothmans International	1.3	31	Churchmans No. 1 (P)	2.3
17	Slim Kings	1.2	31	Gallaher's De Luxe Medium (P)	2.5
17	Winston	1.3	32	Player's No. 3 (P)	2.3
18	Benson and Hedges Sovereign	1.3	34	Pall Mall KS (P)	3.3
18	Embassy American KS	1.4	35	Capstan Full Strength (P)	3.6

(P) indicates plain cigarettes; all other brands have filters

LGC Survey 8
Sampling period December 1976-May 1977

Tar yield mg/cig	Brand	Nicotine yield mg/cig
Low Tar		
under 4	Embassy Ultra Mild	under 0.3
under 4	John Player KS Ultra Mild	under 0.3
under 4	Silk Cut Extra Mild	0.4
7	Piccadilly Mild	0.5
8	John Player KS Extra Mild	0.7
8	Peter Stuyvesant Extra Mild KS	0.7
8	Rothmans Ransom	0.7
9	Embassy Extra Mild	0.8
9	Player's No. 6 Extra Mild	0.7
9	Silk Cut	0.8
9	Silk Cut International	0.9
9	Silk Cut KS	0.9
9	Silk Cut No. 1	0.8
9	Silk Cut No. 3	0.8
9	Silk Cut No. 5	0.8
10	Consulate Menthol	0.8
10	Embassy Extra Mild KS	0.7
10	Embassy Number 5 Extra Mild	0.9
10	Gauloises Filter Mild	0.6
Low to Middle Tar		
11	Belair Menthol Kings	0.8
11	Consulate No. 2	0.7
11	St Moritz	0.9
12	Black Cat Filter	0.8
12	Black Cat No. 9	0.7
12	Piccadilly No. 7	0.7
12	Virginia Slims	1.1
13	Everest Menthol	0.9
13	Gauloises Caporal Filter	0.8
13	Gauloises Longues	0.8
13	Kensitas Club Mild	1.2
13	Kent	1.0
13	Player's No. 10 Extra Mild	0.9
14	Gauloises Disque Bleu	0.8
14	Gitanes Caporal Filter	1.0
14	Kensitas Mild	1.2
14	Peter Stuyvesant KS	1.2
14	Philip Morris International	1.3
15	Benson and Hedges Sovereign Mild	1.3
15	Cadets	1.1
15	Camel Filter Tip	1.1
15	John Player Carlton Long Size	1.4
15	John Player Carlton Premium	1.3
15	Kensitas Corsair Mild	1.3
15	Lark Filter Tip	1.3
15	Marlboro	1.2
16	Cambridge	1.0
16	Chesterfield KS Filter	1.4
16	Guards Select	1.0
16	John Player Carlton KS	1.6
16	Piccadilly No. 3	1.0
16	Three Castles Filter	1.2
Middle Tar		
17	Benson and Hedges Gold Bond	1.2
17	Dunhill KS	1.3
17	Embassy Envoy	1.3
17	Embassy Regal	1.3
17	Rothmans International	1.4
17	Slim Kings	1.3
18	Benson and Hedges Sovereign	1.3
18	Du Maurier	1.4
18	Embassy American KS	1.5

Tar yield mg/cig	Brand	Nicotine yield mg/cig
18	Embassy Filter	1.4
18	John Player KS	1.5
18	Kensitas Corsair	1.3
18	Kensitas 2	1.3
18	Nelson	1.3
18	Park Drive Tipped	1.4
18	Piccadilly Filter De Luxe	1.1
18	Player's No. 6 Filter	1.3
18	Player's No. 6 KS	1.5
18	Sobranie Virginia Intern	1.4
18	Sterling	1.4
18	Winston KS	1.3
19	Benson and Hedges KS	1.5
19	Dunhill International	1.3
19	Embassy American Regular	1.5
19	Embassy Gold	1.4
19	Embassy KS	1.6
19	John Player Special	1.5
19	Kensitas Club	1.3
19	Kensitas KS	1.5
19	Kensitas Tipped	1.4
19	Piccadilly KS	1.3
19	Player's Gold Leaf	1.5
19	Rothmans KS	1.3
19	Senior Service Tipped	1.4
19	Silva Thins	1.5
19	Woodbine Filter	1.4
20	Fribourg and Treyer No. 1 Filter De Luxe	1.7
20	Kensitas Plain (P)	1.7
20	Lambert and Butler Intern Size	1.8
20	More	1.8
20	More Menthol	1.7
20	Player's Filter Virginia	1.5
20	Player's No. 10	1.4
21	Gallaher's De Luxe Mild (P)	1.7
21	Pall Mall Filter	2.4
21	Player's No. 6 Plain (P)	1.6
22	Embassy Plain (P)	1.3
22	Piccadilly No. 1 (P)	1.4
Middle to High Tar		
23	Gauloises Caporal Plain (P)	1.3
23	Gitanes Caporal Plain (P)	1.7
23	Park Drive Plain (P)	1.9
24	Craven 'A' Cork Tipped (P)	1.4
24	Lucky Filters	2.6
24	Weights Plain (P)	1.8
25	Senior Service Plain (P)	2.0
26	Capstan Medium (P)	2.0
26	Lucky Strike Plain (P)	2.0
26	Woodbine Plain (P)	2.2
27	Gold Flake (P)	2.3
27	Player's Medium Navy Cut (P)	2.1
High Tar		
31	Gallaher's De Luxe Medium (P)	2.5
34	Capstan Full Strength (P)	3.7
34	Pall Mall KS (P)	3.5

New brands recently introduced but not yet analysed by the Government Chemist for a period of six months. Estimates by the manufacturers of the tar and nicotine yields for these brands are as follows:

Tar yield mg/cig	Brand	Nicotine yield mg/cig
under 4	Silk Cut Ultra Mild with tobacco substitute	under 0.3
8	Embassy Premier	0.6
8	Peer Extra Mild (with Cytrel)	0.6
8	Silk Cut KS with tobacco subst	0.7
8	Silk Cut No. 3 with tobacco subst	0.6
9	Embassy Premier KS	0.7
9	Player's No. 6 Filter with NSM	0.7
10	Embassy Number 1 Extra Mild	0.8
10	John Player KS with NSM	0.9
10	Player's No. 10 Filter with NSM	0.8
13	Benson and Hedges Sovereign Mild with tobacco substitute	1.0
14	Peer Mild (with Cytrel)	1.0
16	President KS	1.2
17	Embassy Number 3 Standard Size	1.4
18	Embassy Number 1 KS	1.5
19	Imperial International	1.7
19	Nerit	1.6

(P) indicates plain cigarettes; all other brands have filters

LGC Survey 9
Sampling period July 1977-December 1977

Tar yield mg/cig	Brand	Nicotine yield mg/cig
Low Tar		
under 4	Embassy Ultra Mild	under 0.3
under 4	John Player KS Ultra Mild	under 0.3
under 4	Silk Cut Ultra Mild with Subst	under 0.3
7	Embassy Premier	0.5
7	Peter Stuyvesant Extra Mild KS	0.6
8	Embassy Premier KS	0.6
8	Peer Special Extra Mild (with Cytrel)	0.6
8	Piccadilly Mild	0.5
8	Player's No. 6 with NSM	0.6
8	Silk Cut KS with Substitute	0.7
8	Silk Cut No. 3 with Substitute	0.6
8	Silk Cut No. 5	0.7
9	Consulate Menthol	0.5
9	Consulate No. 2	0.5
9	Embassy Extra Mild	0.7
9	Embassy No. 1 Extra Mild	0.7
9	John Player KS Extra Mild	0.7
9	John Player KS with NSM	0.7
9	Player's No. 10 with NSM	0.7
9	Player's No. 6 Extra mild	0.7
9	Silk Cut	0.8
9	Silk Cut International	0.9
9	Silk Cut KS	0.9
9	Silk Cut No. 3	0.8
10	Belair Menthol Kings	0.6
10	Embassy No. 5 Extra Mild	0.8
Low to Middle Tar		
11	Gauloises Filter Mild	0.6
11	St Moritz	0.8
12	Benson and Hedges Sovereign Mild with Substitute	1.0
12	Black Cat No. 9	0.7
12	Gauloises Longues	0.6
12	John Player Carlton KS	1.3
12	John Player Carlton Long Size	1.3
12	John Player Carlton Premium	1.1
12	Player's No. 10 Extra Mild	0.7
12	Virginia Slims	1.0
13	Kensitas Mild	1.2
13	Kent	1.0
13	Peer Special Mild (with Cytrel)	0.9
13	Piccadilly No. 7	0.7
14	Gitanes Caporal Filter	0.8
14	Kensitas Club Mild	1.2
14	Peter Stuyvesant KS	1.0
14	Philip Morris International	1.2
15	Benson and Hedges Sovereign Mild	1.3
15	Gauloises Disque Bleu	0.7
15	Kensitas Corsair Mild	1.3
15	Lark Filter Tip	1.3
15	Marlboro	1.1
15	President KS	1.1
16	Benson and Hedges Gold Bond	1.2
16	Cadets	1.1
16	Camel Filter Tip	1.0
16	Chesterfield KS Filter	1.3
16	Embassy American KS	1.2
16	Guards	1.1
16	Piccadilly Filter De Luxe	1.0
16	Three Castles Filter	1.2
Middle Tar		
17	Kensitas Club	1.3
17	Rothmans International	1.3
18	Benson and Hedges KS	1.5
18	Dunhill KS	1.3
18	Embassy American Regular Size	1.3
18	Embassy Envoy	1.3
18	Embassy Filter	1.3
18	Embassy KS	1.4
18	Embassy No. 1 KS	1.4
18	Embassy No. 3 Standard Size	1.3
18	Embassy Regal	1.2
18	John Player KS	1.3
18	Park Drive Tipped	1.4
18	Player's No. 6 KS	1.3

Tar yield mg/cig	Brand	Nicotine yield mg/cig
Middle Tar		
18	Slim Kings	1.3
18	Winston KS	1.4
19	Benson and Hedges Sovereign	1.3
19	Du Maurier	1.4
19	Dunhill International	1.4
19	Embassy Gold	1.3
19	Kensitas Corsair	1.3
19	Kensitas KS	1.5
19	Kensitas Tipped	1.5
19	Nerit	1.3
19	Piccadilly KS	1.4
19	Player's No. 6 Filter	1.2
19	Rothmans KS	1.4
19	Silva Thins	1.5
19	Sobranie Virginia Intern	1.5
19	Sterling	1.4
19	Woodbine Filter	1.3
20	Craven 'A' Cork Tipped (P)	1.4
20	Fribourg and Treyer No. 1 Filter De Luxe	1.6
20	Imperial International	1.6
20	John Player Special	1.6
20	Player's No. 10	1.3
21	Kensitas Plain (P)	1.7
21	Lambert and Butler Intern Size	1.7
21	More	1.6
21	Pall Mall Filter	2.3
21	Piccadilly No. 1 (P)	1.3
21	Player's Filter Virginia	1.5
21	Player's Gold Leaf	1.6
22	Embassy Plain (P)	1.4
22	Gallaher's De Luxe Mild (P)	1.8
22	More Menthol	1.7
22	Player's No. 6 Plain (P)	1.5

Tar yield mg/cig	Brand	Nicotine yield mg/cig
Middle to High Tar		
23	Gitanes Caporal Plain (P)	1.5
24	Gauloises Caporal Plain (P)	1.2
24	Park Drive Plain (P)	2.0
24	Woodbine Plain (P)	1.9
25	Senior Service Plain (P)	1.9
25	Weights Plain (P)	1.7
26	Capstan Medium (P)	1.9
26	Lucky Filters	2.6
26	Player's Medium Navy Cut (P)	1.9
27	Gold Flake (P)	2.1
27	Lucky Strike Plain (P)	1.9
High Tar		
31	Gallaher's De Luxe Medium (P)	2.4
33	Capstan Full Strength (P)	3.5
34	Pall Mall KS (P)	3.1

New brands recently introduced but not yet analysed by the Government Chemist for a period of six months. Estimates by the manufacturers of the tar and nicotine yields for these brands are as follows:

4	Decade	0.4
18	State Express 555 Filter Kings	1.3
18	Regal KS	1.4
19	Rothmans Royals	1.5
19	State Express 555 Intern	1.5

(P) indicates plain cigarettes; all other brands have filters

LGC Survey 10
Sampling period February 1978-July 1978

Tar yield mg/cig	Brand	Nicotine yield mg/cig
Low Tar		
under 4	Embassy Ultra Mild	under 0.3
under 4	John Player KS Ultra Mild	under 0.3
under 4	Silk Cut Ultra Mild with Subst	under 0.3
8	Embassy Premier KS	0.6
8	Peer Special Extra Mild KS (with Cytrel)	0.6
8	Piccadilly Mild	0.5
8	Silk Cut KS with Substitute	0.7
8	Silk Cut No. 3 with Substitute	0.7
9	Belair Menthol Kings	0.6
9	Embassy No. 1 Extra Mild	0.7
9	Embassy No. 5 Extra Mild	0.8
9	John Player KS Extra Mild	0.7

Tar yield mg/cig	Brand	Nicotine yield mg/cig
9	John Player KS with NSM	0.7
9	Peter Stuyvesant Extra Mild KS	0.8
9	Player's No. 6 Extra mild	0.7
9	Silk Cut	0.9
9	Silk Cut International	0.9
9	Silk Cut KS	1.0
9	Silk Cut No. 3	0.8
9	Silk Cut No. 5	0.8
10	Consulate Menthol	0.6
10	Consulate No. 2	0.6
10	Embassy Extra Mild	0.8
10	Player's No. 6 with NSM	0.7

Tar yield mg/cig	Brand	Nicotine yield mg/cig
Low to Middle Tar		
12	Benson and Hedges Sovereign Mild with Substitute	1.1
12	Gauloises Filter Mild	0.7
12	John Player Carlton Premium	1.1
13	Gauloises Longues	0.8
13	Gitanes International	1.1
13	John Player Carlton Long Size	1.3
13	Player's No. 10 Extra Mild	0.8
13	St Moritz	0.9
14	Black Cat No. 9	1.0
14	John Player Carlton KS	1.5
14	Kent	1.1
14	Peter Stuyvesant KS	1.1
14	Philip Morris International	1.2
14	Piccadilly No. 7	1.0
15	Benson and Hedges Sovereign Mild	1.4
15	Camel Filter Tip	1.0
15	Chesterfield KS Filter	1.3
15	Gauloises Disque Bleu	0.8
15	Gitanes Caporal Filter	0.9
15	Peer Special Mild KS (with Cytrel)	1.1
16	Gauloises Caporal Filter	0.9
16	Guards	1.1
16	Kensitas Club Mild	1.5
16	Kensitas Corsair Mild	1.4
16	Kensitas Mild	1.5
16	Lark Filter Tip	1.4
16	Marlboro	1.2
16	Piccadilly Filter De Luxe	1.2
16	President KS	1.2
16	Three Castles Filter	1.2
Middle Tar		
17	Cadets	1.2
17	Dunhill KS	1.3
17	Embassy Envoy	1.2
18	Benson and Hedges Gold Bond	1.5
18	Dunhill International	1.4
18	Embassy American KS	1.4
18	Embassy Filter	1.4
18	Embassy KS	1.4
18	Embassy No. 3 Standard Size	1.3
18	Embassy Regal	1.3
18	John Player KS	1.3
18	Kensitas Club	1.5
18	Kensitas Club KS	1.6
18	Pall Mall Filter	1.8
18	Piccadilly No. 1 (P)	1.4
18	Regal KS	1.5
18	Rothmans International	1.5
18	State Express 555 Filter Kings	1.4
18	State Express 555 International	1.5
18	Winston KS	1.5
19	Benson and Hedges KS	1.7
19	Benson and Hedges Sovereign	1.5
19	Du Maurier	1.6
19	Embassy Gold	1.4
19	Embassy No. 1 KS	1.4
19	John Player Special	1.6
19	Kensitas Tipped KS	1.7

Tar yield mg/cig	Brand	Nicotine yield mg/cig
19	Piccadilly KS	1.5
19	Player's No. 10	1.3
19	Player's No. 6 Filter	1.3
19	Player's No. 6 KS	1.5
19	Rothmans KS	1.4
19	Rothmans Royals	1.5
19	Slim Kings	1.5
20	Craven 'A' Cork Tipped (P)	1.3
20	Fribourg and Treyer No. 1 Filter De Luxe	1.6
20	Imperial International	1.7
20	Kensitas Corsair	1.6
20	Nerit	1.4
20	Park Drive Tipped	1.7
20	Player's Filter Virginia	1.5
20	Player's Gold Leaf	1.6
20	Silva Thins	1.7
20	Sobranie Virginia Intern	1.7
20	Sterling	1.5
20	Woodbine Filter	1.3
21	Embassy Plain (P)	1.3
21	Kensitas Plain (P)	1.8
21	Lambert and Butler Intern Size	1.7
22	Gallaher's De Luxe Mild (P)	1.8
22	More	1.7
22	More Menthol	1.7
22	Player's No. 6 Plain (P)	1.6
Middle to High Tar		
23	Park Drive Plain (P)	2.0
24	Weights Plain (P)	1.7
24	Woodbine Plain (P)	2.0
25	Capstan Medium (P)	1.9
25	Lucky Filters	2.6
25	Player's Medium Navy Cut (P)	1.9
26	Gitanes Caporal Plain (P)	1.6
26	Gold Flake (P)	2.0
26	Senior Service Plain (P)	2.1
27	Gauloises Caporal Plain (P)	1.4
28	Lucky Strike Plain (P)	2.0
High Tar		
31	Capstan Full Strength (P)	3.5
32	Gallaher's De Luxe Medium (P)	2.6
36	Pall Mall KS (P)	3.5

New brands recently introduced but not yet analysed by the Government Chemist for a period of six months. Estimates by the manufacturers of the tar and nicotine yields for these brands are as follows:

7	Dunhill Intern Superior Mild	0.6
8	Dunhill KS Superior Mild	0.7
12	Merit	1.1
15	Red Label	1.3
18	Emperior KS	1.4
18	State Express 555 Selected Virginia (P)	1.3

(P) indicates plain cigarettes; all other brands have filters

LGC Survey 11
Sampling period September 1978-February 1979

Low Tar

Tar yield mg/cig	Brand	Nicotine yield mg/cig
under 4	Embassy Ultra Mild	under 0.3
under 4	John Player KS Ultra Mild	under 0.3
under 4	Silk Cut Ultra Mild with Subst	under 0.3
8	Dunhill KS Superior Mild	0.7
8	Dunhill Intern Superior Mild	0.7
8	Embassy Premier KS	0.6
8	John Player KS with NSM	0.7
8	Peer Special Extra Mild KS (with Cytrel)	0.7
8	Peter Stuyvesant Extra Mild KS	0.7
8	Piccadilly Mild	0.6
8	Silk Cut KS with Substitute	0.8
9	Belair Menthol Kings	0.6
9	Consulate Menthol	0.6
9	Embassy Extra Mild	0.8
9	Embassy No. 1 Extra Mild	0.7
9	John Player KS Extra Mild	0.7
9	Player's No. 10 with NSM	0.7
9	Player's No. 6 Extra mild	0.7
9	Silk Cut	0.8
9	Silk Cut KS	1.0
9	Silk Cut No. 5	0.7
10	Consulate No. 2	0.6
10	Embassy No. 5 Extra Mild	0.8
10	Silk Cut International	1.0
10	Silk Cut No. 3	0.9

Low to Middle Tar

Tar yield mg/cig	Brand	Nicotine yield mg/cig
12	Gauloises Filter Mild	0.6
12	Gauloises Longues	0.6
12	John Player Carlton Premium	1.1
12	St Moritz	0.9
13	Gitanes International	1.0
13	John Player Carlton KS	1.4
13	John Player Carlton Long Size	1.3
13	Merit	1.1
13	Player's No. 10 Extra Mild	0.8
14	Black Cat No. 9	1.0
14	Kent	1.0
14	Peer Special Mild KS (with Cytrel)	1.2
14	Piccadilly No. 7	1.0
15	Benson and Hedges Sovereign Mild	1.2
15	Gauloises Caporal Filter	0.7
15	Gauloises Disque Bleu	0.7
15	Gitanes Caporal Filter	0.8
15	Kensitas Corsair Mild	1.3
15	Pall Mall Filter	1.4
15	Peter Stuyvesant KS	1.1
15	Philip Morris International	1.3
15	Three Castles Filter	1.1
16	Cadets	1.3
16	Camel Filter Tip	1.1
16	Chesterfield KS Filter	1.5
16	Guards	1.1
16	Kensitas Club Mild	1.4
16	Marlboro	1.2
16	President KS	1.1

Middle Tar

Tar yield mg/cig	Brand	Nicotine yield mg/cig
17	Craven 'A' Cork Tipped (P)	1.3
17	Dunhill International	1.4
17	Dunhill KS	1.4
17	Lark Filter Tip	1.6
17	Lucky Strike KS Filter	1.4
17	More Menthol	1.5
17	Piccadilly Filter De Luxe	1.3
17	Piccadilly KS	1.4
17	Silva Thins	1.5
17	State Express 555 Filter Kings	1.4
17	State Express 555 Intern	1.5
18	Du Maurier	1.5
18	Embassy American KS	1.3
18	Embassy Envoy	1.3
18	Embassy Gold	1.3
18	Embassy No. 3 Standard Size	1.4
18	Embassy Regal	1.4
18	Emperor KS	1.4
18	Fribourg and Treyer No. 1 Filter De Luxe	1.5
18	John Player KS	1.4
18	John Player Special	1.5
18	Kensitas Club KS	1.6
18	Kensitas Tipped KS	1.6
18	Lambert and Butler Intern Size	1.6
18	More	1.6
18	Player's Filter Virginia	1.3
18	Rothmans International	1.6
18	Rothmans Royals	1.7
18	Slim Kings	1.4
18	State Express 555 Selected Virginia (P)	1.3
18	Winston KS	1.4
19	Benson and Hedges Gold Bond	1.5
19	Benson and Hedges KS	1.7
19	Benson and Hedges Sovereign	1.4
19	Capstan Medium (P)	1.4
19	Embassy Filter	1.4
19	Embassy KS	1.4
19	Embassy No. 1 KS	1.4
19	Embassy Plain (P)	1.3
19	Gallaher's De Luxe Green (P)	1.6
19	Imperial International	1.6
19	Kensitas Club	1.5
19	Kensitas Plain (P)	1.6
19	Park Drive Plain (P)	1.6
19	Park Drive Tipped	1.5
19	Player's Gold Leaf	1.6
19	Player's No. 10	1.3
19	Player's No. 6 Filter	1.3
19	Player's No. 6 KS	1.6
19	Player's No. 6 Plain (P)	1.2
19	Regal King Size	1.4
19	Rothmans KS	1.5
19	Senior Service Plain (P)	1.6
19	Sterling	1.6
19	Woodbine Filter	1.3
19	Woodbine Plain (P)	1.6
20	Gold Flake	1.4
20	Kensitas Corsair	1.5
20	Nerit	1.4
20	Piccadilly No. 1 (P)	1.5
20	Sobranie Virginia Intern	1.8
20	Weights Plain (P)	1.2

LGC Survey 11
(*continued*)

Tar yield mg/cig	Brand	Nicotine yield mg/cig
Middle to High Tar		
24	Lucky Strike Plain (P)	1.8
25	Player's Medium Navy Cut (P)	1.9
26	Gauloises Caporal Plain (P)	1.3
26	Gitanes Caporal Plain (P)	1.4
28	Gallaher's De Luxe Blue (P)	2.5
High Tar		
29	Pall Mall KS (P)	2.5
31	Capstan Full Strength (P)	3.6

New brands recently introduced but not yet analysed by the Government Chemist for a period of six months. Estimates by the manufacturers of the tar and nicotine yields for these brands are as follows:

Tar yield mg/cig	Brand	Nicotine yield mg/cig
14	State Express 555 Medium Mild KS	1.2
16	Kensitas Club Mild KS	1.5
17	Benson and Hedges Supreme	1.7
17	Kensitas Mild KS	1.5
19	Benson and Hedges Gold Bond KS	1.6
19	Lambert and Butler KS	1.4

(P) indicates plain cigarettes; all other brands have filters

LGC Survey 12
Sampling period April 1979–September 1979

Tar yield mg/cig	Brand	Nicotine yield mg/cig
Low Tar		
under 4	Embassy Ultra Mild	under 0.3
under 4	John Player KS Ultra Mild	under 0.3
under 4	Silk Cut Ultra Mild with Subst	under 0.3
7	Silk Cut KS with Substitute	0.8
8	Consulate Menthol	0.6
8	Dunhill Intern Superior Mild	0.7
8	Embassy Premier KS	0.5
8	Peter Stuyvesant Extra Mild KS	0.7
8	Piccadilly Mild	0.5
9	Consulate No. 2	0.5
9	Dunhill KS Superior Mild	0.7
9	Embassy Extra Mild	0.8
9	Embassy No. 1 Extra Mild	0.7
9	John Player KS Extra Mild	0.7
9	John Player KS with NSM	0.8
9	Peer Special Extra Mild KS (with Cytrel)	0.7
9	Player's No. 6 Extra mild	0.7
9	Silk Cut	0.8
9	Silk Cut International	0.9
9	Silk Cut KS	0.9
9	Silk Cut No. 5	0.8
10	Belair Menthol Kings	0.7
10	Embassy No. 5 Extra Mild	0.8
10	Player's No. 10 with NSM	0.7
10	Silk Cut No. 3	0.8
Low to Middle Tar		
11	Gauloises Filter Mild	0.5
11	Gauloises Longues	0.6
11	St Moritz	0.8
12	Gitanes International	1.0
12	John Player Carlton Premium	1.2
12	Player's No. 10 Extra Mild	0.8

Tar yield mg/cig	Brand	Nicotine yield mg/cig
13	John Player Carlton KS	1.5
13	John Player Carlton Long Size	1.4
13	Peer Special Mild KS (with Cytrel)	1.2
14	Gauloises Disque Bleu	0.7
14	Gitanes Caporal Filter	0.7
14	Kensitas Club Mild KS	1.4
14	Merit	1.2
14	Peter Stuyvesant KS	1.1
14	Piccadilly No. 7	1.0
14	State Express 555 Medium Mild KS	1.2
15	Benson and Hedges Sovereign Mild	1.3
15	Black Cat No. 9	1.1
15	Cadets	1.2
15	Camel Filter Tip	1.1
15	Chesterfield KS Filter	1.2
15	Craven 'A' Cork Tipped (P)	1.2
15	Dunhill KS	1.3
15	Gauloises Caporal Filter	0.7
15	Kensitas Club Mild	1.3
15	Kensitas Mild KS	1.4
15	Kent	1.1
15	L and M Filter	1.2
15	More Menthol	1.5
15	Pall Mall Filter	1.4
15	Rothmans International	1.3
15	Three Castles Filter	1.1
16	Guards	1.1
16	Kensitas Corsair Mild	1.3
16	Lark Filter Tip	1.5
16	Marlboro	1.3
16	More	1.6
16	Philip Morris International	1.3
16	Piccadilly Filter De Luxe	1.3
16	Rothmans Royal	1.4

Tar yield mg/cig	Brand	Nicotine yield mg/cig
Middle Tar		
17	Du Maurier	1.5
17	Dunhill International	1.5
17	Lucky Strike KS Filter	1.4
17	Piccadilly KS	1.5
17	Silva Thins	1.6
17	State Express 555 Filter Kings	1.4
17	State Express 555 Selected Virginia (P)	1.3
18	Benson and Hedges Gold Bond	1.5
18	Benson and Hedges Gold Bond KS	1.7
18	Benson and Hedges KS	1.7
18	Benson and Hedges Supremes	1.8
18	Embassy Envoy	1.4
18	Embassy Filter	1.5
18	Embassy No. 1 KS	1.4
18	Embassy No. 3 Standard Size	1.5
18	Embassy Regal	1.5
18	Emperor KS	1.4
18	Fribourg and Treyer No. 1 Filter De Luxe	1.5
18	Imperial International	1.6
18	John Player KS	1.5
18	John Player Special	1.6
18	Kensitas Club KS	1.6
18	Kensitas Tipped KS	1.6
18	Lambert and Butler Intern Size	1.5
18	Lambert and Butler KS	1.5
18	Piccadilly No. 1 (P)	1.4
18	Player's Filter Virginia	1.4
18	Player's Gold Leaf	1.5
18	Player's Medium Navy Cut (P)	1.4
18	Player's No. 6 Filter	1.3
18	Player's No. 6 KS	1.6
18	Player's No. 6 Plain (P)	1.2
18	Regal KS	1.4
18	Rothmans KS	1.4
18	Slim Kings	1.4
18	Sobranie Virginia Intern	1.6
18	State Express 555 Intern	1.6

Tar yield mg/cig	Brand	Nicotine yield mg/cig
18	Weights Plain (P)	1.2
18	Woodbine Plain (P)	1.6
19	Benson and Hedges Sovereign	1.5
19	Capstan Medium (P)	1.4
19	Embassy Gold	1.4
19	Embassy KS	1.4
19	Embassy Plain (P)	1.4
19	Gallaher's De Luxe Green (P)	1.5
19	Gold Flake	1.4
19	Kensitas Club	1.5
19	Kensitas Corsair	1.4
19	Kensitas Plain (P)	1.6
19	Nerit	1.6
19	Park Drive Plain (P)	1.6
19	Park Drive Tipped	1.5
19	Player's No. 10	1.3
19	Senior Service Plain (P)	1.5
19	Sterling	1.6
19	Winston KS	1.5
19	Woodbine Filter	1.3
Middle to High Tar		
24	Lucky Strike Plain (P)	1.7
25	Gitanes Caporal Plain (P)	1.4
26	Gallaher's De Luxe Blue (P)	2.3
26	Gauloises Caporal Plain (P)	1.3
28	Capstan Full Strength (P)	3.1
28	Pall Mall KS (P)	2.4

New brands recently introduced but not yet analysed by the Government Chemist for a period of six months. Estimates by the manufacturers of the tar and nicotine yields for these brands are as follows:

6	Silk Cut Extra Mild	0.7
8	Craven A KS Special Mild	0.6
17	Craven A KS	1.4
17	Kent De Luxe Length	1.3

(P) indicates plain cigarettes; all other brands have filters

Tar yield mg/cig	Brand	Nicotine yield mg/cig
Low Tar		
under 4	Embassy Ultra Mild	under 0.3
under 4	John Player KS Ultra Mild	under 0.3
under 4	Silk Cut Ultra Mild with Subst	under 0.3
6	Silk Cut Extra Mild	0.7
7	Silk Cut KS with Substitute	0.7
8	Embassy Premier KS	0.6
8	John Player KS with NSM	0.7
8	Piccadilly Mild	0.5
9	Consulate Menthol	0.6
9	Craven A KS Special Mild	0.7
9	Dunhill Intern Superior Mild	0.8
9	Dunhill KS Superior Mild	0.7
9	Embassy No. 5 Extra Mild	0.7
9	John Player KS Extra Mild	0.7
9	Lambert and Butler KS Mild	0.7
9	Peer Special Extra Mild KS (with Cytrel)	0.7
9	Silk Cut	0.8
9	Silk Cut International	0.9
9	Silk Cut No. 5	0.7
10	Belair Menthol Kings	0.6
10	Consulate No. 2	0.6
10	Embassy Extra Mild	0.8
10	Embassy No. 1 Extra Mild	0.8
10	Peter Stuyvesant Extra Mild KS	0.8
10	Player's No. 10 with NSM	0.7
10	Player's No. 6 Extra mild	0.7
10	Silk Cut KS	0.9
10	Silk Cut No. 3	0.8
Low to Middle Tar		
11	Gauloises Longues	0.6
12	Gauloises Filter Mild	0.6
12	Gitanes International	0.9
12	Rothmans KS Mild	0.9
12	St Moritz	0.9
13	Gitanes Caporal Filter	0.7
13	John Player Carlton KS	1.5
13	John Player Carlton Long Size	1.4
13	John Player Carlton Premium	1.2
13	Player's No. 10 Extra Mild	0.8
14	Black Cat No. 9	1.0
14	Dunhill International Menthol	1.0
14	Gauloises Disque Bleu	0.6
14	Kensitas Mild KS	1.4
14	Kent	1.0
14	Lark Filter Tip	1.1
14	Peer Special Mild KS (with Cytrel)	1.2
14	Peter Stuyvesant KS	1.2
14	Piccadilly No. 7	1.1
15	Benson and Hedges Sovereign Mild	1.2
15	Chesterfield KS Filter	1.1
15	Gauloises Caporal Filter	0.7
15	Kensitas Club Mild KS	1.4
15	Kensitas Corsair Mild	1.1
15	L and M Filter	1.1
15	Merit	1.2
15	More	1.5
15	More Menthol	1.5
15	Pall Mall Filter	1.4

Tar yield mg/cig	Brand	Nicotine yield mg/cig
15	Three Fives Medium Mild KS	1.3
15	Three Castles Filter	1.0
16	Cadets	1.2
16	Camel Filter Tip	1.1
16	Carroll's No. 1	1.2
16	Carroll's No. 1 KS	1.3
16	Dunhill International	1.4
16	Dunhill KS	1.3
16	Guards	1.1
16	Kensitas Club Mild	1.3
16	Marlboro	1.3
16	Philip Morris International	1.4
16	Piccadilly Filter De Luxe	1.4
16	Piccadilly KS	1.3
16	Rothmans International	1.5
Middle Tar		
17	Craven 'A' Cork Tipped (P)	1.3
17	Craven 'A' KS	1.3
17	Kent De Luxe Length	1.2
17	Lucky Strike KS Filter	1.4
17	MS Filter	1.3
17	Rothmans Royal	1.5
17	Silva Thins	1.5
17	Sobranie Virginia Intern	1.5
18	Benson and Hedges Gold Bond	1.5
18	Benson and Hedges Gold Bond KS	1.5
18	Benson and Hedges KS	1.6
18	Benson and Hedges Supremes	1.7
18	Du Maurier	1.5
18	Embassy Envoy	1.2
18	Embassy Filter	1.4
18	Embassy Gold	1.3
18	Embassy KS	1.4
18	Embassy No. 3 Standard Size	1.4
18	Embassy Regal	1.4
18	Emperor KS	1.4
18	Fribourg and Treyer No. 1 Filter De Luxe	1.5
18	Imperial International	1.6
18	John Player Special	1.5
18	Kensitas Club KS	1.5
18	Kensitas Corsair	1.3
18	Kensitas Tipped KS	1.5
18	Piccadilly No. 1 (P)	1.4
18	Player's Medium Navy Cut (P)	1.4
18	Rothmans KS	1.4
18	Slim Kings	1.4
18	Three Fives Filter Kings	1.5
18	Weights Plain (P)	1.2
18	Winston KS	1.4
18	Woodbine Plain (P)	1.5
19	Benson and Hedges Sovereign	1.4
19	Capstan Medium (P)	1.3
19	Embassy No. 1 KS	1.4
19	Embassy Plain (P)	1.3
19	Gallaher's De Luxe Green (P)	1.5
19	Gold Flake	1.3
19	John Player KS	1.5
19	Kensitas Club	1.5
19	Lambert and Butler Intern Size	1.5

LGC Survey 13
(*continued*)

Middle Tar

Tar yield mg/cig	Brand	Nicotine yield mg/cig
19	Lambert and Butler KS	1.5
19	Major Extra Size	1.3
19	Park Drive Plain (P)	1.5
19	Park Drive Tipped	1.5
19	Player's Filter Virginia	1.4
19	Player's Gold Leaf	1.5
19	Player's No. 6 Filter	1.3
19	Player's No. 6 KS	1.6
19	Player's No. 6 Plain (P)	1.2
19	Player's No. 10	1.3
19	Regal KS	1.4
19	Senior Service Plain (P)	1.6
19	Sterling	1.6
19	Woodbine Filter	1.3
20	Kensitas Plain (P)	1.6
20	Nerit	1.5
20	Three Fives International	1.7
20	Three Fives Selected Virginia (P)	1.4
22	Sweet Afton Bank Size Plain (P)	1.9

Middle to High Tar

Tar yield mg/cig	Brand	Nicotine yield mg/cig
24	Lucky Strike Plain (P)	1.8
25	Gallaher's De Luxe Blue (P)	2.1
25	Gauloises Caporal Plain (P)	1.2
25	Gitanes Caporal Plain (P)	1.4
26	Capstan Full Strength (P)	2.7
27	Pall Mall KS (P)	2.2

New brands recently introduced but not yet analysed by the Government Chemist for a period of six months. Estimates by the manufacturers of the tar and nicotine yields for these brands are as follows:

Tar yield mg/cig	Brand	Nicotine yield mg/cig
14	Du Maurier KS	1.2
15	Benson and Hedges Sovereign KS	1.3
18	Benson and Hedges Academy	1.8
19	John Player Special KS	1.4

(P) indicates plain cigarettes; all other brands have filters

LGC Survey 14
Sampling period June 1980-November 1980

Low Tar

Tar yield mg/cig	Brand	Nicotine yield mg/cig
under 4	Embassy Ultra Mild	under 0.3
under 4	John Player KS Ultra Mild	under 0.3
under 4	Silk Cut Ultra Mild with Subst	under 0.3
4	Silk Cut Extra Mild	0.5
7	Silk Cut KS with Substitute	0.7
8	Embassy Premier KS	0.6
8	Piccadilly Mild	0.5
9	Belair Menthol Kings	0.6
9	Consulate Menthol	0.6
9	Consulate No. 2	0.6
9	Dunhill KS Superior Mild	0.7
9	Embassy Extra Mild	0.7
9	John Player KS Extra Mild	0.8
9	John Player KS with NSM	0.8
9	John Player Vanguard KS	1.0
9	Lambert and Butler Special Mild KS	0.8
9	Peer Special Extra Mild KS (with Cytrel)	0.8
9	Silk Cut	0.7
9	Silk Cut International	0.8
9	Silk Cut KS	0.9
9	Silk Cut No. 5	0.6
10	Craven A Special Mild KS Filter	0.8
10	Dunhill Intern Superior Mild	0.9
10	Embassy No. 1 Extra Mild	0.8
10	Embassy No. 5 Extra Mild	0.7
10	Peter Stuyvesant Extra Mild KS	0.8
10	Peter Stuyvesant Luxury Length Extra Mild	0.9
10	Player's No. 6 Extra mild	0.7
10	Player's No. 10 with NSM	0.7
10	Silk Cut No. 3	0.8

Low to Middle Tar

Tar yield mg/cig	Brand	Nicotine yield mg/cig
11	Gauloises Filter Mild	0.6
11	Gauloises Longues	0.5
11	St Moritz	0.8
12	Rothmans KS Mild	0.9
13	Du Maurier KS	1.1
13	Gauloises Caporal Filter	0.6
13	Gitanes Caporal Filter	0.7
13	Gitanes International	0.9
13	John Player Carlton Long Size	1.4
13	John Player Carlton Premium	1.2
13	Player's No. 10 Extra Mild F	0.8
14	Benson and Hedges Sovereign Mild	1.1
14	Black Cat No. 9	1.0
14	Dunhill Intern Menthol	1.0
14	Gauloises Disque Bleu	0.6
14	Kensitas Club Mild KS	1.3
14	Kensitas Corsair Mild	1.1
14	Kensitas Mild KS	1.3
14	L and M Filter Box	1.1

Tar yield mg/cig	Brand	Nicotine yield mg/cig
Low to Middle Tar		
14	Peer Special Mild KS (with Cytrel)	1.2
14	Peter Stuyvesant KS	1.2
14	Piccadilly No. 7	1.0
14	Three Fives Medium Mild KS	1.2
15	Cadets Filter Virginia	1.1
15	Carroll's No. 1 KS	1.2
15	Chesterfield KS Filter	1.1
15	Lark Filter Tip	1.2
15	Pall Mall Filter Tipped	1.4
15	Three Castles Filter	1.0
16	Camel Filter Tip	1.0
16	Carreras Guards	1.1
16	Carroll's No. 1 Virginia	1.0
16	Dunhill International	1.3
16	Dunhill KS	1.3
16	Kensitas Club Mild	1.2
16	Kent De Luxe Length	1.2
16	Lucky Strike KS Filter	1.2
16	Marlboro Filter	1.2
16	More Menthol Filter 120s	1.4
16	MS Filter KS	1.1
16	Philip Morris International	1.3
16	Piccadilly Filter De Luxe	1.3
16	Piccadilly KS	1.4
16	Rothmans International	1.5
16	Silva Thins Filter 100s	1.4
Middle Tar		
17	Benson and Hedges Supreme International	1.7
17	Craven 'A' KS	1.3
17	Embassy Envoy	1.2
17	Embassy Regal	1.3
17	Imperial Intern F Virginia	1.4
17	Kensitas Club KS	1.4
17	Kensitas Corsair F Virginia	1.2
17	More Filter 120s	1.5
17	Piccadilly No. 1 (P)	1.3
17	Rothmans KS	1.4
17	Rothmans Royals	1.4
17	Slim Kings Special Virginia F	1.3
17	Sobranie Virginia Intern	1.6
17	Three Fives Filter Kings	1.3
17	Three Fives International	1.5
17	Three Fives Selected Virginia (P)	1.2
18	Benson and Hedges Academy Intern	1.8
18	Benson and Hedges Gold Bond F	1.4
18	Benson and Hedges Gold Bond KS	1.6
18	Benson and Hedges Sovereign F	1.3
18	Benson and Hedges Special F KS	1.6
18	Craven 'A' Cork Tipped (P)	1.4
18	Du Maurier	1.4
18	Embassy Filter	1.3
18	Embassy KS	1.3
18	Embassy No. 1 KS	1.3
18	Embassy No. 3 Standard Size	1.4
18	Emperor KS	1.3
18	Fribourg and Treyer No. 1 Filter De Luxe	1.4
18	Gold Flake (P)	1.2
18	Gold Leaf Filter Virginia	1.4
18	John Player KS	1.4
18	John Player Special	1.5
18	John Player Special KS	1.4
18	Kensitas Filter Virginia KS	1.5
18	Lambert and Butler Intern Size	1.4
18	Lambert and Butler KS	1.4
18	Major Virginia Filter Extra Size	1.2
18	Park Drive Special Virginia (P)	1.4
18	Player's Medium Navy Cut Filter	1.4
18	Player's Medium Navy Cut (P)	1.4
18	Player's No. 10 Filter Virginia	1.2
18	Player's No. 6 Filter Virginia	1.3
18	Player's No. 6 Finest Virginia (P)	1.1
18	Player's Weights Finest Virginia (P)	1.2
18	Regal KS	1.4
18	Winston KS	1.3
18	Woodbine Filter Virginia	1.3
18	Woodbine Virginia (P)	1.4
19	Benson and Hedges Sterling F	1.5
19	Capstan Medium (P)	1.2
19	Embassy Gold	1.3
19	Embassy Virginia (P)	1.3
19	Gallaher's De Luxe Green (P)	1.5
19	Kensitas Club Filter Virginia	1.4
19	Kensitas Fine Virginia (P)	1.6
19	Nerit Filter	1.4
19	Park Drive Tipped	1.4
19	Player's No. 6 KS	1.5
19	Senior Service Fine Virginia (P)	1.5
21	Lucky Strike Plain (P)	1.5
22	Sweet Afton Virginia (P)	1.8
Middle to High Tar		
23	Gauloises Caporal Plain (P)	1.1
24	Capstan Full Strength (P)	2.4
24	Gitanes Caporal Plain (P)	1.4
25	Gallaher's De Luxe Blue (P)	2.0
27	Pall Mall (P)	2.1

New brands recently introduced but not yet analysed by the Government Chemist for a period of six months. Estimates by the manufacturers of the tar and nicotine yields for these brands are as follows:

8	Kent KS	0.7
9	Merit Extra Mild	0.8
15	Benson and Hedges Sovereign KS	1.2

(P) indicates plain cigarettes; all other brands have filters

LGC Survey 15
Sampling period January 1981-June 1981

Tar yield mg/cig	Brand	Nicotine yield mg/cig
Low Tar		
under 4	Embassy Ultra Mild KS	under 0.3
under 4	John Player KS Ultra Mild	under 0.3
under 4	Silk Cut KS Ultra Low	under 0.3
under 4	Silk Cut KS Ultra Mild with substitute	0.5
4	Silk Cut KS Extra Mild	0.6
7	Silk Cut KS with Substitute	0.8
8	Barclay KS	0.8
8	Dunhill KS Superior Mild	0.8
8	Kent KS	0.8
8	Merit Extra Mild	0.8
8	Peer Special Extra Mild KS (with Cytrel)	0.8
8	Peter Stuyvesant Extra Mild KS	0.8
8	Silk Cut International	0.7
9	Belair Menthol Kings	0.6
9	Berkeley KS Extra Mild	1.0
9	Consulate Menthol	0.7
9	Consulate No. 2	0.6
9	Craven 'A' Special Mild KS	0.7
9	Embassy No. 1 Extra Mild	0.9
9	John Player KS Extra Mild	0.8
9	John Player Vanguard KS	1.0
9	Lambert and Butler Special Mild KS	0.9
9	Silk Cut KS	1.0
9	Silk Cut No. 5	0.7
9	State Express 555 Special Mild KS	0.9
10	Dunhill Intern Superior Mild	0.9
10	Embassy Extra Mild	0.8
10	Embassy No. 5 Extra Mild	0.8
10	Gauloises Longues Caporal Filter	0.5
10	Peter Stuyvesant Lux Length Extra M	0.9
10	Player's No. 6 Extra mild	0.7
10	Silk Cut	0.9
10	Silk Cut No. 3	0.8
Low to Middle Tar		
12	Gauloises Caporal Filter	0.6
12	Gauloises Filter Mild	0.6
12	Gitanes International	1.1
12	Rothmans KS Special Mild	1.0
12	St Moritz Lux Length Menthol	0.9
13	Dunhill International Menthol	1.1
13	Gauloises Disque Bleu Caporal F	0.7
13	Gitanes Caporal Filter	0.7
13	John Player Carlton Long Size	1.4
13	Kensitas Mild KS	1.3
13	Peer Special Mild KS (with Cytrel)	1.1
13	Player's No. 10 Extra Mild F Virg	0.8
14	Du Maurier KS	1.2
14	John Player Carlton Premium	1.2
14	Kensitas Club Mild KS	1.3
14	Peter Stuyvesant KS	1.2
14	Piccadilly No. 7	1.1
14	State Express 555 Medium Mild KS	1.2
15	Benson and Hedges Sovereign KS	1.3
15	Benson and Hedges Sovereign Mild	1.2
15	Camel Filter Tip	1.2
15	Carroll's No. 1 Virginia	1.1
15	Chesterfield KS Filter	1.2
15	Dunhill KS	1.3

Tar yield mg/cig	Brand	Nicotine yield mg/cig
15	Kensitas Club Mild	1.3
15	Kent De Luxe Length	1.2
15	L and M Filter Box	1.2
15	More Filter 120s	1.4
15	Pall Mall Filter Tipped	1.4
15	Peter Stuyvesant Lux Length	1.4
15	Piccadilly KS	1.3
15	Royal Standard KS	1.2
15	Three Castles Filter	1.1
16	Benson and Hedges Academy Intern	1.6
16	Carroll's No. 1 KS	1.4
16	Craven 'A' KS	1.3
16	Guards	1.2
16	Lark Filter Tip	1.3
16	Marlboro	1.3
16	More Menthol Filter 120s	1.5
16	Philip Morris International	1.4
Middle Tar		
17	Benson and Hedges Gold Bond KS	1.5
17	Benson and Hedges Special F KS	1.5
17	Benson and Hedges Supreme Intern	1.6
17	Dunhill International	1.5
17	Embassy Filter	1.4
17	Embassy No. 3 Standard Size	1.4
17	Embassy Regal	1.3
17	Emperor KS	1.5
17	Fribourg and Treyer No. 1 Filter De Luxe	1.4
17	Gold Leaf Filter Virginia	1.4
17	John Player KS	1.4
17	John Player Special Intern	1.5
17	Kensitas Club KS	1.4
17	Kensitas Filter Virginia KS	1.5
17	Lucky Strike KS Filter	1.4
17	MS Filter KS	1.2
17	Park Drive Tipped KS	1.5
17	Piccadilly Filter De Luxe	1.5
17	Player's No. 6 KS	1.5
17	Player's No. 10 Filter Virginia	1.2
17	Rothmans International	1.6
17	Rothmans KS Filter	1.4
17	Silva Thins Filter 100s	1.5
17	Slim Kings Special Virginia F	1.3
17	Winston KS	1.4
17	State Express 555 Filter Kings	1.4
17	State Express 555 International	1.5
18	Benson and Hedges Gold Bond F	1.4
18	Benson and Hedges Sovereign F	1.3
18	Du Maurier	1.4
18	Embassy KS	1.4
18	Embassy No. 1 KS	1.5
18	Imperial Intern Filter Virginia	1.5
18	John Player Special KS	1.4
18	Kensitas Club Filter Virginia	1.4
18	Kensitas Corsair Filter Virginia	1.3
18	Lambert and Butler Intern Size	1.5
18	Lambert and Butler KS	1.5
18	Major Virginia Filter Extra Size	1.3
18	Park Drive Special Virginia (P)	1.5
18	Piccadilly No. 1 (P)	1.6

LGC Survey 15
(*continued*)

Tar yield mg/cig	Brand	Nicotine yield mg/cig
Middle Tar		
18	Player's Medium Navy Cut Filter	1.5
18	Player's No. 6 Filter Virginia	1.4
18	Player's No. 6 Finest Virginia (P)	1.2
18	Player's Weights Finest Virginia (P)	1.2
18	Regal KS	1.5
18	Rothmans Royals 120s	1.6
18	Woodbine Filter Virginia	1.4
18	Woodbine Virginia (P)	1.5
18	State Express 555 Selected Virginia (P)	1.3
19	Capstan Medium (P)	1.4
19	Craven 'A' Cork Tipped (P)	1.6
19	Embassy Gold	1.4
19	Embassy Virginia (P)	1.3
19	Gold Flake (P)	1.3
19	Kensitas Fine Virginia (P)	1.6
19	London KS	1.7
19	Player's Medium Navy Cut (P)	1.4
19	Senior Service Fine Virginia (P)	1.6
20	Gallaher's De Luxe Green (P)	1.7
22	Sweet Afton Virginia (P)	2.0

Tar yield mg/cig	Brand	Nicotine yield mg/cig
Middle to High Tar		
23	Gauloises Caporal (P)	1.2
24	Gallaher's De Luxe Blue (P)	2.0
24	Gitanes Caporal (P)	1.4
26	Capstan Full Strength (P)	2.7

New brands recently introduced but not yet analysed by the Government Chemist for a period of six months. Estimates by the manufacturers of the tar and nicotine yields for these brands are as follows:

8	Cartier Intern Luxury Mild	0.8
9	Benson and Hedges Sovereign Mild KS	1.1
14	Marlboro 100s	1.5
15	Benson and Hedges Sterling KS	1.3
15	Senior Service Cadets KS	1.3
15	United Filter Virginia	1.1

(P) indicates plain cigarettes; all other brands have filters

LGC Survey 16
Sampling period August 1981-January 1982

Tar yield mg/cig	Brand	Carbon monoxide yield mg/cig	Nicotine yield mg/cig
Low Tar			
under 4	Embassy Ultra Mild Ks	under 3	under 0.3
under 4	John Player KS Ultra Mild	under 3	under 0.3
under 4	Silk Cut KS Ultra Low	under 3	under 0.3
under 4	Silk Cut KS Ultra Mild with substitute	under 3	0.5
6	Silk Cut KS Extra Mild	6	0.7
7	Silk Cut KS with Substitute	8	0.7
8	Barclay KS	8	0.7
8	Cartier Intern Lux Mild	9	0.8
8	Kent KS	9	0.7
8	Merit Extra Mild	9	0.8
8	Peter Stuyvesant Extra Mild KS	7	0.9
9	Benson and Hedges Sovereign Mild KS	12	0.9
9	Berkeley KS Extra Mild	9	0.9
9	Consulate No. 2	8	0.7
9	Dunhill KS Superior Mild	8	0.8
9	Embassy Extra Mild	10	0.7
9	Embassy No. 1 Extra Mild	10	0.8
9	Embassy No. 5 Extra Mild	10	0.7
9	John Player KS Extra Mild	9	1.0
9	John Player Vanguard KS	13	1.0
9	Lambert and Butler Special Mild KS	10	0.8
9	Silk Cut	10	0.9
9	Silk Cut KS	10	0.9
9	State Express 555 Special Mild KS	10	0.9
10	Belair Menthol Kings	14	0.7
10	Consulate Menthol	10	0.9
10	Dunhill Intern Superior Mild	9	1.0
10	Peer Special KS Extra Mild (with Cytrel)	14	0.9
10	Peter Stuyvesant Luxury Length Extra Mild	10	1.0
10	Player's No. 6 Extra mild	11	0.7
10	Silk Cut International	14	0.9
10	Silk Cut No. 3	9	0.8
10	Silk Cut No. 5	10	0.7
Low to Middle Tar			
11	Gauloises Filter Mild	17	0.6
11	Gauloises Longues Caporal F	17	0.6
11	Gitanes International	15	1.0
12	Du Maurier KS	12	1.1
12	Gauloises Caporal Filter	16	0.6
12	Player's No. 10 Extra Mild Filter Virginia	12	0.8
13	Gauloises Disque Bleu Caporal Filter	17	0.7
13	Gitanes Caporal Filter	17	0.7
13	John Player Carlton Long Size	11	1.3
13	John Player Carlton Premium	11	1.2

Tar yield mg/cig	Brand	Carbon monoxide yield mg/cig	Nicotine yield mg/cig
Low to Middle Tar			
13	St Moritz Lux Length Menthol	15	1.1
14	Benson and Hedges Sterling KS	15	1.3
14	Kensitas Club Mild KS	12	1.2
14	Kensitas Mild KS	12	1.2
14	Peter Stuyvesant KS	14	1.3
14	Peter Stuyvesant Lux Length	15	1.4
14	State Express 555 Medium Mild KS	13	1.2
15	Benson and Hedges Sovereign KS	15	1.2
15	Benson and Hedges Sovereign Mild	10	1.1
15	Camel Filter Tip	14	1.1
15	Carroll's No. 1 KS	16	1.3
15	Dunhill Intern Menthol	15	1.2
15	Dunhill KS	14	1.2
15	Kensitas Club Mild	13	1.2
15	L and M Filter Box	14	1.2
15	Marlboro 100s	13	1.4
15	More Filter 120s	16	1.3
15	More Menthol Filter 120s	16	1.3
15	Park Drive Tipped KS	15	1.3
15	Peer Special Mild KS (with Cytrel)	13	1.5
15	Piccadilly KS	14	1.2
15	Piccadilly No. 7	13	1.1
15	Senior Service Cadets KS	15	1.2
15	Three Castles Filter	16	1.1
15	United Filter Virginia	15	1.1
15	Winston KS	14	1.2
16	Benson and Hedges Academy International	13	1.6
16	Carroll's No. 1 Virginia	16	1.2
16	Chesterfield KS Filter	14	1.3
16	Dunhill International	15	1.5
16	Embassy KS	15	1.3
16	Embassy No. 3 Standard Size	17	1.3
16	Embassy Regal	16	1.3
16	Fribourg and Treyer No. 1 Filter De Luxe	19	1.3
16	John Player Special Intern	15	1.4
16	Kent De Luxe Length	13	1.3
16	Lark Filter Tip	13	1.3
16	Marlboro KS	15	1.3
16	Pall Mall Filter Tipped	14	1.6
16	Philip Morris International	15	1.4
16	Rothmans International	15	1.6
Middle Tar			
17	Benson and Hedges Gold Bond KS	16	1.4
17	Benson and Hedges Special Filter KS	17	1.5
17	Benson and Hedges Supreme International	13	1.7
17	Du Maurier	17	1.3
17	Embassy Filter	17	1.4
17	Embassy No. 1 KS	16	1.4
17	Gold Leaf Filter Virginia	17	1.4
17	Guards	16	1.3
17	John Player KS	18	1.4
17	Kensitas Club KS	17	1.3
17	Kensitas Corsair F Virginia	14	1.2
17	Kensitas Filter Virginia KS	17	1.4
17	Lambert and Butler KS	17	1.4
17	Lucky Strike KS Filter	16	1.3
17	MS Filter KS	15	1.2
17	Piccadilly Filter De Luxe	14	1.4
17	Player's Medium Navy Cut F	17	1.4
17	Player's No. 6 KS	17	1.4
17	Player's No. 10 F Virginia	15	1.2
17	Player's Weights Finest Virginia (P)	11	1.1
17	Regal KS	17	1.4
17	Rothmans KS Filter	15	1.5
17	Slim Kings Special Virginia F	17	1.3
17	State Express 555 Selected Virginia (P)	11	1.2
18	State Express 555 F Kings	16	1.3
18	Benson and Hedges Gold Bond Filter	16	1.4
18	Benson and Hedges Sovereign Filter	14	1.3
18	Embassy Gold	14	1.3
18	Embassy Virginia (P)	11	1.3
18	Imperial International Filter Virginia	17	1.5
18	John Player Special KS	19	1.4
18	Lambert and Butler Intern Size	17	1.4
18	Major Virginia F Extra Size	17	1.2
18	Park Drive Special Virginia (P)	12	1.5
18	Piccadilly No. 1 (P)	11	1.5
18	Player's Medium Navy Cut (P)	11	1.4
18	Player's No. 6 F Virginia	18	1.4
18	Player's No. 6 Finest Virginia (P)	11	1.1
18	Rothmans Royals 120s	15	1.8
18	Silva Thins Filter 100s	18	1.5
18	Woodbine Filter Virginia	14	1.4
19	Capstan Medium (P)	11	1.3
19	Gallaher's De Luxe Green (P)	11	1.5
19	Gold Flake (P)	11	1.3
19	Kensitas Club Filter Virginia	16	1.4
19	Kensitas Fine Virginia (P)	11	1.5
19	Senior Service Fine Virginia (P)	11	1.5
19	Woodbine Virginia (P)	10	1.5
20	London KS	17	1.9
20	Royal Standard KS	16	1.6
20	Sweet Afton Virginia (P)	11	1.7
22	Gitanes Caporal (P)	17	1.3
Middle to High Tar			
24	Gallaher's De Luxe Blue (P)	15	2.0
24	Gauloises Caporal (P)	19	1.3
26	Capstan Full Strength (P)	14	2.6

New brands recently introduced but not yet analysed by the Government Chemist for a period of six months. Estimates by the manufacturers of the tar and nicotine yields for these brands are as follows:

6	Philip Morris Super Lights	6	0.5
9	Craven 'A' Luxury Length Special Mild	9	0.9
14	Craven 'A' Luxury Length	16	1.4
15	Sobranie Virginia Blend	13	1.4
18	Fine 120 Super Length	17	1.6

(P) indicates plain cigarettes; all other brands have filters

LGC Survey 17
Sampling period March 1982-August 1982

Tar yield mg/cig	Brand	Carbon monoxide yield mg/cig	Nicotine yield mg/cig
Low Tar			
under 4	Embassy Ultra Mild KS	under 3	0.4
under 4	John Player KS Ultra Mild	under 3	under 0.3
under 4	Silk Cut KS Ultra Low	under 3	under 0.3
under 4	Silk Cut KS Ultra Mild with substitute	under 3	0.4
5	Philip Morris Super Lights	7	0.5
5	Silk Cut KS Extra Mild	5	0.6
7	Barclay KS	8	0.7
7	Kent KS	9	0.7
7	Silk Cut KS with Substitute	9	0.7
8	Dunhill KS Superior Mild	8	0.8
8	Peer Special KS Extra Mild (with Cytrel)	8	0.8
8	Peter Stuyvesant Extra Mild KS	7	0.9
9	Belair Menthol Kings	13	0.6
9	Berkeley KS Extra Mild	9	0.9
9	Cartier Intern Luxury Mild	9	0.8
9	Consulate Menthol	9	0.8
9	Consulate No. 2	8	0.8
9	Embassy Extra Mild	10	0.7
9	Embassy No. 1 Extra Mild	10	0.8
9	Embassy No. 5 Extra Mild	9	0.7
9	John Player KS Extra Mild	10	1.0
9	John Player Vanguard KS	13	1.0
9	Lambert and Butler Special Mild KS	10	0.8
9	Merit Extra Mild	9	0.8
9	Silk Cut	10	0.8
9	Silk Cut International	12	0.9
9	Silk Cut King Size	10	0.9
10	Craven 'A' Luxury Length Special Mild	10	0.9
10	Du Maurier KS	10	0.9
10	Dunhill Intern Superior Mild	10	0.9
10	Gauloises Filter Mild	14	0.6
10	Gauloises Longues Caporal F	17	0.6
10	Peter Stuyvesant Luxury Length Extra Mild	10	0.9
10	Player's No. 6 Extra mild	11	0.8
10	Silk Cut No. 3	10	0.8
10	Silk Cut No. 5	10	0.7
10	State Express 555 Special Mild KS	10	0.9
Low to Middle Tar			
11	Gauloises Caporal Filter	16	0.6
11	Gitanes International	16	0.9
12	Gauloises Disque Bleu Caporal Filter	16	0.6
12	Gitanes Caporal Filter	17	0.7
12	St Moritz Lux Length Menthol	15	0.9
13	Dunhill International Menthol	15	1.1
13	John Player Carlton Long Size	12	1.3
13	John Player Carlton Premium	12	1.1
13	Jubilee KS	12	1.2
13	Kensitas Club Mild KS	12	1.2
13	Kensitas Mild KS	12	1.2
13	Peer Special Mild KS (with Cytrel)	14	1.3
13	Peter Stuyvesant Lux Length	16	1.3
13	Piccadilly KS	14	1.1
13	Player's No. 10 Extra Mild Filter Virginia	13	0.9
14	Carroll's No. 1 KS	16	1.3
14	Craven 'A' Luxury Length	16	1.3
14	Dunhill KS	14	1.2
14	Kensitas Club Mild	13	1.2
14	More Filter 120s	16	1.2
14	More Menthol Filter 120s	16	1.2
14	Sobranie Virginia Blend	13	1.3
14	State Express 555 Medium Mild KS	14	1.2
15	Benson and Hedges Sovereign Mild	11	1.2
15	Camel Filter Tip	14	1.2
15	Carroll's No. 1 Virginia	17	1.2
15	Guards	15	1.1
15	Kent De Luxe Length	14	1.2
15	L and M Filter Box	13	1.2
15	Marlboro	16	1.3
15	Marlboro 100s	14	1.3
15	Park Drive Tipped KS	16	1.4
15	Peter Stuyvesant KS	15	1.3
15	Philip Morris International	15	1.3
15	Winston King Size	14	1.2
16	Benson and Hedges Sovereign KS	18	1.4
16	Benson and Hedges Sterling KS	18	1.4
16	Chesterfield KS Filter	15	1.3
16	Du Maurier	17	1.4
16	Dunhill International	15	1.4
16	Embassy Filter	15	1.4
16	Embassy No. 1 KS	16	1.3
16	Embassy No. 3 Standard Size	15	1.4
16	Embassy Regal	14	1.4
16	Fribourg and Treyer No. 1 Filter De Luxe	18	1.3
16	John Player KS	16	1.4
16	John Player Special Intern	16	1.4
16	Lambert and Butler KS	16	1.4
16	Lark Filter Tip	14	1.3
16	Pall Mall Filter Tipped	14	1.6
16	Piccadilly Filter De Luxe	15	1.3
16	Piccadilly No. 1 (P)	10	1.4
16	Player's No. 6 KS	16	1.5
16	Player's No. 10 F Virginia	15	1.2
16	Rothmans KS Filter	15	1.4
16	Rothmans Royals 120s	14	1.5
16	Senior Service Cadets KS	19	1.3
16	Silva Thins Filter 100s	18	1.4
16	Slim Kings Special Virginia F	16	1.2
16	State Express 555 Filter Kings	17	1.3
16	State Express 555 Selected Virginia (P)	11	1.2
16	United Filter Virginia	16	1.2

LGC Survey 17
(*continued*)

Tar yield mg/cig	Brand	Carbon monoxide yield mg/cig	Nicotine yield mg/cig
Middle Tar			
17	Benson and Hedges Academy International	14	1.6
17	Benson and Hedges Gold Bond KS	19	1.5
17	Benson and Hedges Sovereign Filter	14	1.3
17	Benson and Hedges Supreme International	14	1.7
17	Embassy Gold	15	1.3
17	Fine 120 Super Length	17	1.5
17	Gold Leaf Filter Virginia	17	1.4
17	John Player Special KS	18	1.4
17	Kensitas Club KS	18	1.4
17	Kensitas Corsair F Virginia	14	1.3
17	Kensitas Filter Virginia KS	18	1.4
17	MS Filter KS	15	1.2
17	Major Virginia F Extra Size	17	1.2
17	Player's Medium Navy Cut F	17	1.4
17	Player's No. 6 Filter Virginia	17	1.4
17	Player's No. 6 Finest Virginia (P)	11	1.1
17	Player's Weights Finest Virginia (P)	12	1.1
17	Regal KS	16	1.4
17	Rothmans International	17	1.5
17	Woodbine Filter Virginia	14	1.3
18	Benson and Hedges Gold Bond Filter	16	1.4
18	Benson and Hedges Special Filter KS	19	1.5
18	Capstan Medium (P)	11	1.3
18	Embassy Virginia (P)	11	1.2
18	Gallaher's De Luxe Green (P)	11	1.5
18	Gold Flake (P)	11	1.3
18	Kensitas Club Filter Virginia	16	1.4
18	Kensitas Fine Virginia (P)	11	1.5
18	Lambert and Butler International Size	18	1.5
18	Park Drive Special Virginia (P)	12	1.5
18	Player's Medium Navy Cut (P)	12	1.3
18	Royal Standard KS	16	1.5
18	Senior Service Fine Virginia (P)	11	1.5
18	Woodbine Virginia (P)	11	1.4
19	London KS	16	1.6
21	Sweet Afton Virginia (P)	12	1.8
22	Gitanes Caporal (P)	17	1.4
Middle to High Tar			
23	Gallaher's De Luxe Blue (P)	15	1.9
23	Gauloises Caporal (P)	19	1.3
25	Capstan Full Strength (P)	14	2.6

New brands recently introduced but not yet analysed by the Government Chemist for a period of six months. Estimates by the manufacturers of the tar and nicotine yields for these brands are as follows:

Tar yield mg/cig	Brand	Carbon monoxide yield mg/cig	Nicotine yield mg/cig
13	Dunhill Luxury Length	16	1.3
13	Kim	17	1.1
15	Berkeley Luxury Length	14	1.4
16	Ardath KS	17	1.3

LGC Survey 18
Sampling period October 1982-March 1983

Tar yield mg/cig	Brand	Carbon monoxide yield mg/cig	Nicotine yield mg/cig
Low Tar			
under 4	Embassy Ultra Mild KS	under 3	under 0.3
under 4	John Player KS Ultra Mild	under 3	under 0.3
under 4	Silk Cut Ultra Low KS	under 3	under 0.3
4	Silk Cut Extra Mild KS	4	0.5
7	Barclay KS	7	0.7
7	Peer Special KS Extra Mild (with Cytrel)	7	0.8
8	Cartier Intern Luxury Mild	9	0.8
8	Kent KS	8	0.7
8	Peter Stuyvesant Extra Mild KS	6	0.8
9	Berkeley KS Extra Mild	9	0.9
9	Consulate Menthol	8	0.8
9	Consulate No. 2	8	0.8
9	Du Maurier KS	10	0.9
9	Dunhill Intern Superior Mild	9	0.8
9	Dunhill KS Superior Mild	8	0.8
9	Embassy Extra Mild	10	0.8
9	Embassy No. 1 Extra Mild	10	0.8
9	John Player Vanguard KS	13	0.9
9	Merit Extra Mild	9	0.8
9	Peter Stuyvesant Luxury Length Extra Mild	9	0.8
9	Player's No. 6 Extra mild	9	0.7
9	Silk Cut	10	0.8

Tar yield mg/cig	Brand	Carbon monoxide yield mg/cig	Nicotine yield mg/cig

Low Tar

Tar yield mg/cig	Brand	Carbon monoxide yield mg/cig	Nicotine yield mg/cig
9	Silk Cut International	9	0.9
9	Silk Cut KS	10	0.9
9	Target KS Filter	8	0.8
10	Belair Menthol Kings	13	0.6
10	Craven 'A' Luxury Length Special Mild	10	0.9
10	Embassy No. 5 Extra Mild	9	0.8
10	Gauloises Filter Mild	14	0.6
10	Gauloises Longues Caporal F	17	0.5
10	John Player KS Extra Mild	10	1.0
10	Lambert and Butler Special Mild KS	11	0.9
10	Silk Cut No. 3	9	0.8
10	Silk Cut No. 5	10	0.8
10	State Express 555 Special Mild KS	10	0.9

Low to Middle Tar

Tar yield mg/cig	Brand	Carbon monoxide yield mg/cig	Nicotine yield mg/cig
11	St Moritz Lux Length Menthol	14	1.0
12	Dunhill Intern Menthol	15	1.1
12	Gauloises Caporal Filter	18	0.6
12	Gitanes International	17	1.0
13	Gauloises Disque Bleu Caporal Filter	20	0.7
13	Gitanes Caporal Filter	18	0.7
13	John Player Carlton Long Size	10	1.2
13	John Player Carlton Premium	11	1.1
13	Jubilee KS	11	1.2
13	Kensitas Club Mild KS	12	1.2
13	Kensitas Mild KS	11	1.2
13	Peer Special Mild KS (with Cytrel)	12	1.1
13	Peter Stuyvesant KS	13	1.2
13	Peter Stuyvesant Lux Length	15	1.2
13	Player's No. 10 Extra Mild Filter Virginia	13	0.9
14	Benson and Hedges Sovereign Mild	10	1.2
14	Carroll's No. 1 KS	16	1.2
14	Craven 'A' Luxury Length	16	1.3
14	Dunhill KS	14	1.2
14	Dunhill Luxury Length	16	1.3
14	Kensitas Club Mild	13	1.2
14	Kim	13	1.2
14	Marlboro 100s	13	1.3
14	More Filter 120s	15	1.3
14	More Menthol Filter 120s	15	1.3
14	State Express 555 Medium Mild KS	14	1.1
15	Benson and Hedges Sovereign KS	16	1.3
15	Benson and Hedges Sterling KS	16	1.3
15	Camel Filter Tip	15	1.2
15	Dunhill International	15	1.4
15	Fine 120 Super Length	15	1.4
15	Guards	15	1.1
15	Lambert and Butler KS	15	1.3
15	Pall Mall Filter Tipped	13	1.3

Tar yield mg/cig	Brand	Carbon monoxide yield mg/cig	Nicotine yield mg/cig
15	Piccadilly Filter De Luxe	14	1.3
15	Rothmans International	15	1.3
15	Senior Service Cadets KS	16	1.3
15	Sobranie Virginia Blend	13	1.4
15	United Filter Virginia	17	1.1
15	Winston KS	15	1.2
16	Benson and Hedges Gold Bond KS	17	1.4
16	Benson and Hedges Longer Length	14	1.5
16	Benson and Hedges Sovereign Filter	14	1.1
16	Benson and Hedges Supreme International	13	1.5
16	Berkeley Luxury Length	15	1.4
16	Carrolls No. 1 Virginia	17	1.2
16	Du Maurier	16	1.2
16	Embassy Filter	15	1.3
16	Embassy No. 1 KS	15	1.3
16	Embassy No. 3 Standard Size	15	1.3
16	Embassy Regal	14	1.3
16	Fribourg and Treyer No. 1 Filter De Luxe	17	1.4
16	John Player KS	15	1.3
16	Kent De Luxe Length	14	1.2
16	L and M Filter Box	14	1.3
16	Marlboro	16	1.3
16	Park Drive Tipped KS	18	1.4
16	Piccadilly KS	15	1.2
16	Piccadilly No. 1 (P)	10	1.4
16	Player's Medium Navy Cut F	15	1.3
16	Player's No. 6 Filter Virginia	15	1.4
16	Player's No. 6 KS	16	1.4
16	Regal KS	16	1.4
16	Rothmans Royals 120s	14	1.5
16	Silva Thins Filter 100s	17	1.4
16	Slim Kings Special Virginia F	17	1.2

Middle Tar

Tar yield mg/cig	Brand	Carbon monoxide yield mg/cig	Nicotine yield mg/cig
17	Ardath KS	17	1.3
17	Benson and Hedges Academy International	14	1.6
17	Capstan Medium (P)	11	1.3
17	Embassy Gold	14	1.4
17	Gold Leaf Filter Virginia	16	1.3
17	John Player Special Intern	14	1.4
17	John Player Special KS	16	1.5
17	Kensitas Club F Virginia	15	1.4
17	Kensitas Corsair F Virginia	15	1.3
17	Kensitas Filter Virginia KS	18	1.4
17	Lambert and Butler International Size	18	1.5
17	Lark Filter Tip	14	1.5
17	MS Filter KS	15	1.3
17	Major Virginia Filter Extra Size	17	1.3
17	Player's Medium Navy Cut (P)	11	1.3
17	Player's No. 6 Finest Virginia (P)	11	1.1
17	Player's No. 10 Filter Virginia	15	1.2
17	Player's Weights Finest Virginia (P)	11	1.1

LGC Survey 18
(*continued*)

Middle Tar

Tar yield mg/cig	Brand	Carbon monoxide yield mg/cig	Nicotine yield mg/cig
17	Rothmans KS Filter	16	1.4
17	State Express 555 Filter Kings	17	1.2
17	Woodbine Filter Virginia	13	1.4
18	Benson and Hedges Gold Bond Filter	16	1.4
18	Benson and Hedges Special Filter KS	19	1.5
18	Camel Plain (P)	11	1.2
18	Embassy Virginia (P)	11	1.3
18	Gallaher's De Luxe Green (P)	11	1.4
18	Gold Flake (P)	11	1.3
18	Kensitas Club KS	18	1.4
18	Kensitas Fine Virginia (P)	11	1.5
18	London KS	16	1.2
18	Park Drive Special Virginia (P)	12	1.5
18	Royal Standard KS	16	1.3
18	Senior Service Fine Virginia (P)	11	1.4
18	State Express 555 Selected Virginia (P)	11	1.4
18	Woodbine Virginia (P)	11	1.5
22	Gallaher's De Luxe Blue (P)	14	1.8
22	Sweet Afton Virginia (P)	11	1.9

Middle to High Tar

Tar yield mg/cig	Brand	Carbon monoxide yield mg/cig	Nicotine yield mg/cig
23	Gitanes Caporal (P)	18	1.3
24	Gauloises Caporal (P)	20	1.3
25	Capstan Full Strength (P)	14	2.4

New brands recently introduced but not yet analysed by the Government Chemist for a period of six months. Estimates by the manufacturers of the tar and nicotine yields for these brands are as follows:

9	More Special Mild 120s	8	1.0
9	More Special Mild Menthol 120s	8	0.9
16	Chesterfield KS	16	1.4
16	Fribourg and Treyer Superkings	15	1.6
16	John Player Superkings	15	1.6
16	Kings Filter Virginia	18	1.2

(P) indicates plain cigarettes; all other brands have filters

LGC Survey 19
Sampling period May 1983-October 1983

Low Tar

Tar yield mg/cig	Brand	Carbon monoxide yield mg/cig	Nicotine yield mg/cig
under 4	Embassy Ultra Mild KS	under 3	under 0.3
under 4	John Player KS Ultra Mild	under 3	under 0.3
under 4	Silk Cut Ultra Low KS	under 3	under 0.3
4	Silk Cut Extra Mild KS	4	0.5
6	Lambert and Butler Special Mild KS	7	0.6
7	Peer Special KS Extra Mild (with Cytrel)	7	0.7
7	Peter Stuyvesant Extra Mild KS	6	0.8
8	Cartier Intern Luxury Mild	8	0.7
8	Consulate Menthol	8	0.8
8	Consulate No. 2	7	0.8
8	Dunhill Intern Superior Mild	9	0.8
8	Kent KS	9	0.7
8	Merit Extra Mild	9	0.8
8	Silk Cut KS	9	0.9
9	Berkeley KS Extra Mild	9	0.9
9	Craven 'A' Luxury Length Special Mild	9	0.8
9	Du Maurier KS	9	0.9
9	Dunhill KS Superior Mild	9	0.9
9	Embassy Extra Mild	10	0.8
9	Embassy No. 1 Extra Mild	11	0.9
9	Embassy No. 5 Extra Mild	9	0.7
9	John Player KS Extra Mild	8	1.0
9	John Player Vanguard KS	13	0.9
9	Peter Stuyvesant Luxury Length Extra Mild	10	0.8
9	Silk Cut	9	0.8
9	Silk Cut No. 3	9	0.8
9	State Express 555 Special Mild KS	9	0.9
10	Belair Menthol Kings	13	0.6
10	Gauloises Longues Caporal F	18	0.5
10	Player's No. 6 Extra mild	10	0.8
10	Silk Cut No. 5	10	0.8

Low to Middle Tar

Tar yield mg/cig	Brand	Carbon monoxide yield mg/cig	Nicotine yield mg/cig
11	St Moritz Lux Length Menthol	14	0.9
12	Gauloises Caporal Filter	18	0.6
12	Gauloises Disque Bleu Caporal Filter	18	0.6
12	Gitanes Caporal Filter	17	0.7
12	Gitanes International	16	1.0
12	John Player Carlton Long Size	11	1.2
12	Peer Special Mild KS (with Cytrel)	12	1.1
12	Player's No. 10 Extra Mild Special Filter Virginia	12	0.8

Low to Middle Tar

Tar yield mg/cig	Brand	Carbon monoxide yield mg/cig	Nicotine yield mg/cig
13	Craven 'A' Lux Length	15	1.3
13	Dunhill Intern Menthol	15	1.1
13	John Player Carlton Premium	11	1.1
13	More Filter 120s	15	1.2
13	Peter Stuyvesant KS	14	1.1
13	Peter Stuyvesant Lux Length	15	1.3
13	State Express 555 Medium Mild KS	14	1.2
14	Acclaim KS	17	1.0
14	Benson and Hedges Sovereign Mild	10	1.2
14	Dunhill KS	14	1.2
14	Embassy No. 3 Standard Size	13	1.3
14	Embassy Regal	13	1.3
14	John Player KS	15	1.3
14	Kensitas Club Mild KS	12	1.3
14	Kensitas Mild KS	12	1.3
14	Kim	12	1.2
14	Marlboro 100s	12	1.2
14	More Menthol Filter 120s	16	1.2
14	Pall Mall Filter Tipped	12	1.2
14	Piccadilly Filter De Luxe	14	1.3
14	Sobranie Virginia Blend	13	1.4
15	Berkeley Luxury Length	13	1.3
15	Carrolls No. 1 Virginia	16	1.2
15	Chesterfield KS	14	1.2
15	Du Maurier	15	1.2
15	Dunhill Luxury Length	16	1.3
15	Embassy Filter	14	1.3
15	Embassy No. 1 KS	15	1.3
15	Fribourg and Treyer No. 1 Filter De Luxe	17	1.3
15	Fribourg and Treyer Superkings	15	1.6
15	Guards	15	1.2
15	John Player Superkings	15	1.5
15	Kensitas Club Mild	14	1.3
15	Lambert and Butler KS	15	1.3
15	London KS	17	0.9
15	Park Drive Tipped KS	15	1.4
15	Piccadilly KS	15	1.3
15	Player's No. 6 KS	14	1.3
15	Regal King Size	15	1.3
15	Rothmans International	16	1.4
15	Rothmans Royals 120s	14	1.4
15	Senior Service Cadets KS	16	1.3
15	Winston KS	14	1.3
16	Ardath KS	16	1.3
16	Benson and Hedges Longer Length	14	1.5
16	Benson and Hedges Sovereign Filter	14	1.1
16	Benson and Hedges Sovereign KS	16	1.4
16	Benson and Hedges Sterling KS	17	1.4
16	Camel Filter Tip	15	1.3
16	Dunhill International	16	1.4
16	Embassy Gold	13	1.3
16	Fine 120 Super Length	16	1.4
16	John Player Special Intern	13	1.4
16	Kent De Luxe Length	14	1.4
16	Kings Filter Virginia	17	1.1
16	L and M Filter Box	16	1.3
16	Lark Filter Tip	16	1.4
16	Marlboro	15	1.3
16	Piccadilly No. 1 (P)	10	1.4
16	Player's Medium Navy Cut F	16	1.3
16	Player's No. 6 F Virginia	14	1.3
16	Senior Service Superkings	14	1.5
16	Slim Kings Special Virginia F	17	1.3
16	State Express 555 Filter Kings	15	1.2
16	Woodbine Filter Virginia	13	1.4

Middle Tar

Tar yield mg/cig	Brand	Carbon monoxide yield mg/cig	Nicotine yield mg/cig
17	Benson and Hedges Supreme International	13	1.6
17	Capstan Medium (P)	11	1.3
17	Gold Flake (P)	11	1.3
17	Gold Leaf F Virginia	15	1.4
17	John Player Special KS	15	1.4
17	Kensitas Corsair F Virginia	13	1.3
17	Kensitas F Virginia KS	18	1.4
17	Kensitas Fine Virginia (P)	10	1.4
17	Lambert and Butler International Size	18	1.5
17	MS Filter KS	16	1.3
17	Player's Medium Navy Cut (P)	11	1.2
17	Player's No. 6 Finest Virginia (P)	11	1.1
17	Player's No. 10 F Virginia	15	1.2
17	Player's Weights Finest Virginia (P)	11	1.1
17	Rothmans KS Filter	17	1.4
17	United Filter Virginia	19	1.2
17	Woodbine Virginia (P)	11	1.3
18	Benson and Hedges Gold Bond Filter	17	1.5
18	Benson and Hedges Special Filter KS	19	1.5
18	Camel Plain (P)	11	1.3
18	Embassy Virginia (P)	12	1.3
18	Gallaher's De Luxe Green (P)	11	1.4
18	Kensitas Club F Virginia	16	1.5
18	Kensitas Club KS	18	1.5
18	Major Virginia F Extra Size	17	1.3
18	Park Drive Special Virginia (P)	12	1.5
18	Royal Standard KS	16	1.2
18	Senior Service Fine Virginia (P)	11	1.4
19	Benson and Hedges Gold Bond Filter	17	1.5
19	State Express 555 Selected Virginia (P)	11	1.5
21	Sweet Afton Virginia (P)	11	1.9

Middle to High Tar

Tar yield mg/cig	Brand	Carbon monoxide yield mg/cig	Nicotine yield mg/cig
23	Gallaher's De Luxe Blue (P)	14	2.0
23	Gauloises Caporal (P)	19	1.2
23	Gitanes Caporal (P)	18	1.4
25	Capstan Full Strength (P)	14	2.5

New brands recently introduced but not yet analysed by the Government Chemist for a period of six months. Estimates by the manufacturers of the tar and nicotine yields for these brands are as follows:

14	Victoria Wine KS	19	0.9
16	National Luxury Length	16	1.2
16	Hyde Park KS	17	1.2

(P) indicates plain cigarettes; all other brands have filters

LGC Survey 20
Sampling period December 1983-May 1984

Low Tar

Tar yield mg/cig	Brand	Carbon monoxide yield mg/cig	Nicotine yield mg/cig
under 4	Embassy Ultra Mild KS	under 3	under 0.3
under 4	John Player KS Ultra Mild	under 3	0.3
under 4	Silk Cut Ultra Low KS	under 3	under 0.3
4	Lambert and Butler Special Mild KS	6	0.6
4	Silk Cut Extra Mild KS	4	0.5
6	Peer Special KS Extra Mild (with Cytrel)	6	0.7
7	Cartier Intern Luxury Mild	8	0.7
7	Kent KS	8	0.7
7	Merit Extra Mild	9	0.6
7	Peter Stuyvesant Extra Mild KS	6	0.8
8	Consulate KS Menthol	8	0.8
8	Craven 'A' Luxury Length Special Mild	9	0.8
8	Dunhill Intern Superior Mild	9	0.8
8	Dunhill KS Superior Mild	8	0.8
8	Silk Cut	9	0.8
9	Belair Menthol Kings	13	0.6
9	Berkeley KS Extra Mild	9	0.9
9	Consulate No. 2 Menthol	8	0.8
9	Craven 'A' KS Special Mild	8	0.7
9	Du Maurier KS	10	1.0
9	Embassy Extra Mild	9	0.9
9	Embassy No. 5 Extra Mild	8	0.7
9	John Player KS Extra Mild	9	0.9
9	John Player Vanguard KS	12	0.9
9	Peter Stuyvesant Luxury Length Extra Mild	10	0.8
10	Embassy No. 1 Extra Mild	11	0.9
10	Player's No. 6 Extra mild	9	0.8
10	Player's No. 10 Extra Mild Filter Virginia	9	0.7
10	Silk Cut KS	10	1.0
10	Silk Cut No. 3	10	0.8
10	Silk Cut No. 5	10	0.8

Low to Middle Tar

Tar yield mg/cig	Brand	Carbon monoxide yield mg/cig	Nicotine yield mg/cig
11	Gauloises Disque Bleu Caporal Filter	17	0.6
11	Gauloises Longues Caporal F	18	0.6
11	Gitanes International	15	1.0
11	Peer Special Mild KS (with Cytrel)	12	1.0
11	St Moritz Lux Length Menthol	14	0.9
12	Gauloises Caporal Filter	17	0.6
12	Gitanes Caporal Filter	17	0.8
12	John Player Carlton Long Size	10	1.2
12	Peter Stuyvesant KS	13	1.0
13	Craven 'A' Luxury Length	14	1.2
13	Dunhill Intern Menthol	14	1.0
13	John Player Carlton Premium	11	1.1
13	Victoria Wine KS	17	0.9
14	Acclaim KS	17	1.0
14	Embassy Regal	13	1.3
14	Guards	15	1.1
14	John Player KS	13	1.3
14	Kensitas Club Mild KS	12	1.3
14	Kensitas Mild KS	13	1.3
14	Kim	11	1.2
14	London KS	16	0.9
14	Pall Mall Filter Tipped	12	1.2
14	Player's No. 6 KS	14	1.3
15	Benson and Hedges Sovereign KS	15	1.3
15	Benson and Hedges Sterling KS	16	1.3
15	Berkeley Luxury Length	13	1.4
15	Carrolls No. 1 Virginia	16	1.2
15	Dunhill Luxury Length	17	1.3
15	Embassy Filter	13	1.3
15	Embassy No. 1 KS	14	1.3
15	Embassy No. 3 Standard Size	13	1.3
15	Fribourg and Treyer Superkings	15	1.5
15	John Player Special Intern	12	1.3
15	John Player Superkings	15	1.6
15	Kensitas Club Mild	13	1.3
15	Kent De Luxe Length	14	1.3
15	Kings Filter Virginia	17	1.0
15	Lambert and Butler KS	14	1.3
15	Marlboro	14	1.1
15	More Filter 120s	16	1.3
15	More Menthol Filter 120s	17	1.3
15	Peter Stuyvesant Lux Length	16	1.3
15	Piccadilly Filter De Luxe	13	1.3
15	Raffles 100s	16	1.4
15	Regal KS	14	1.3
15	Rothmans International	16	1.4
15	Rothmans Royals 120s	14	1.4
15	Royal Standard KS	16	1.0
15	Senior Service Cadets KS	15	1.3
15	Sobranie Virginia Blend	14	1.4
15	United Filter Virginia	17	1.0
16	Benson and Hedges Longer Length	14	1.5
16	Benson and Hedges Sovereign Mild	11	1.2
16	Camel Filter Tip	15	1.3
16	Chesterfield KS	14	1.2
16	Dunhill International	16	1.4
16	Dunhill KS	15	1.3
16	Fine 120 Super Length	16	1.4
16	John Player Special KS	15	1.4
16	L and M Filter Box	14	1.2
16	Lark Filter Tip	14	1.4
16	Park Drive Tipped KS	16	1.4
16	Piccadilly KS	15	1.3
16	Player's Medium Navy Cut F	15	1.3
16	Player's No. 6 F Virginia	14	1.4
16	Player's No. 10 F Virginia	15	1.2
16	Senior Service Superkings	14	1.6
16	Slim Kings Special Virginia F	15	1.2
16	State Express 555 Filter Kings	16	1.3
16	Winston KS	15	1.3

Middle Tar

Tar yield mg/cig	Brand	Carbon monoxide yield mg/cig	Nicotine yield mg/cig
17	Ardath KS	17	1.3
17	Benson and Hedges Sovereign Filter	14	1.3

LGC Survey 20
(*continued*)

Tar yield mg/cig	Brand	Carbon monoxide yield mg/cig	Nicotine yield mg/cig
Middle Tar			
17	Benson and Hedges Special Filter KS	18	1.5
17	Benson and Hedges Supreme International	13	1.7
17	Dorchester Filter	19	1.2
17	Embassy Gold	14	1.4
17	Fribourg and Treyer No. 1 Filter De Luxe	17	1.4
17	Gold Leaf Filter Virginia	16	1.3
17	Kensitas Corsair F Virginia	14	1.3
17	Lambert and Butler International Size	17	1.5
17	MS Filter KS	15	1.3
17	Piccadilly No. 1 (P)	11	1.4
17	Player's Medium Navy Cut (P)	11	1.3
17	Rothmans KS Filter	15	1.4
17	Woodbine Filter Virginia	14	1.4
17	Woodbine Virginia (P)	11	1.3
18	Benson and Hedges Gold Bond Filter	16	1.5
18	Benson and Hedges Gold Bond KS	17	1.5
18	Camel Plain (P)	11	1.3
18	Capstan Medium (P)	12	1.3
18	Craven 'A' KS	17	1.4
18	Embassy Virginia (P)	11	1.3
18	Gallaher's De Luxe Green (P)	11	1.5

Tar yield mg/cig	Brand	Carbon monoxide yield mg/cig	Nicotine yield mg/cig
18	Gold Flake (P)	11	1.3
18	Kensitas Club F Virginia	16	1.5
18	Kensitas Club KS	18	1.4
18	Kensitas Filter Virginia KS	19	1.5
18	Major Virginia Filter Extra Size	17	1.3
18	Park Drive Special Virginia (P)	12	1.4
19	Kensitas Fine Virginia (P)	11	1.4
19	Player's No. 6 Finest Virginia (P)	11	1.2
19	Player's Weights Finest Virginia (P)	12	1.2
19	Senior Service Fine Virginia (P)	11	1.4
22	Gauloises Caporal (P)	19	1.1
Middle to High Tar			
23	Gitanes Caporal (P)	17	1.4
23	Sweet Afton Virginia (P)	12	2.1
24	Gallaher's De Luxe Blue (P)	14	1.9
25	Capstan Full Strength (P)	14	2.5

New brands recently introduced but not yet analysed by the Government Chemist for a period of six months. Estimates by the manufacturers of the tar and nicotine yields for these brands are as follows:

13	Marlboro 100s	15	1.0

(P) indicates plain cigarettes; all other brands have filters

LGC Survey 21
Sampling period July 1984-December 1984

Tar yield mg/cig	Brand	Carbon monoxide yield mg/cig	Nicotine yield mg/cig
Low Tar			
under 4	Embassy Ultra Mild KS	under 3	under 0.3
under 4	John Player KS Ultra Mild	under 3	under 0.3
under 4	Silk Cut Ultra Low KS	under 3	under 0.3
4	Lambert and Butler Special Mild KS	5	0.5
4	Silk Cut Extra Mild KS	4	0.5
7	Consulate No. 2	6	0.7
7	Merit Extra Mild	9	0.6
8	Cartier Intern Luxury Mild	8	0.8
8	Consulate Menthol	7	0.8
8	Craven 'A' KS Special Mild	8	0.7
8	Dunhill Intern Superior Mild	9	0.8
8	Dunhill KS Superior Mild	8	0.7
8	John Player Superkings Low Tar	8	0.9
8	Kent KS	8	0.7
8	Peter Stuyvesant Extra Mild KS	7	0.7
8	Silk Cut	9	0.8
9	Belair Menthol Kings	13	0.6

Tar yield mg/cig	Brand	Carbon monoxide yield mg/cig	Nicotine yield mg/cig
9	Berkeley KS Extra Mild	9	0.9
9	Craven 'A' Luxury Length Special Mild	10	0.8
9	Du Maurier KS	9	0.8
9	Embassy Extra Mild	9	0.8
9	Embassy No. 1 Extra Mild KS	9	0.9
9	Embassy No. 5 Extra Mild	8	0.8
9	John Player KS Extra Mild	9	0.9
9	Peter Stuyvesant Luxury Length Extra Mild	10	0.8
9	Player's No. 6 Extra mild	9	0.8
9	Player's No. 10 Extra Mild Filter Virginia	9	0.7
9	Silk Cut KS	9	0.9
9	Silk Cut No. 3	9	0.7
9	Vanguard KS	13	0.9
10	Gauloises Longues Caporal F	16	0.5
10	Silk Cut No. 5	9	0.7
10	St Moritz Lux Length Menthol	13	0.9

Low to Middle Tar

Tar yield mg/cig	Brand	Carbon monoxide yield mg/cig	Nicotine yield mg/cig
11	Gauloises Disque Bleu Caporal Filter	17	0.6
12	Carlton Long Size	10	1.2
12	Carlton Premium	10	1.1
12	Craven 'A' Luxury Length	13	1.1
12	Dunhill Intern Menthol	14	1.0
12	Gauloises Caporal Filter	17	0.6
12	Gitanes Caporal Filter	16	0.7
12	Peter Stuyvesant KS	13	1.1
13	Gitanes International	16	1.1
13	John Player KS	13	1.3
13	London KS	16	0.8
13	Marlboro 100s	13	1.0
14	Acclaim KS	16	1.0
14	Cartier KS	13	1.2
14	Dunhill Lux Length	16	1.2
14	Embassy No. 1 KS	14	1.3
14	Embassy No. 3 Standard Size	13	1.3
14	Guards	14	1.1
14	Hyde Park KS	16	0.9
14	Kensitas Club Mild KS	12	1.3
14	Kensitas Mild KS	12	1.3
14	Kim	11	1.2
14	Lambert and Butler KS	15	1.3
14	Lark Filter Tip	14	1.2
14	Marlboro KS	13	0.9
14	More Filter 120s	15	1.2
14	Piccadilly Filter De Luxe	13	1.2
14	Player's No. 6 KS	14	1.3
14	Raffles 100s	15	1.3
14	Regal KS	14	1.3
15	Ardath KS	15	1.2
15	Benson and Hedges Sovereign KS	16	1.3
15	Benson and Hedges Sovereign Mild	10	1.2
15	Benson and Hedges Sterling KS	16	1.3
15	Camel Filter Tip	14	1.3
15	Carrolls No. 1 Virginia	15	1.2
15	Dunhill KS	15	1.3
15	Embassy Filter	14	1.3
15	Embassy Regal	13	1.3
15	Fine 120 Super Length	14	1.3
15	Fribourg and Treyer Superkings	14	1.5
15	John Player Special Filter	12	1.3
15	John Player Superkings	14	1.5
15	Kensitas Club Mild	13	1.3
15	Kent De Luxe Length	14	1.4
15	L and M Filter Box	14	1.2
15	More Menthol Filter 120s	16	1.2
15	Pall Mall Filter Tipped	12	1.4
15	Park Drive Tipped KS	16	1.3
15	Peter Stuyvesant Lux Length	17	1.4
15	Piccadilly KS	15	1.2
15	Player's No. 6 Filter	13	1.3
15	Senior Service Cadets KS	15	1.3
15	Sobranie Virginia Blend	14	1.4
15	State Express 555 Filter Kings	14	1.2
15	Victoria Wine KS	16	1.0
15	Winston KS	15	1.3
16	Benson and Hedges Longer Length	14	1.5
16	Dorchester Filter	17	1.1
16	Dunhill International	16	1.4
16	Embassy Gold	13	1.3
16	Gold Leaf F Virginia	15	1.3
16	John Player Special KS	15	1.4
16	Kings Filter Virginia	16	1.0
16	Piccadilly No. 1 (P)	11	1.4
16	Player's Medium Navy Cut F	15	1.3
16	Player's No. 10 Filter	15	1.2
16	Rothmans International	16	1.5
16	Rothmans Royals 120s	15	1.5
16	Senior Service Superkings	15	1.5
16	Woodbine Filter Virginia	13	1.4

Middle Tar

Tar yield mg/cig	Brand	Carbon monoxide yield mg/cig	Nicotine yield mg/cig
17	Benson and Hedges Gold Bond KS	17	1.4
17	Benson and Hedges Special Filter KS	16	1.5
17	Benson and Hedges Supreme International	13	1.6
17	Capstan Medium (P)	10	1.3
17	Craven 'A' KS	15	1.3
17	Fribourg and Treyer No. 1 Filter De Luxe	17	1.5
17	Gold Flake (P)	11	1.3
17	Kensitas Club F Virginia	15	1.4
17	Kensitas Club KS	17	1.4
17	Kensitas Corsair F Virginia	14	1.3
17	Kensitas F Virginia KS	18	1.5
17	Lambert and Butler International Size	17	1.5
17	Player's Medium Navy Cut (P)	11	1.3
17	Player's No. 6 Plain (P)	10	1.3
17	Rothmans KS Filter	15	1.5
17	United Filter Virginia	17	1.1
17	Weights Plain (P)	10	1.3
17	Woodbine Plain (P)	10	1.3
18	Benson and Hedges Gold Bond Filter	16	1.5
18	Benson and Hedges Sovereign Filter	14	1.4
18	Camel Plain (P)	11	1.3
18	Embassy Plain (P)	11	1.3
18	Gallaher's De Luxe Green (P)	11	1.5
18	Kensitas Fine Virginia (P)	11	1.5
18	Park Drive Special Virginia (P)	11	1.4
18	Senior Service Fine Virginia (P)	11	1.5
19	Major Virginia F Extra Size	17	1.5
22	Gauloises Caporal (P)	18	1.1
22	Gitanes Caporal (P)	17	1.3
22	Sweet Afton Virginia (P)	12	2.0

Middle to High Tar

Tar yield mg/cig	Brand	Carbon monoxide yield mg/cig	Nicotine yield mg/cig
24	Gallaher's De Luxe Blue (P)	14	1.9
25	Capstan Full Strength (P)	14	2.6

New brands recently introduced but not yet analysed by the Government Chemist for a period of six months. Estimates by the manufacturers of the tar and nicotine yields for these brands are as follows:

15	Ronson KS	18	1.3

(P) indicates plain cigarettes; all other brands have filters

LGC Survey 22
Sampling period February 1985-July 1985

Tar yield mg/cig	Brand	Carbon monoxide yield mg/cig	Nicotine yield mg/cig	Tar yield mg/cig	Brand	Carbon monoxide yield mg/cig	Nicotine yield mg/cig
Low Tar				13	Kensitas Mild KS	12	1.2
under 4	Embassy Ultra Mild KS	under 3	under 0.3	13	Kings Filter Virginia	13	0.9
under 4	John Player KS Ultra Mild	under 3	under 0.3	13	Lambert and Butler KS	15	1.2
under 4	Silk Cut Ultra Low KS	under 3	under 0.3	13	Marlboro 100s	14	0.9
4	Lambert and Butler Special Mild KS	6	0.5	13	Marlboro KS	13	0.8
4	Silk Cut Extra Mild KS	5	0.5	13	More Filter 120s	16	1.2
7	Cartier Intern Luxury Mild	9	0.7	13	More Menthol Filter 120s	15	1.2
7	Consulate Menthol	8	0.7	13	Piccadilly Filter De Luxe	13	1.3
7	Consulate No. 2	7	0.6	13	Player's No. 6 KS	14	1.3
7	Du Maurier KS	8	0.7	13	Regal KS	15	1.2
7	Dunhill KS Superior Mild	7	0.7	13	United Filter Virginia	13	1.0
7	Merit Extra Mild	9	0.5	13	Victoria Wine KS	12	0.9
7	Peter Stuyvesant Extra Mild KS	7	0.7	13	Winston KS	15	1.2
8	Belair Menthol Kings	14	0.6	14	Ardath KS	15	1.2
8	Berkeley KS Extra Mild	9	0.8	14	Benson and Hedges Longer Length	14	1.3
8	Craven 'A' KS Special Mild	8	0.7	14	Benson and Hedges Sovereign KS	15	1.2
8	Craven 'A' Luxury Length Special Mild	10	0.7	14	Benson and Hedges Sterling KS	15	1.2
8	Dunhill Intern Superior Mild	9	0.7	14	Berkeley Superkings	13	1.3
8	Embassy Extra Mild	9	0.8	14	Carrolls No. 1 Virginia	14	1.2
8	Embassy No. 1 Extra Mild	9	0.9	14	Chesterfield KS	14	1.2
8	Embassy No. 5 Extra Mild	8	0.7	14	Dunhill Luxury Length	16	1.2
8	John Player Superkings (Low Tar)	8	0.9	14	Embassy Filter	13	1.3
8	John Player KS Extra Mild	9	0.8	14	Embassy No. 3 Standard Size	13	1.3
8	Peter Stuyvesant Luxury Length Extra Mild	9	0.7	14	Embassy Regal	13	1.2
8	Player's No. 10 Extra Mild	9	0.6	14	Fribourg and Treyer Superkings	14	1.4
8	Silk Cut	9	0.7	14	Kim	11	1.1
8	Silk Cut No. 3	9	0.7	14	Lark Filter Tip	14	1.1
8	Silk Cut No. 5	9	0.7	14	London KS	16	0.9
8	Vanguard KS	11	0.8	14	Park Drive Tipped KS	15	1.2
9	Gauloises Longues Caporal F	16	0.5	14	Piccadilly KS	15	1.1
9	Kent KS	7	0.8	14	Raffles 100s	15	1.3
9	Player's No. 6 Extra mild	9	0.8	14	Senior Service Cadets KS	15	1.2
9	Silk Cut KS	10	0.9	14	Senior Service Superkings	13	1.4
Low to Middle Tar				**Middle Tar**			
10	Gauloises Disque Bleu Caporal Filter	17	0.6	15	Camel Filter Tip	14	1.2
10	St Moritz Lux Length Menthol	13	0.9	15	Dorchester Filter	17	1.0
11	Dunhill Intern Menthol	14	1.0	15	Dunhill KS	14	1.3
11	Gauloises Caporal Filter	18	0.6	15	Embassy Gold	13	1.3
11	Peter Stuyvesant KS	13	1.0	15	Fine 120 Super Length	14	1.3
12	Acclaim KS	15	1.0	15	Hyde Park KS	17	1.1
12	Benson and Hedges Sovereign Mild	9	1.0	15	John Player Superkings	15	1.5
12	Carlton Long Size	11	1.1	15	John Player Special F	13	1.4
12	Carlton Premium	11	1.1	15	Kensitas Club F Virginia	15	1.3
12	Gitanes Caporal Filter	16	0.7	15	Kent De Luxe Length	15	1.2
12	John Player KS	13	1.2	15	L and M Filter Box	14	1.3
12	Kensitas Club Mild	11	1.1	15	Pall Mall Filter Tipped	12	1.3
13	Craven 'A' Luxury Length	14	1.2	15	Peter Stuyvesant Lux Length	16	1.4
13	Crown Crest KS	12	0.9	15	Player's Medium Navy Cut F	15	1.3
13	Embassy No. 1 KS	14	1.2	15	Player's No. 6 Filter	14	1.3
13	Gitanes International	17	1.1	15	Rothmans KS	17	1.2
13	Guards	15	1.1	15	Rothmans Royals 120s	15	1.5
13	Kensitas Club Mild KS	13	1.2	15	State Express 555 F Kings	15	1.3
				15	Woodbine Filter	13	1.3
				16	Benson and Hedges Gold Bond Filter	15	1.3
				16	Benson and Hedges Sovereign Filter	13	1.3

LGC Survey 22
(*continued*)

Middle Tar

Tar yield mg/cig	Brand	Carbon monoxide yield mg/cig	Nicotine yield mg/cig
16	Benson and Hedges Special Filter KS	17	1.4
16	Craven 'A' KS	15	1.3
16	Dunhill International	16	1.5
16	Fribourg and Treyer No. 1 Filter De Luxe	18	1.4
16	Gold Flake (P)	11	1.2
16	Gold Leaf Filter Virginia	15	1.3
16	John Player Special KS	15	1.4
16	Kensitas Club KS	17	1.4
16	Kensitas Corsair F Virginia	14	1.2
16	Kensitas F Virginia KS	17	1.4
16	Kingsmen F Virginia	16	1.2
16	Lambert and Butler International Size	16	1.4
16	Major Virginia F Extra Size	17	1.4
16	Park Drive Special Virginia (P)	11	1.4
16	Piccadilly No. 1 (P)	11	1.3
16	Player's Medium Navy Cut (P)	11	1.3
16	Player's No. 6 Plain (P)	10	1.3
16	Player's No. 10 Filter	16	1.2
16	Rothmans International	16	1.5
16	Rothmans KS Filter	15	1.6
16	Royal Standard KS	17	1.1
16	Spar KS	17	1.2
16	Weights Plain (P)	10	1.3
16	Woodbine Plain (P)	10	1.3
17	Benson and Hedges Gold Bond KS	17	1.5
17	Benson and Hedges Supreme International	14	1.6
17	Camel (P)	10	1.3
17	Capstan Medium (P)	11	1.3
17	Gallaher's De Luxe Green (P)	10	1.4
17	Kensitas Fine Virginia (P)	11	1.4
17	Senior Service Fine Virginia (P)	10	1.4

High Tar

Tar yield mg/cig	Brand	Carbon monoxide yield mg/cig	Nicotine yield mg/cig
21	Gauloises Caporal (P)	18	1.2
22	Gitanes Caporal (P)	17	1.3
22	Sweet Afton Virginia (P)	12	1.9
23	Gallaher's De Luxe Blue (P)	14	1.9
25	Capstan Full Strength (P)	14	2.6

New brands recently introduced but not yet analysed by the Government Chemist for a period of six months. Estimates by the manufacturers of the tar and nicotine yields for these brands are as follows:

Tar yield mg/cig	Brand	Carbon monoxide yield mg/cig	Nicotine yield mg/cig
9	Silk Cut Extra	9	1.0
9	Dorchester Extra Mild	10	1.0
14	Embassy President	14	1.4
14	Regal 100s	14	1.4

(P) indicates plain cigarettes; all other brands have filters

LGC Survey 23
Sampling period September 1985-February 1986

Low Tar

Tar yield mg/cig	Brand	Carbon monoxide yield mg/cig	Nicotine yield mg/cig
under 4	Embassy Ultra Mild KS	under 3	under 0.3
under 4	John Player KS Ultra Mild	under 3	under 0.3
under 4	Silk Cut Ultra Low KS	under 3	under 0.3
4	Lambert and Butler Special Mild KS	6	0.5
4	Silk Cut Extra Mild KS	4	0.5
7	Embassy Extra Mild	9	0.8
7	Merit Extra Mild	9	0.5
7	Peter Stuyvesant Extra Mild KS	6	0.7
8	Belair Menthol Kings	14	0.6
8	Berkeley KS Mild	9	0.9
8	Cartier Intern Luxury Mild	9	0.8
8	Consulate Menthol	7	0.8
8	Consulate No. 2	7	0.8
8	Craven 'A' Luxury Length Special Mild	10	0.7
8	Dorchester Extra Mild	9	0.8
8	Dunhill Intern Superior Mild	9	0.8
8	Dunhill KS Superior Mild	8	0.8
8	Embassy No. 5 Extra Mild	8	0.7
8	John Player KS Extra Mild	9	0.9
8	Player's No. 10 Extra Mild	8	0.7
8	Silk Cut	9	0.8
8	Silk Cut No. 5	8	0.8
8	Vanguard KS	11	0.9
9	Craven 'A' KS Special Mild	9	0.8
9	Du Maurier KS	10	0.9
9	Embassy No. 1 Extra Mild	9	0.9
9	John Player Superkings (Low Tar)	8	1.0
9	Peter Stuyvesant Lux Length Extra Mild	10	0.8
9	Player's No. 6 Extra mild	9	0.9
9	Silk Cut Extra	9	1.0
9	Silk Cut KS	9	0.9
9	Silk Cut No. 3	9	0.7
9	Victoria Wine Low Tar	9	0.9

Low to Middle Tar

Tar yield mg/cig	Brand	Carbon monoxide yield mg/cig	Nicotine yield mg/cig
11	Dunhill Intern Menthol	14	1.1
11	Kensitas Club Mild	10	1.1
11	Peter Stuyvesant KS	13	1.0
11	St Moritz Lux Length Menthol	15	1.0
12	Acclaim KS	14	1.0
12	Benson and Hedges Sovereign Mild	9	1.1
12	Carlton Premium	11	1.1
12	Carrolls No. 1 Virginia	13	1.1
12	Gauloises Disque Bleu Caporal Filter	19	0.7
12	Gitanes International	17	1.0
13	Carlton Long Size	12	1.3
13	Craven 'A' Luxury Length	14	1.2
13	Embassy No. 1 KS	15	1.2
13	Embassy No. 3 Standard Size	13	1.3
13	Gauloises Caporal Filter	20	0.8
13	Gitanes Caporal Filter	18	0.8
13	Guards	16	1.2
13	John Player Superkings	14	1.4
13	John Player KS	14	1.2
13	Kensitas Club Mild KS	13	1.3
13	Kensitas Mild KS	13	1.3
13	Lambert and Butler KS	16	1.3
13	Marlboro 100s	13	1.0
13	Marlboro KS	13	0.9
13	Piccadilly Filter De Luxe	13	1.4
13	Regal 100s	14	1.4
13	Regal KS	15	1.3
13	Winston KS	15	1.1
14	Benson and Hedges Longer Length	14	1.4
14	Benson and Hedges Sterling KS	16	1.3
14	Berkeley Superkings	14	1.4
14	Chesterfield KS	14	1.2
14	Crown Crest KS	13	1.3
14	Dunhill KS	15	1.3
14	Embassy Filter	14	1.3
14	Embassy President	14	1.6
14	Embassy Regal	14	1.3
14	Fribourg and Treyer Superkings	14	1.5
14	Kim	12	1.2
14	Kings Filter Virginia	14	1.0
14	More Filter 120s	17	1.3
14	More Menthol Filter 120s	16	1.3
14	Park Drive Tipped KS	15	1.4
14	Peter Stuyvesant Lux Length	15	1.4
14	Piccadilly KS	15	1.4
14	Player's No. 6 KS	15	1.3
14	Raffles 100s	16	1.4
14	Red Band KS	16	1.2
14	Rothmans Royals 120s	13	1.5
14	Senior Service Cadets KS	15	1.3
14	Senior Service Superkings	14	1.4
14	Spar KS	16	1.2
14	United Filter Virginia	13	1.2

Middle Tar

Tar yield mg/cig	Brand	Carbon monoxide yield mg/cig	Nicotine yield mg/cig
15	Ardath KS	15	1.3
15	Benson and Hedges Sovereign KS	16	1.3
15	Camel Filter Tip	15	1.3
15	Dorchester Filter	17	1.1
15	Dunhill Luxury Length	16	1.4
15	Embassy Gold	14	1.3
15	Fine 120 Super Length	15	1.3
15	Hyde Park KS	16	1.0
15	Kensitas Club F Virginia	15	1.3
15	Kingsmen Filter Virginia	16	1.3
15	Pall Mall Filter Tipped	13	1.5
15	Player's No. 6 Filter	15	1.4
15	State Express 555 F Kings	15	1.3
15	Victoria Wine KS	14	1.2
15	Woodbine Filter	13	1.3
16	Benson and Hedges Gold Bond Filter	16	1.4
16	Benson and Hedges Special Filter KS	17	1.5
16	Dunhill International	16	1.7
16	Fribourg and Treyer No. 1 Filter De Luxe	18	1.4
16	Gold Leaf F Virginia	15	1.4
16	John Player Special F	13	1.5
16	John Player Special KS	16	1.4
16	Kensitas Club KS	17	1.4
16	Kensitas Filter Virginia KS	17	1.5
16	Lambert and Butler International Size	17	1.4
16	London KS	16	1.1
16	Major Virginia F Extra Size	17	1.4
16	Piccadilly No. 1 (P)	11	1.4
16	Player's Medium Navy Cut F	15	1.4
16	Player's No. 6 Plain (P)	10	1.3
16	Player's No. 10 Filter	16	1.3
16	Rothmans International	16	1.7
16	Rothmans KS Filter	15	1.6
16	Royal Standard KS	16	1.1
16	Weights Plain (P)	10	1.3
16	Woodbine Plain (P)	10	1.3
17	Benson and Hedges Sovereign Filter	14	1.3
17	Camel (P)	10	1.3
17	Craven 'A' KS	17	1.5
17	Kensitas Corsair F Virginia	15	1.3
17	Park Drive Special Virginia (P)	11	1.5
17	Player's Medium Navy Cut (P)	11	1.4

High Tar

Tar yield mg/cig	Brand	Carbon monoxide yield mg/cig	Nicotine yield mg/cig
18	Capstan Medium (P)	11	1.5
18	Gallaher's De Luxe Green (P)	11	1.5
18	Gold Flake (P)	11	1.4
18	Senior Service Fine Virginia (P)	11	1.5
19	Kensitas Fine Virginia (P)	11	1.6
22	Gitanes Caporal (P)	18	1.5
22	Sweet Afton Virginia (P)	12	1.9
23	Gauloises Caporal (P)	20	1.4
24	Gallaher's De Luxe Blue (P)	14	2.1
25	Capstan Full Strength (P)	14	2.7

New brands recently introduced but not yet analysed by the Government Chemist for a period of six months. Estimates by the manufacturers of the tar and nicotine yields for these brands are as follows:

Tar yield mg/cig	Brand	Carbon monoxide yield mg/cig	Nicotine yield mg/cig
7	More Special Mild 120s	6	0.9
7	Royal Standard Mild	7	0.6
8	More Special Mild Menthol 120s	7	1.0
9	Gauloises Legeres	10	0.7
9	Rothmans Special	9	1.3
11	Hyde Park Superkings	16	1.0
14	Tesco Virginia KS	15	1.1

(P) indicates plain cigarettes; all other brands have filters

Low Tar

Tar yield mg/cig	Brand	Carbon monoxide yield mg/cig	Nicotine yield mg/cig
under 4	Embassy Ultra Mild KS	under 3	under 0.3
under 4	John Player KS Ultra Mild	under 3	under 0.3
under 4	Silk Cut Ultra Low KS	under 3	under 0.3
4	Lambert and Butler Special Mild KS	5	0.5
4	Silk Cut Extra Mild KS	4	0.4
6	Peter Stuyvesant Extra Mild KS	6	0.5
7	Belair Menthol Kings	13	0.5
7	Consulate Menthol	8	0.8
7	Consulate No. 2	8	0.7
7	Embassy Extra Mild	9	0.7
7	Merit Extra Mild	9	0.6
7	More Special Mild 120s	6	0.9
7	Royal Standard Mild	7	0.6
7	Silk Cut No. 5	7	0.7
7	Vanguard KS	11	0.8
8	Berkeley KS Mild	9	0.8
8	Cartier Intern Luxury Mild	10	0.8
8	Craven 'A' KS Special Mild	8	0.8
8	Dorchester Extra Mild	9	0.8
8	Dunhill Intern Superior Mild	10	0.8
8	Embassy No. 1 Extra Mild	9	0.9
8	John Player Superkings (Low Tar)	8	0.9
8	John Player KS Extra Mild	9	0.9
8	More Special Mild Menthol 120s	8	1.0
8	Player's No. 6 Extra mild	8	0.7
8	Player's No. 10 Extra Mild	8	0.7
8	Silk Cut	10	0.8
8	Silk Cut Extra	9	0.9
8	Silk Cut KS	9	0.9
8	Silk Cut No. 3	7	0.8
9	Craven 'A' Luxury Length Special Mild	11	0.9
9	Dunhill KS Superior Mild	8	0.9
9	Embassy No. 5 Extra Mild	9	0.9
9	Gauloises Legeres	11	0.6
9	Peter Stuyvesant Luxury Length Extra Mild	10	0.8
9	Victoria Wine Low Tar	10	0.8

Low to Middle Tar

Tar yield mg/cig	Brand	Carbon monoxide yield mg/cig	Nicotine yield mg/cig
10	Peter Stuyvesant KS	12	0.8
10	Rothmans Special	9	1.1
10	St Moritz Lux Length Menthol	15	0.9
11	Dunhill Intern Menthol	14	1.1
11	Gauloises Caporal Filter	19	0.7
11	Gauloises Disque Bleu Caporal Filter	19	0.7
11	Gitanes International	17	1.0
11	Kensitas Club Mild	12	1.0
12	Benson and Hedges Sovereign Mild	9	1.1
12	Carlton Long Size	12	1.1
12	Carlton Premium	11	1.0
12	Carrolls No. 1 Virginia	13	1.1
12	Gitanes Caporal Filter	18	0.8
12	Hyde Park Superkings	15	1.0
12	Independent No. 3 KS	16	1.0
12	John Player KS	13	1.1
12	King George KS	17	1.0
12	Piccadilly Filter De Luxe	13	1.2
13	Acclaim KS	14	0.9
13	Benson and Hedges Sterling KS	15	1.3
13	Classic KS	16	1.0
13	Embassy Filter	13	1.2
13	Embassy No. 1 KS	15	1.2
13	Embassy No. 3 Standard Size	13	1.2
13	Embassy Regal	13	1.2
13	Fine Fare Grey	17	1.1
13	Guards	16	1.1
13	Hyde Park KS	16	0.8
13	John Player Superkings	14	1.4
13	Kensitas Club Mild KS	13	1.3
13	Kingsmen Filter Virginia	16	1.0
13	Lambert and Butler KS	15	1.2
13	Marlboro KS	14	0.9
13	Park Drive Tipped KS	15	1.3
13	Peter Stuyvesant Lux Length	15	1.4
13	Red Band KS	16	1.0
13	Regal 100s	14	1.4
13	Regal KS	15	1.2
13	Rothmans Royals 120s	12	1.5
13	Senior Service Cadets KS	16	1.2
13	Spar KS	17	1.0
13	Winston KS	15	1.1
14	Benson and Hedges 100s	15	1.4
14	Benson and Hedges Sovereign KS	16	1.3
14	Berkeley Superkings	14	1.4
14	Concord KS	15	1.4
14	Craven 'A' Luxury Length	16	1.3
14	Dunhill KS	15	1.3
14	Dunhill Luxury Length	16	1.3
14	Fine 120 Super Length	15	1.2
14	John Player Special Filter	12	1.4
14	Kensitas Mild KS	13	1.3
14	Kings Filter Virginia	14	1.1
14	Lambert and Butler International Size	17	1.3
14	Marlboro 100s	13	1.1
14	More Menthol F 120s	18	1.3
14	Piccadilly KS	15	1.3
14	Player's No. 6 Filter	14	1.4
14	Player's No. 6 KS	14	1.3
14	Raffles 100s	16	1.3
14	Ronson KS	18	1.2
14	Senior Service Superkings	14	1.3
14	Tesco Virginia KS	15	1.2

Middle Tar

Tar yield mg/cig	Brand	Carbon monoxide yield mg/cig	Nicotine yield mg/cig
15	Camel Filter Tip	15	1.3
15	Crown Crest KS	14	1.3
15	Dorchester Filter	17	1.1
15	Embassy Gold	13	1.3
15	Fribourg and Treyer Superkings	18	1.4
15	John Player Special KS	16	1.4
15	London KS	15	1.0
15	Pall Mall Filter Tipped	13	1.4

LGC Survey 24
(*continued*)

Middle Tar

Tar yield mg/cig	Brand	Carbon monoxide yield mg/cig	Nicotine yield mg/cig
15	Player's Medium Navy Cut F	15	1.3
15	Player's No. 10 Filter	15	1.2
15	Rothmans International	16	1.5
15	Royal Standard KS	16	1.1
15	Victoria Wine KiS	16	1.2
15	Weights Plain (P)	10	1.2
15	Woodbine Filter	13	1.2
16	Benson and Hedges Gold Bond Filter	17	1.4
16	Benson and Hedges Sovereign Filter	14	1.4
16	Benson and Hedges Special Filter KS	17	1.5
16	Capstan Medium (P)	11	1.2
16	Chesterfield KS	16	1.3
16	Craven 'A' KS	17	1.4
16	Dunhill International	16	1.5
16	Gold Flake (P)	11	1.3
16	Gold Leaf F Virginia	16	1.4
16	Kensitas Club F Virginia	17	1.4
16	Kensitas Club KS	17	1.5
16	Kensitas Corsair F Virginia	14	1.4
16	Kensitas F Virginia KS	17	1.4
16	Major Virginia F Extra Size	18	1.4
16	More Menthol Filter 120s	19	1.4
16	Park Drive Special Virginia (P)	11	1.4
16	Piccadilly No. 1 (P)	11	1.4

Tar yield mg/cig	Brand	Carbon monoxide yield mg/cig	Nicotine yield mg/cig
16	Player's Medium Navy Cut (P)	11	1.2
16	Player's No. 6 Plain (P)	10	1.3
16	Rothmans KS Filter	16	1.5
16	United Filter Virginia	17	1.3
16	Woodbine Plain (P)	10	1.3
17	Camel (P)	10	1.2
17	Kensitas Fine Virginia (P)	11	1.4

High Tar

Tar yield mg/cig	Brand	Carbon monoxide yield mg/cig	Nicotine yield mg/cig
18	Gallaher's De Luxe Green (P)	11	1.5
18	Senior Service Fine Virginia (P)	11	1.5
22	Gallaher's De Luxe Blue (P)	14	1.8
22	Sweet Afton Virginia (P)	12	2.0
24	Capstan Full Strength (P)	14	2.5
24	Gauloises Caporal (P)	22	1.4
24	Gitanes Caporal (P)	21	1.6

New brands recently introduced but not yet analysed by the Government Chemist for a period of six months. Estimates by the manufacturers of the tar and nicotine yields for these brands are as follows:

Tar yield mg/cig	Brand	Carbon monoxide yield mg/cig	Nicotine yield mg/cig
8	Dorchester Menthol KS	10	0.7
12	Red Band Superkings	15	1.0
13	Lambert and Butler 100s	14	1.3
14	Gold Mark KS	16	1.1

(P) indicates plain cigarettes; all other brands have filters

LGC Survey 25
Sampling period November 1986-April 1987

Low Tar

Tar yield mg/cig	Brand	Carbon monoxide yield mg/cig	Nicotine yield mg/cig
under 4	Embassy Ultra Mild KS	under 3	under 0.3
under 4	John Player KS Ultra Mild	under 3	under 0.3
under 4	Silk Cut Ultra Low KS	under 3	under 0.3
4	Lambert and Butler Special Mild KS	5	0.5
5	Silk Cut Extra Mild KS	5	0.6
7	Belair Menthol Kings	12	0.5
7	Consulate No. 2	7	0.7
7	Embassy Extra Mild	9	0.8
7	Marlboro Lights KS	9	0.6
7	Peter Stuyvesant Extra Mild KS	7	0.7
7	Red Band KS Mild	8	0.6
7	Silk Cut Extra DeLuxe Mild	8	0.8
8	Berkeley KS Mild	9	0.8
8	Consulate Menthol	8	0.8
8	Craven 'A' KS Special Mild	8	0.7

Tar yield mg/cig	Brand	Carbon monoxide yield mg/cig	Nicotine yield mg/cig
8	Craven 'A' Luxury Length Special Mild	10	0.8
8	Dorchester Extra Mild	10	0.9
8	Dorchester Menthol KS	9	0.7
8	Dunhill Intern Superior Mild	10	0.8
8	Embassy No. 1 Extra Mild	8	0.8
8	Embassy No. 5 Extra Mild	8	0.7
8	John Player Superkings (Low Tar)	8	0.9
8	John Player KS Extra Mild	9	0.8
8	Marlboro Lights 100s	8	0.6
8	More Special Mild 120s	8	1.0
8	More Special Mild Menthol 120s	8	1.0
8	Peter Stuyvesant Luxury Length Extra Mild	9	0.8
8	Player's No. 6 Extra mild	8	0.7
8	Player's No. 10 Extra Mild	8	0.7
8	Silk Cut	9	0.8

Tar yield mg/cig	Brand	Carbon monoxide yield mg/cig	Nicotine yield mg/cig
Low Tar			
8	Silk Cut No. 3	9	0.8
8	Silk Cut No. 5	8	0.8
8	Vanguard KS	11	0.8
9	Cartier Intern Luxury Mild	10	0.8
9	Dunhill KS Superior Mild	8	0.8
9	Gauloises Legeres	10	0.7
9	Rothmans Special	8	1.1
9	Silk Cut Extra	9	1.0
9	Silk Cut KS	9	1.0
Low to Middle Tar			
10	Kensitas Club Mild	11	1.0
10	St Moritz Lux Length Menthol	14	0.9
10	Victoria Wine Low Tar	12	0.8
11	Dunhill Intern Menthol	13	1.1
11	Gauloises Caporal Filter	18	0.6
11	Gauloises Disque Bleu Caporal Filter	18	0.7
11	Gitanes International	15	1.0
11	Peter Stuyvesant KS	12	0.9
11	Spar Superkings	14	1.0
12	Carlton Long Size	11	1.2
12	Carlton Premium	10	1.0
12	Carrolls No. 1 Virginia	13	1.1
12	Gitanes Caporal Filter	18	0.8
12	Hyde Park Superkings	15	1.1
12	John Player KS	13	1.1
12	More Filter 120s	14	1.1
12	Peter Stuyvesant Lux Length	14	1.3
12	Piccadilly Filter De Luxe	12	1.2
12	Red Band Superkings	14	1.0
12	Ronson 100s	14	1.1
12	VG King Size	16	0.9
13	Benson and Hedges 100s	15	1.4
13	Benson and Hedges Sovereign KS	16	1.2
13	Berkeley Superkings	14	1.3
13	Embassy Filter	13	1.2
13	Embassy No. 1 KS	15	1.2
13	Embassy No. 3 Standard Size	13	1.2
13	Embassy Regal	13	1.3
13	Gold Mark KS	16	1.0
13	Guards	15	1.1
13	Independent No. 3 KS	16	1.0
13	John Player Superkings	14	1.4
13	Kensitas Club Mild KS	12	1.3
13	Kensitas Corsair F Virginia	12	1.1
13	Kensitas Mild KS	12	1.2
13	Lambert and Butler 100s	13	1.3
13	Lambert and Butler KS	15	1.2
13	Marlboro 100s	12	1.0
13	Marlboro KS	13	0.9
13	Park Drive Tipped KS	15	1.2
13	Piccadilly KS	14	1.2
13	Raffles 100s	16	1.2
13	Red Band KS	16	1.0
13	Regal 100s	13	1.4
13	Rothmans Royals 120s	11	1.4
13	Senior Service Cadets KS	15	1.2
13	Spar KS	16	1.0

Tar yield mg/cig	Brand	Carbon monoxide yield mg/cig	Nicotine yield mg/cig
13	Winston KS	16	1.1
14	Benson and Hedges Gold Bond Filter	16	1.3
14	Benson and Hedges Sovereign Filter	13	1.2
14	Benson and Hedges Sovereign Mild	11	1.2
14	Benson and Hedges Sterling KS	16	1.2
14	Craven 'A' Luxury Length	15	1.3
14	Dunhill KS	14	1.3
14	Dunhill Luxury Length	15	1.3
14	Fine 120 Super Length	14	1.2
14	Hyde Park KS	15	1.0
14	King George KS	16	1.0
14	Kingsmen F Virginia	16	1.1
14	More Menthol F 120s	17	1.3
14	Pall Mall Filter Tipped	12	1.4
14	Player's No. 6 KS	15	1.3
14	Regal KS	15	1.3
14	Ronson KS	17	1.1
14	Senior Service Superkings	14	1.4
14	Solo KS	16	1.0
Middle Tar			
15	Camel Filter Tip	14	1.2
15	Dorchester Filter	16	1.1
15	Dunhill International	15	1.5
15	Embassy Gold	14	1.3
15	John Player Special KS	15	1.4
15	Kensitas Club F Virginia	16	1.3
15	Kensitas Club KS	16	1.4
15	Player's No. 6 Filter	14	1.4
15	Player's No. 10 Filter	14	1.2
15	Rothmans International	15	1.5
15	Royal Standard KS	15	1.2
15	United Filter Virginia	16	1.1
15	Weights Plain (P)	10	1.3
15	Woodbine Filter	13	1.3
16	Balmoral KS	15	1.2
16	Benson and Hedges Special Filter KS	16	1.5
16	Craven 'A' KS	16	1.3
16	Fribourg and Treyer No. 1 Filter De Luxe	17	1.4
16	Gold Flake (P)	10	1.3
16	Gold Leaf Filter Virginia	15	1.3
16	John Player Special F	13	1.5
16	Kensitas F Virginia KS	16	1.5
16	Kings 100s	18	1.3
16	Lambert and Butler International Size	17	1.4
16	London KS	15	1.2
16	Major Virginia F Extra Size	17	1.4
16	Nisa KS	15	1.4
16	Park Drive Special Virginia (P)	11	1.5
16	Piccadilly No. 1 (P)	11	1.5
16	Player's Medium Navy Cut (P)	11	1.3
16	Player's No. 6 Plain (P)	10	1.3
16	Rothmans KS Filter	14	1.5

LGC Survey 25
(*continued*)

Tar yield mg/cig	Brand	Carbon monoxide yield mg/cig	Nicotine yield mg/cig
Middle Tar			
16	Victoria Wine KS	15	1.3
16	Woodbine Plain (P)	10	1.3
17	Kingsway Plain (P)	15	1.4
17	Player's Medium Navy Cut F	15	1.6
High Tar			
18	Capstan Medium (P)	11	1.4
18	Gallaher's De Luxe Green (P)	11	1.5
18	Kensitas Fine Virginia (P)	10	1.5
18	Senior Service Fine Virginia (P)	11	1.5
21	Gallaher's De Luxe Blue (P)	14	1.6
23	Capstan Full Strength (P)	13	2.5

New brands recently introduced but not yet analysed by the Government Chemist for a period of six months. Estimates by the manufacturers of the tar and nicotine yields for these brands are as follows:

9	Berkeley Superkings Mild	9	1.0
13	Benson and Hedges XL	13	1.5
15	John Player Special 100s	16	1.6

(P) indicates plain cigarettes; all other brands have filters

LGC Survey 26
Sampling period June 1987 November 1987

Tar yield mg/cig	Brand	Carbon monoxide yield mg/cig	Nicotine yield mg/cig
Low Tar			
under 4	Embassy Ultra Mild KS	under 3	under 0.3
under 4	John Player KS Ultra Mild	under 3	under 0.3
under 4	Silk Cut Ultra Low KS	under 3	under 0.3
4	Lambert and Butler Special Mild KS	4	0.4
5	Silk Cut KS DeLuxe Mild	5	0.5
6	Silk Cut Extra DeLuxe Mild	8	0.7
7	Consulate No. 2	7	0.7
7	Craven 'A' KS Special Mild	7	0.7
7	Peter Stuyvesant Extra Mild KS	6	0.6
7	Player's No. 6 Extra mild	7	0.6
7	Red Band KS Mild	8	0.6
7	Silk Cut	9	0.7
8	Belair Menthol Kings	13	0.5
8	Consulate Menthol	8	0.8
8	Dorchester Extra Mild	10	0.8
8	Embassy Extra Mild	10	0.8
8	Embassy No. 1 Extra Mild	9	0.9
8	John Player KS Extra Mild	9	0.8
8	Marlboro Lights 100s	8	0.6
8	Marlboro Lights KS	10	0.6
8	More Special Mild 120s	7	0.9
8	More Special Mild Menthol 120s	8	0.9
8	Peter Stuyvesant Luxury Length Extra Mild	9	0.6
8	Player's No. 10 Extra Mild	7	0.7
8	Silk Cut No. 3	9	0.8
8	Silk Cut No. 5	8	0.7
8	Vanguard KS	11	0.8
9	Berkeley KS Mild	10	0.9
9	Berkeley Superkings Mild	9	1.0
9	Cartier Intern Luxury Mild	10	0.8
9	Craven 'A' Luxury Length Special Mild	10	0.8
9	Dorchester Menthol KS	10	0.7
9	Dunhill Intern Superior Mild	10	0.8
9	Dunhill KS Superior Mild	8	0.8
9	Embassy No. 5 Extra Mild	9	0.8
9	Gauloises Legeres	10	0.7
9	John Player Superkings (Low Tar)	9	0.9
9	Knights (Low Tar)	12	0.7
9	Rothmans Special	8	1.1
9	Silk Cut Extra	9	0.9
9	Silk Cut KS	10	0.9
9	Victoria Wine Low Tar	12	0.7
Low to Middle Tar			
10	Kensitas Club Mild	11	0.9
10	St Moritz Lux Length Menthol	15	1.0
11	Dunhill Intern Menthol	13	1.0
11	Gauloises Disque Bleu Caporal Filter	18	0.7
11	Gitanes International	16	0.9
11	Peter Stuyvesant KS	13	0.9
12	Carlton Long Size	12	1.1
12	Carlton Premium	10	1.0
12	Gold Mark Superkings	14	1.0
12	Independent No. 3 KS	14	1.0
12	John Player KS	13	1.1
12	Kensitas Club Mild KS	13	1.1
12	Peter Stuyvesant Lux Length	14	1.3

Tar yield mg/cig	Brand	Carbon monoxide yield mg/cig	Nicotine yield mg/cig
12	Ronson 100s	15	1.1
12	Spar Superkings	14	1.0
13	Benson and Hedges Sovereign KS	16	1.2
13	Benson and Hedges Sovereign Mild	11	1.1
13	Benson and Hedges Sterling KS	15	1.2
13	Benson and Hedges XL	13	1.4
13	Berkeley Superkings	14	1.2
13	Dunhill Luxury Length	15	1.2
13	Embassy Filter	14	1.2
13	Embassy No. 3 Standard Size	14	1.2
13	Embassy Regal	14	1.2
13	Gold Mark KS	15	1.0
13	Guards	15	1.1
13	Hyde Park Superkings	14	1.1
13	John Player Superkings	14	1.4
13	Kensitas Mild KS	13	1.2
13	King George KS	15	1.0
13	Knights KS	12	1.0
13	Lambert and Butler KS	15	1.2
13	Maceline KS	14	1.2
13	Marlboro 100s	13	1.1
13	Marlboro KS	13	0.9
13	More Filter 120s	16	1.2
13	Piccadilly Filter De Luxe	12	1.2
13	Red Band KS	15	1.0
13	Red Band Superkings	15	1.1
13	Regal 100s	14	1.4
13	Richmond KS	15	1.1
13	Ronson KS	17	1.1
13	Rothmans Royals 120s	12	1.4
13	Senior Service Superkings	13	1.2
13	Spar KS	16	1.0
13	VG KS	15	1.1
13	Winston KS	16	1.1
14	Belmont KS	13	1.2
14	Benson and Hedges 100s	16	1.4
14	Benson and Hedges Gold Bond Filter	15	1.1
14	Benson and Hedges Special Filter KS	15	1.2
14	Camel Filter Tip	14	1.2
14	Classic KS	17	1.1
14	Craven 'A' Luxury Length	16	1.3
14	Dunhill KS	13	1.2
14	Embassy No. 1 KS	16	1.3
14	Fine 120 Super Length	15	1.1
14	First KS	15	1.2
14	Independent No. 3 KS	16	1.0
14	John Player Special 100s	16	1.5
14	Kensitas Club F Virginia	15	1.2
14	Kensitas Corsair F Virginia	13	1.1
14	Kings KS	14	1.1
14	Kingsmen F Virginia	15	1.1
14	Lambert and Butler 100s	14	1.4
14	More Menthol Filter 120s	17	1.3
14	Park Drive Tipped KS	17	1.3
14	Piccadilly KS	14	1.2

Tar yield mg/cig	Brand	Carbon monoxide yield mg/cig	Nicotine yield mg/cig
14	Player's No. 6 KS	15	1.3
14	Raffles 100s	16	1.3
14	Regal KS	16	1.3
14	Senior Service Cadets KS	17	1.3
14	Solo KS	16	1.0

Middle Tar

15	Balmoral KS	15	1.2
15	Benson and Hedges Sovereign Filter	14	1.2
15	Dorchester Filter	17	1.2
15	Dunhill International	15	1.4
15	Embassy Gold	13	1.3
15	Gold Flake (P)	10	1.2
15	John Player Special F	15	1.3
15	John Player Special KS	16	1.4
15	Kensitas Club KS	17	1.4
15	Kensitas Filter Virginia KS	16	1.3
15	Player's Medium Navy Cut F	16	1.4
15	Player's No. 6 Filter	15	1.3
15	Player's No. 6 Plain (P)	10	1.2
15	Player's No. 10 Filter	13	1.2
15	Rothmans International	15	1.4
15	Rothmans KS Filter	14	1.4
15	Victoria Wine KS	14	1.2
15	Weights Plain (P)	10	1.2
15	Woodbine Filter	13	1.3
16	Capstan Medium (P)	11	1.2
16	Craven 'A' KS	15	1.2
16	Fribourg and Treyer No. 1 Filter De Luxe	17	1.5
16	Gold Leaf Filter Virginia	16	1.4
16	Kensitas Fine Virginia (P)	10	1.3
16	Lambert and Butler International Size	17	1.4
16	Major Virginia F Extra Size	16	1.4
16	Park Drive Special Virginia (P)	11	1.4
16	Piccadilly No. 1 (P)	10	1.4
16	Player's Medium Navy Cut (P)	10	1.2
16	Royal Standard KS	15	1.2
16	Woodbine Plain (P)	10	1.2
17	Gallaher's De Luxe Green (P)	10	1.3
17	London KS	15	1.2
17	Senior Service Fine Virginia (P)	10	1.4

High Tar

21	Gallaher's De Luxe Blue (P)	14	1.6
24	Capstan Full Strength (P)	14	2.4

New brands recently introduced but not yet analysed by the Government Chemist for a period of six months. Estimates by the manufacturers of the tar and nicotine yields for these brands are as follows:

7	Craven 'A' Superkings Mild	7	0.6
9	Berkeley Superkings Menthol	8	0.9
13	Craven 'A' Superkings	16	1.1
13	Rothmans 100s	16	1.3

(P) indicates plain cigarettes; all other brands have filters

Low Tar

Tar yield mg/cig	Brand	Carbon monoxide yield mg/cig	Nicotine yield mg/cig
under 4	John Player KS Ultra Mild	under 3	under 0.3
under 4	Silk Cut Ultra Low KS	under 3	under 0.3
4	Lambert and Butler Special Mild KS	5	0.4
6	Silk Cut KS DeLuxe Mild	6	0.6
7	Craven 'A' Superkings Mild	6	0.6
7	Peter Stuyvesant Extra Mild KS	6	0.7
7	Player's No. 6 Extra mild	8	0.7
7	Red Band KS Mild	8	0.6
7	Solo Extra Mild KS	8	0.6
8	Belair Menthol Kings	13	0.6
8	Cartier Intern Luxury Mild	8	0.7
8	Consulate Menthol	7	0.8
8	Consulate No. 2	7	0.7
8	Craven 'A' KS Special Mild	8	0.7
8	Dorchester Extra Mild	9	0.9
8	Dorchester Menthol KS	9	0.7
8	Dunhill Intern Superior Mild	8	0.7
8	Embassy Extra Mild	9	0.8
8	Embassy No. 1 Extra Mild	9	0.8
8	John Player KS Extra Mild	9	0.8
8	Marlboro Lights 100s	8	0.7
8	Marlboro Lights KS	9	0.6
8	Peter Stuyvesant Luxury Length Extra Mild	9	0.7
8	Rothmans Special	7	0.8
8	Silk Cut	9	0.7
8	Silk Cut Extra DeLuxe Mild	9	0.8
8	Silk Cut No. 3	9	0.8
8	Silk Cut No. 5	9	0.7
8	Vanguard KS	11	0.7
9	Berkeley Superkings Menthol	9	0.9
9	Berkeley Superkings Mild	10	0.9
9	Consulate 100s	9	0.9
9	Dunhill KS Superior Mild	8	0.8
9	John Player Superkings (Low Tar)	9	0.9
9	Silk Cut Extra	9	0.8
9	Silk Cut KS	10	0.8

Low to Middle Tar

Tar yield mg/cig	Brand	Carbon monoxide yield mg/cig	Nicotine yield mg/cig
10	Gauloises Legeres	11	0.7
10	Kensitas Club Mild	11	0.9
10	Knights (Low Tar)	12	0.9
10	St Moritz Lux Length Menthol	15	0.9
10	Victoria Wine Low Tar	13	0.9
11	Benson and Hedges Sovereign Mild	10	1.0
11	Carlton Premium	10	0.9
11	Gauloises Disque Bleu Caporal Filter	18	0.7
11	Peter Stuyvesant KS	13	0.9
11	Red Band Superkings	14	0.9
12	Carlton Long Size	11	1.1
12	Dunhill Intern Menthol	14	1.1
12	Embassy No. 3 Standard Size	14	1.1
12	Gold Mark Superkings	14	1.0
12	Independent No. 3 KS	14	1.0
12	John Player KS	13	1.1
12	More Menthol Filter 120s	13	1.1
12	Solo Superkings	14	1.0
12	Spar Superkings	14	1.0
13	Benson and Hedges Sovereign KS	17	1.2
13	Benson and Hedges Sterling KS	15	1.2
13	Benson and Hedges XL	13	1.4
13	Berkeley Superkings	14	1.2
13	Classic KS	15	1.0
13	Craven 'A' Superkings	16	1.1
13	Embassy Filter	13	1.2
13	Embassy Regal	13	1.2
13	Gold Mark KS	16	1.0
13	Guards	15	1.0
13	Hyde Park Superkings	15	1.0
13	Independent No. 3 KS	15	0.9
13	John Player Superkings	13	1.3
13	Kensitas Club Mild KS	14	1.2
13	Kensitas Mild KS	13	1.2
13	King George KS	15	1.0
13	Kingsmen Filter Virginia	16	1.0
13	Knights 100s	10	1.3
13	Knights KS	13	1.2
13	Lambert and Butler 100s	14	1.3
13	Lambert and Butler KS	15	1.2
13	Maceline KS	15	1.2
13	Marlboro KS	12	1.0
13	Peter Stuyvesant Lux Length	14	1.3
13	Piccadilly Filter De Luxe	12	1.2
13	Player's No. 6 KS	15	1.2
13	Raffles 100s	15	1.1
13	Red Band KS	15	1.0
13	Regal 100s	13	1.3
13	Richmond KS	15	0.9
13	Rothmans Royals 120s	12	1.1
13	Senior Service Cadets KS	17	1.2
13	Senior Service Superkings	15	1.3
13	Solo KS	15	0.9
13	Spar KS	15	1.0
13	Style KS	16	1.0
13	Winston KS	17	1.1
14	Benson and Hedges 100s	17	1.3
14	Benson and Hedges Gold Bond Filter	15	1.2
14	Benson and Hedges Special Filter KS	15	1.2
14	Camel Filter Tip	14	1.2
14	Dorchester Superkings	17	1.0
14	Dunhill KS	14	1.2
14	Dunhill Luxury Length	16	1.2
14	Embassy No. 1 KS	16	1.3
14	First KS	15	1.1
14	Globe KS	16	1.0
14	Kensitas Club F Virginia	15	1.2
14	Kensitas Corsair F Virginia	14	1.2
14	Kensitas F Virginia KS	15	1.2
14	Marlboro 100s	14	1.1
14	More Filter 120s	17	1.3

Tar yield mg/cig	Brand	Carbon monoxide yield mg/cig	Nicotine yield mg/cig
Low to Middle Tar			
14	Park Drive Tipped KS	17	1.3
14	Piccadilly KS	14	1.2
14	Player's No. 6 Filter	15	1.3
14	Regal KS	16	1.2
14	Rothmans 100s	15	1.3
14	Woodbine Filter	12	1.1
Middle Tar			
15	Benson and Hedges Sovereign Filter	14	1.2
15	Dorchester Filter	17	1.1
15	Dunhill International	15	1.5
15	Embassy Gold	12	1.2
15	Fribourg and Treyer No. 1 Filter De Luxe	18	1.3
15	John Player Special 100s	16	1.5
15	John Player Special Filter	15	1.3
15	John Player Special KS	16	1.3
15	Kensitas Club KS	17	1.3
15	Player's No. 10 Filter	13	1.1
15	Ronson KS	16	1.3
15	Rothmans International	15	1.4
16	Belmont KS	14	1.5
16	Craven 'A' KS	15	1.3
16	Gold Leaf F Virginia	16	1.3
16	Kings KS	13	1.5
16	Lambert and Butler International Size	17	1.3
16	London KS	15	1.3

Tar yield mg/cig	Brand	Carbon monoxide yield mg/cig	Nicotine yield mg/cig
16	Park Drive Special Virginia (P)	11	1.3
16	Piccadilly No. 1 (P)	11	1.3
16	Player's Medium Navy Cut (P)	11	1.2
16	Player's Medium Navy Cut F	17	1.4
16	Player's No. 6 Plain (P)	10	1.2
16	Rothmans KS Filter	15	1.5
16	Royal Standard KS	15	1.3
16	Weights Plain (P)	10	1.2
16	Woodbine Plain (P)	10	1.2
17	Balmoral KS	14	1.5
17	Capstan Medium (P)	11	1.4
17	Gold Flake (P)	10	1.3
17	Kensitas Fine Virginia (P)	10	1.4
17	Senior Service Fine Virginia (P)	10	1.4
17	Victoria Wine KS	14	1.6
High Tar			
18	Gallaher's De Luxe Green (P)	10	1.4
20	Gallaher's De Luxe Blue (P)	13	1.6
23	Capstan Full Strength (P)	14	2.3

New brands recently introduced but not yet analysed by the Government Chemist for a period of six months. Estimates by the manufacturers of the tar and nicotine yields for these brands are as follows:

8	Craven 'A' Menthol	7	0.7
8	Vogue Superslims 100s	5	0.7
14	Berkeley Special KS	15	1.1
14	Blackcat Superkings	16	1.1

(P) indicates plain cigarettes; all other brands have filters

LGC Survey 28
Sampling period August 1988-January 1989

Tar yield mg/cig	Brand	Carbon monoxide yield mg/cig	Nicotine yield mg/cig
Low Tar			
under 4	Silk Cut Ultra Low KS	under 3	under 0.3
4	Lambert and Butler KS Low Tar	5	0.4
5	Silk Cut KS DeLuxe Mild	6	0.5
7	Cartier Intern Luxury Mild	8	0.7
7	Craven 100s Superkings Mild	6	0.7
7	Embassy Extra Mild	9	0.7
7	Peter Stuyvesant Extra Mild KS	6	0.6
7	Red Band KS Mild	8	0.6
7	Silk Cut	9	0.7
7	Silk Cut Extra DeLuxe Mild	8	0.7
7	Solo Extra Mild KS	8	0.6
7	Vogue Superslim's 100s	5	0.7

Tar yield mg/cig	Brand	Carbon monoxide yield mg/cig	Nicotine yield mg/cig
8	Belair Menthol Kings	13	0.6
8	Berkeley Superkings Mild	8	0.8
8	Consulate 100s	8	0.8
8	Consulate No. 2	7	0.7
8	Craven 'A' KS Menthol	8	0.8
8	Craven 'A' KS Special Mild	8	0.7
8	Dorchester Extra Mild KS	9	0.8
8	Dorchester Menthol KS	10	0.7
8	Dunhill Intern Superior Mild	9	0.7
8	Embassy No. 1 Extra Mild	9	0.8
8	John Player KS Extra Mild	9	0.8
8	Marlboro Lights 100s	8	0.7
8	Marlboro Lights KS	9	0.6

Tar yield mg/cig	Brand	Carbon monoxide yield mg/cig	Nicotine yield mg/cig
Low Tar			
8	Peter Stuyvesant Luxury Length Extra Mild	9	0.7
8	Rothmans Special	8	0.9
8	Silk Cut No. 3	9	0.7
8	Silk Cut No. 5	8	0.7
9	Berkeley Superkings Menthol	8	0.9
9	Consulate Menthol	8	0.8
9	Dunhill KS Superior Mild	8	0.8
9	Gauloises Legeres	10	0.6
9	John Player Superkings (Low Tar)	9	0.9
9	Knights (Low Tar)	13	0.7
9	Silk Cut Extra	10	0.9
9	Silk Cut KS	10	0.8
9	Victoria Wine Special Mild	12	0.7
Low to Middle Tar			
10	Kensitas Club Mild	11	0.9
10	St Moritz Lux Length Menthol	14	1.0
11	Benson and Hedges Sovereign Mild	9	0.9
11	Gitanes Caporal Filter	17	0.7
11	Gold Mark Superkings	13	1.0
11	Independent No. 3 Superkings	13	0.9
11	Peter Stuyvesant KS	13	1.0
11	Red Band Superkings	14	1.0
11	Solo Superkings	13	1.0
11	Spar Superkings	13	1.0
12	Berkeley Superkings	13	1.1
12	Gauloises Disque Bleu Caporal Filter	18	0.7
12	John Player KS	13	1.0
12	Kensitas Club Mild KS	14	1.0
12	Kensitas Mild KS	13	1.0
12	King George KS	15	0.9
12	Knights KS	13	1.0
12	More Filter 120s	14	1.2
12	More Menthol Filter 120s	14	1.1
12	Richmond KS	15	0.9
12	Senior Service Superkings	14	1.1
13	Benson and Hedges 100s	15	1.2
13	Benson and Hedges Gold Bond Filter	15	1.1
13	Bentley KS	14	1.1
13	Berkeley Special KS	14	1.1
13	Blackcat Superkings	16	1.2
13	Choice KS	14	1.1
13	Classic KS	16	0.9
13	Craven 'A' Superkings	16	1.2
13	Dunhill Intern Menthol	15	1.2
13	Embassy Filter	13	1.1
13	Gold Leaf F Virginia	14	1.1
13	Gold Mark KS	15	0.9
13	Guards	14	1.1
13	Hyde Park Superkings	15	0.9
13	Independent No. 3 KS	15	0.9
13	John Player Superkings	14	1.3
13	Kensitas Club	15	1.1
13	Kingsmen KS	15	0.9
13	Knights 100s	9	1.3
13	Lambert and Butler 100s	14	1.2
13	Lambert and Butler KS	15	1.1
13	London Superkings	15	1.1
13	Marlboro KS	13	1.0
13	Park Drive Tipped KS	17	1.2
13	Peter Stuyvesant Lux Length	13	1.4
13	Piccadilly Filter De Luxe	12	1.2
13	Player's No. 6 KS	15	1.2
13	Raffles Kings	14	1.1
13	Red Band KS	15	1.0
13	Regal Filter	13	1.1
13	Regal KS	15	1.2
13	Regatta KS	13	1.0
13	Rothmans 100s	15	1.2
13	Rothmans Royals 120s	13	1.1
13	Senior Service Cadets KS	18	1.1
13	Solo KS	16	0.9
13	Spar KS	15	0.9
13	Style KS	15	1.0
13	Winston KS	16	1.0
14	Benson and Hedges Sovereign Filter	13	1.1
14	Benson and Hedges Sovereign KS	17	1.2
14	Benson and Hedges Special Filter KS	15	1.2
14	Benson and Hedges Sterling KS	16	1.3
14	Benson and Hedges XL	14	1.3
14	Dorchester KS	16	1.0
14	Dorchester Superkings	16	1.0
14	Embassy No. 1 KS	16	1.2
14	First KS	15	1.1
14	Globe KS	17	1.2
14	Kensitas Club KS	17	1.2
14	Kensitas Corsair F Virginia	13	1.2
14	Kensitas Filter Virginia KS	17	1.2
14	Maceline KS	15	1.2
14	Marlboro 100s	14	1.2
14	Piccadilly KS	14	1.2
14	Raffles 100s	16	1.3
14	Ronson KS	16	1.3
Middle Tar			
15	Balmoral KS	13	1.4
15	Camel Filters	14	1.2
15	Dunhill KS	15	1.3
15	Dunhill Luxury Length	16	1.3
15	John Player Special KS	16	1.3
15	London KS	14	1.2
15	Player's No. 6 Filter	15	1.3
15	Player's No. 10 F Virginia	13	1.1
15	Rothmans International	15	1.5
15	Weights Plain (P)	10	1.2
15	Woodbine Plain (P)	10	1.2
16	Belmont KS	13	1.4
16	Dunhill International	15	1.5
16	Kings 100s	14	1.5
16	Kings KS	14	1.4

LGC Survey 28
(*continued*)

Middle Tar

Tar yield mg/cig	Brand	Carbon monoxide yield mg/cig	Nicotine yield mg/cig
16	Major Extra Size	16	1.3
16	Park Drive Special Virginia (P)	10	1.3
16	Piccadilly No. 1 (P)	10	1.4
16	Rothmans KS Filter	14	1.5
16	Royal Standard KS	15	1.3
16	Victoria Wine Special F	13	1.4
17	Capstan Medium (P)	11	1.3
17	Craven 'A' KS	16	1.4
17	Kensitas Fine Virginia (P)	11	1.3
17	Player's Medium Navy Cut (P)	11	1.2

High Tar

Tar yield mg/cig	Brand	Carbon monoxide yield mg/cig	Nicotine yield mg/cig
18	Gallaher's De Luxe Green (P)	11	1.4
18	Senior Service Fine Virginia (P)	11	1.3
21	Gallaher's De Luxe Blue (P)	13	1.5
23	Capstan Full Strength (P)	14	2.3

(P) indicates plain cigarettes; all other brands have filters

LGC Survey 29
Sampling period March 1989–August 1989

Low Tar

Tar yield mg/cig	Brand	Carbon monoxide yield mg/cig	Nicotine yield mg/cig
under 4	Silk Cut Ultra Low KS	under 3	under 0.3
4	Lambert and Butler KS Low Tar	5	0.4
5	Silk Cut KS DeLuxe Mild	6	0.5
6	Craven 100s Superkings Mild	6	0.7
7	Consulate No. 2	7	0.7
7	Dorchester Superkings Mild	7	0.8
7	Embassy Extra Mild	9	0.7
7	Embassy No. 1 Extra Mild	8	0.8
7	John Player KS Extra Mild	8	0.8
7	Peter Stuyvesant Extra Mild KS	6	0.6
7	Red Band KS Mild	8	0.6
7	Silk Cut	9	0.7
7	Silk Cut Extra DeLuxe Mild	9	0.7
7	Silk Cut No. 5	8	0.7
7	Vogue Superslim's 100s	5	0.7
8	Berkeley Superkings Mild	8	0.8
8	Cartier Intern Luxury Mild	8	0.7
8	Consulate 100s	8	0.8
8	Craven 'A' KS Special Mild	8	0.8
8	Dorchester Extra Mild KS	9	0.8
8	Dorchester Menthol KS	9	0.6
8	Dunhill Intern Superior Mild	9	0.8
8	John Player Superkings (Low Tar)	8	0.8
8	Marlboro Lights 100s	9	0.7
8	Marlboro Lights KS	10	0.7
8	Peter Stuyvesant Lux Length Extra Mild	8	0.7
8	Rothmans Special	7	0.9
8	Silk Cut Extra	9	0.8
8	Silk Cut KS	10	0.8
8	Silk Cut No. 3	9	0.8
8	Windsor Blue Low Tar	13	0.6
9	Berkeley Superkings Menthol	9	0.9
9	Consulate Menthol	8	0.9
9	Craven 'A' KS Menthol	8	0.9
9	Dunhill KS Superior Mild	8	0.8
9	Gauloises Legeres	11	0.6
9	Knights (Low Tar)	12	0.7
9	Victoria Wine Special Mild	12	0.7

Low to Middle Tar

Tar yield mg/cig	Brand	Carbon monoxide yield mg/cig	Nicotine yield mg/cig
10	Benson and Hedges Sovereign Mild	9	0.9
10	Kensitas Club Mild	11	1.0
10	York Superkings	9	0.9
11	Gauloises Disque Bleu Caporal Filter	19	0.7
11	Gitanes Caporal Filter	18	0.8
11	Kensitas Mild KS	13	0.9
11	Peter Stuyvesant KS	13	0.9
11	Regatta KS	13	0.9
11	Windsor Blue KS	13	0.9
11	Windsor Blue Lux Length	10	1.1
11	Winston KS	16	0.8
12	Benson and Hedges Sovereign Filter	12	0.9
12	Berkeley Superkings	13	1.1
12	Choice KS	15	0.9
12	Embassy Filter	13	1.1
12	Globe 100s	15	0.9
12	Globe KS	16	0.8

Tar yield mg/cig	Brand	Carbon monoxide yield mg/cig	Nicotine yield mg/cig
Low to Middle Tar			
12	Gold Mark Superkings	13	1.0
12	Independent No. 3 KS	15	0.9
12	Kensitas Club Mild KS	13	1.0
12	Kensitas Corsair F Virginia	12	0.9
12	Knights 100s	9	1.2
12	Knights KS	13	1.0
12	Lambert and Butler KS	15	1.1
12	More Filter 120s	15	1.1
12	Red Band KS	15	0.9
12	Red Band Superkings	13	1.1
12	Regal Filter	13	1.1
12	Rothmans Royals 120s	13	1.1
12	Senior Service Cadets KS	18	1.0
12	Senior Service Superkings	13	1.1
12	Solo Superkings	13	1.0
12	Spar Superkings	13	1.0
12	Style KS	15	0.9
12	Supreme KS	14	1.0
13	Benson and Hedges 100s	16	1.2
13	Benson and Hedges Sovereign KS	17	1.2
13	Benson and Hedges Sterling KS	15	1.1
13	Bentley KS	14	1.0
13	Blackcat Superkings	16	1.2
13	Classic KS	15	0.9
13	Craven 100s Superkings	16	1.2
13	Dorchester Superkings	16	1.0
13	Dunhill Intern Menthol	15	1.2
13	Embassy No. 1 KS	14	1.1
13	First KS	14	1.0
13	Gold Leaf F Virginia	13	1.1
13	Gold Mark KS	16	1.0
13	Guards	15	1.1
13	Hyde Park Superkings	16	0.9
13	John Player Superkings	14	1.4
13	John Player KS	15	1.1
13	King George KS	15	0.9
13	Kingsmen KS	15	1.0
13	Knightsbridge	15	1.0
13	Lambert and Butler 100s	14	1.2
13	Lambeth KS	15	1.0
13	London KS	14	0.9
13	Marlboro KS	12	1.0
13	More Menthol Filter 120s	15	1.2
13	Park Drive Tipped KS	17	1.1
13	Peter Stuyvesant Lux Length	13	1.3
13	Piccadilly Filter De Luxe	12	1.2
13	Player's No. 6 KS	15	1.2
13	Raffles Kings	14	1.1
13	Regal KS	15	1.2
13	Solo KS	15	0.9
13	Spar KS	15	1.0
13	St Moritz Lux Length Menthol	15	1.2
14	Balmoral KS	13	1.3
14	Benson and Hedges Gold Bond Filter	15	1.1
14	Benson and Hedges Special Filter KS	16	1.2
14	Benson and Hedges XL	14	1.4
14	Camel Filters	14	1.1
14	Dunhill KS	14	1.2
14	Elite KS	13	1.3
14	John Player Special KS	15	1.2
14	Kensitas Club	14	1.2
14	Kensitas Club KS	17	1.2
14	Kensitas Filter Virginia KS	17	1.2
14	Kings 100s	14	1.4
14	Maceline KS	15	1.3
14	Maceline Super KS	17	1.3
14	Marlboro 100s	15	1.1
14	Piccadilly KS	14	1.2
14	Player's No. 6 Filter	14	1.2
14	Player's No. 10 F Virginia	13	1.0
14	Raffles 100s	15	1.3
14	Rothmans 100s	15	1.4
14	Victoria Wine Special F	13	1.3
Middle Tar			
15	Dorchester KS	16	1.1
15	Dunhill Luxury Length	16	1.3
15	Major Extra Size	16	1.2
15	Park Drive Special Virginia (P)	10	1.2
15	Rothmans International	15	1.5
15	Woodbine Plain (P)	9	1.1
16	Belvedere International	17	1.3
16	Craven 'A' KS	16	1.4
16	Dunhill International	15	1.5
16	Piccadilly No. 1 (P)	11	1.4
16	Ronson KS	16	1.4
16	Rothmans KS Filter	14	1.6
17	Gallaher's De Luxe Green (P)	11	1.3
17	Kensitas Fine Virginia (P)	10	1.3
17	Player's Medium Navy Cut (P)	11	1.3
17	Senior Service Fine Virginia (P)	10	1.3
High Tar			
21	Gallaher's De Luxe Blue (P)	15	1.5
23	Capstan Full Strength (P)	14	2.3

New brands recently introduced but not yet analysed by the Government Chemist for a period of six months. Estimates by the manufacturers of the tar and nicotine yields for these brands are as follows:

11	Viva 100s	15	0.7

(P) indicates plain cigarettes; all other brands have filters